Technologies of Mind and Body in the Soviet Union and the Eastern Bloc

Technologies of Mind and Body in the Soviet Union and the Eastern Bloc

Edited by
Anna Toropova and Claire Shaw

BLOOMSBURY ACADEMIC
LONDON • NEW YORK • OXFORD • NEW DELHI • SYDNEY

BLOOMSBURY ACADEMIC

Bloomsbury Publishing Plc, 50 Bedford Square, London, WC1B 3DP, UK
Bloomsbury Publishing Inc, 1385 Broadway, New York, NY 10018, USA
Bloomsbury Publishing Ireland, 29 Earlsfort Terrace, Dublin 2, D02 AY28, Ireland

BLOOMSBURY, BLOOMSBURY ACADEMIC and the Diana logo are trademarks of
Bloomsbury Publishing Plc

First published in Great Britain 2024
Paperback edition published 2025

Copyright © Claire Shaw and Anna Toropova, 2024

Claire Shaw and Anna Toropova have asserted their right under the Copyright, Designs
and Patents Act, 1988, to be identified as Editor of this work.

Cover image: Soviet health resort workers undergoing quartz and
sun-ray treatment in the light therapy room of the skala sanatorium
at kislovodsk, May 1951 © Sovfoto/Getty Images

All rights reserved. No part of this publication may be: i) reproduced or transmitted
in any form, electronic or mechanical, including photocopying, recording or by means
of any information storage or retrieval system without prior permission in writing from
the publishers; or ii) used or reproduced in any way for the training, development or
operation of artificial intelligence (AI) technologies, including generative AI technologies.
The rights holders expressly reserve this publication from the text and data mining
exception as per Article 4(3) of the Digital Single Market Directive (EU) 2019/790.

Bloomsbury Publishing Plc does not have any control over, or responsibility for, any third-
party websites referred to or in this book. All internet addresses given in this book were
correct at the time of going to press. The author and publisher regret any inconvenience
caused if addresses have changed or sites have ceased to exist, but can accept no
responsibility for any such changes.

Every effort has been made to trace the copyright holders and obtain permission
to reproduce the copyright material. Please do get in touch with any enquiries or
any information relating to such material or the rights holder. We would be pleased
to rectify any omissions in subsequent editions of this publication should they
be drawn to our attention.

A catalogue record for this book is available from the British Library.

A catalog record for this book is available from the Library of Congress.

ISBN: HB: 978-1-3502-7126-5
PB: 978-1-3502-7130-2
ePDF: 978-1-3502-7127-2
eBook: 978-1-3502-7128-9

Typeset by Integra Software Services Pvt. Ltd.

For product safety related questions contact productsafety@bloomsbury.com.

To find out more about our authors and books visit www.bloomsbury.com
and sign up for our newsletters.

In memory of Philippa Hetherington, 1984–2022

Contents

List of illustrations	viii
List of contributors	ix
Acknowledgements	xi
Note on Transliteration	xii
Introduction *Anna Toropova and Claire Shaw*	1

Part 1 Knowledges

1. 'Rest for the brain' or 'technology of the unconscious?': Hypnosis in early Soviet medicine and culture *Anna Toropova* 29
2. From psychosis to psychopathy: Psychiatry and crime in communist Czechoslovakia (1948–70) *Jakub Střelec* 51
3. Broadcasting communist morality: Sex education in Soviet Latvia *Siobhán Hearne* 65
4. Health and heroism: Shifting patterns in late socialist Central Europe *Jan Arend* 83

Part 2 Practices

5. Work and therapy: Two visions of the Bulgarian New Man *Julian Chehirian* 101
6. 'Human capabilities are limitless': Will and self-improvement in postwar Soviet psychotherapy *Aleksandra Brokman* 121
7. Soviet pioneers in smoking cessation: From group therapy in the 1920s to Cytisine in the 1970s *Tricia Starks* 139

Part 3 *Artefacts*

8. Illuminating microbes: Preventing infectious diseases with bactericidal lamps in Soviet medicine, 1917–53 *Johanna Conterio* 157
9. Embodied technologies: Lilya Brik's *The Glass Eye* (1929) and Esfir Shub's *Today* (1930) *Lilya Kaganovsky* 177
10. Arm race: The Cold War story of a bionic arm *Frances Bernstein* 197
11. Dreams of a synaesthetic future: Technologies of deafness in late Soviet socialism *Claire Shaw* 217

Index 237

List of Illustrations

1.1	Hypnosis on screen: Film still from *To Your Health* (1929)	33
1.2	Paralysed consciousness: Film still from *To Your Health* (1929)	33
1.3	'Wax-like plasticity': Illustration of Hypnotic Catalepsy, 1924	35
1.4	From 'Ania' to 'Anichka': Illustration of age regression under hypnosis, 1923	39
5.1	Dimitar Kazakov and Nikola Kazakov before the fire, 1979/80	104
5.2	Work therapy with patients at the Karlukovo Hospital, 1960s	112
5.3	Work therapy by patients at Regional Psychoneurological Hospital in Lovech, 1966	114
5.4	Nikola Kazakov a year after discharge, 1994	115
8.1	Physical culture practitioners in the sports sector of the Central House of the Red Army in Moscow undergoing treatment in the Great Quartz Hall, 1933	161
8.2	Patients on the 'beach' of the Great Quartz Hall, 1933	163
9.1	Director Lilya Brik, courtesy of Heritage Images/Getty Images	179
9.2	Cameraman Anatoly Golovnya with an adjustable iris diaphragm: Film still from *The Glass Eye*, dir. Brik, 1929	181
9.3	Director Esfir Shub at flatbed with celluloid-strip, 1931	185
9.4a and 9.4b	Children at play: Film still from *Today*, dir. Shub, 1930	190
10.1	'Electronic hand made by Reds for amputees': Illustration, *Tribune News Service*, 1965	197
10.2	The Russia Arm prosthesis: Photograph, 1965	198
10.3	The second model of the bioelectric control system: Photograph, Institute of Machine Research and Central Scientific-Research Institute of Prosthetics and Prosthetics Manufacturing, 1960	201
10.4	'Morning Shave': Film still from 'Bioelectricheskaia ruka', 1961	202
11.1	Veniamin Tsukerman, Irina Tsukerman and Leonid Galynker, Moscow, 1956	219
11.2	Sensory devices for deaf people: Illustration by Irina Tsukerman, 1973	221
11.3	Irina Tsukerman with her Morse code telephone adapter, 1967	222

List of Contributors

Jan Arend is Lecturer at the Institute for Eastern European History and Area Studies at the University of Tübingen. His research focuses on the social and cultural history of Russia and East Central Europe since the late nineteenth century, with a special focus on the history of science and emotions. He is currently writing a book on the conceptual and social history of mental stress in Czechoslovakia/Czech Republic since the 1960s.

Frances Bernstein is Associate Professor of History at Drew University. She has published numerous articles in the history of sexuality and the history of disability in the USSR. Her most recent publication is 'The History of Disability during Stalinism', in Cornelis Boterbloem, ed., *Life in Stalin's Soviet Union, 1929–1953* (2019), 115–37. She is completing a manuscript on the bureaucratic, representational, and physical erasure of disabled soldiers from Soviet life during and after the Second World War.

Aleksandra Brokman is an independent scholar, currently working in mental health policy. In 2018 she received a PhD from the University of East Anglia and subsequently worked as Postdoctoral Research Fellow on the 'Growing Old in the USSR, 1945–1991' project at Liverpool John Moores University. Her academic research focuses on psychotherapy and psychiatry in the post-war USSR.

Julian Chehirian is a PhD candidate in the History of Science at Princeton University and Fellow in its Interdisciplinary Doctoral Program in the Humanities. He writes on the history of psychotherapy and the psychological sciences across the twentieth century in transnational contexts. His research has taken the form of scholarly writing, public history exhibitions, art installations and documentary film.

Johanna Conterio is Associate Professor of Environmental History in the Department of Archaeology, Conservation and History at the University of Oslo. She is a historian of Modern Russia and the Soviet Union, especially focusing on the 'subtropical' south and Black Sea region. Her research examines questions at the intersection of environment, health, nature protection, urban planning and maritime environments, in transnational and international context. She is the curator of a special forum on the Black Sea world published in *Kritika: Explorations in Russian and Eurasian Studies* in 2018.

Siobhán Hearne is a historian of the Russian Empire and the Soviet Union, with particular expertise on the Baltic region. She is currently a Wellcome Trust Research Fellow at the University of Manchester. Her research broadly focuses on gender, sexuality and medicine, and she is the author of *Policing Prostitution: Regulating the Lower Classes in Late Imperial Russia* (2021).

Lilya Kaganovsky is Professor of Slavic, East European and Eurasian Languages and Cultures at UCLA. Her publications include *The Voice of Technology: Soviet Cinema's Transition to Sound, 1928–1935* (2018), *How the Soviet Man Was Unmade* (2008), three edited volumes, and articles on Russian and Soviet cinema. She is a member of the editorial board of the journal *Studies in Russian and Soviet Cinema* and the Associate Editor for film and media at *The Russian Review*.

Claire Shaw is Associate Professor in the History of Modern Russia at the University of Warwick. Her research focuses on the history of disability, the senses and the body under Soviet socialism. She is the author of *Deaf in the USSR: Marginality, Community, and Soviet Identity, 1917–1991* (2017), and a member of the editorial board of the *Slavonic and East European Review*.

Tricia Starks is Professor of History at the University of Arkansas and director of their Humanities Center. She researches public health in the Soviet Union and its successor states with particular attention to gender, the lived experience and behaviour modification. Her most recent book is *Cigarettes and Soviets: Tobacco in the USSR* (2022).

Jakub Střelec is a PhD candidate at the Institute of International Studies, Charles University in Prague. In 2020–1, he was PhD Fellow at the French Research Centre in Humanities and Social Sciences (CEFRES) in Prague. His research interests focus on the social and cultural history of violence, crime and psychiatry in Central and Eastern Europe after 1945.

Anna Toropova is Research Fellow at the Centre for Culture and the Mind at the University of Copenhagen. Her current project explores the interchanges between cinema and medicine in the early Soviet Union. She is the author of *Feeling Revolution: Cinema, Genre and the Politics of Affect under Stalin* (2020) and articles on Soviet cinema, biopolitics, medicine and spectatorship.

Acknowledgements

The majority of the chapters in this volume began life as papers presented at a two-day international symposium at the University of Nottingham in May 2019. We would like to thank the institutions and the people that made this conference such a lively and fruitful exchange of ideas. The event was generously supported by the Wellcome Trust [grant number 203372/Z/16/Z], the Centre for the History of Medicine, the European History Research Centre and the Global History and Culture Centre at the University of Warwick, as well as the University of Nottingham. Alongside the wonderful scholars whose chapters appear in this volume, we would like to sincerely thank the conference participants for their invaluable insights, including Ben Krupp, Ana Hedberg Olenina, Nick Baron, Ken Pinnow, Ben Zajicek, Susan Grant, Andy Byford, Pavel Vasilyev, Anna Ozhiganova, Diana Kurkovsky West, Anja Werner, Michael Rasell, Frank Henschel, Oksana Sarkisova, Ekaterina Vikulina, Zhipeng Gao, Natalia Savelyeva, Anna Kozlova, Jessica Werneke, Polly McMichael, Susan Read, Simon Huxtable and Julia Sutton-Mattocks. Special thanks are reserved for Sarah Marks and Simon Pawley, who participated not only in the Nottingham symposium but also in the 2015 British Association of Slavonic and East European Studies (BASEES) conference panel where the 'technologies of mind and body' concept first originated. Our ideas for the volume have benefitted from discussion with Sarah and Simon, as well as with Miriam Dobson and the participants of the University of Sheffield's History Department seminar. We are also grateful to Sophie Mann for her very helpful comments on the volume introduction.

Invaluable research assistance was provided by Irina Makhalova as well as the staff at the SSEES and Bodleian libraries. We are also grateful for the administrative support of staff at the University of Oxford, especially Hazel Cook, the University of Nottingham and the University of Warwick, and to the Wellcome Trust for financial assistance with the image licensing fees for the volume. We would like to thank our editors at Bloomsbury, Gabriella Cox, Laura Reeves and Rhodri Mogford, for their faith in the project, and our anonymous reviewer for their helpful comments. Thanks in particular to Sean Dyde for his work on the index. We are indebted to our colleagues at Oxford, Nottingham and Warwick for all their help and support during this project's life span, especially Sarah Badcock, Anna Greenwood, Roberta Bivins and Dan Healey. Finally, we both would like to thank our families and friends for their invaluable support during the production of this volume.

Our thinking about techniques of human transformation was greatly inspired by the conference on the *Borders of Biopolitics: Gender, Population and Power in Modern Russia* that the late Philippa Hetherington organized at SSEES, UCL in 2016. Philippa's participation at the 2019 Nottingham symposium was tragically disrupted by her cancer diagnosis. We deeply miss her intellectual power, unique insight and endless positivity. This book is dedicated to her memory.

Note on Transliteration

In transliterating terms from Russian, Ukrainian, and Bulgarian, the authors in this volume use the Library of Congress system, with the exception of names that have a commonly accepted English spelling; that is, Maksim Gorky rather than Gor'kii. The Ukrainian capital is rendered as Kyiv, rather than Kiev.

Introduction

Anna Toropova and Claire Shaw

The project to create a 'New Man' and 'New Woman' initiated in the Soviet Union and the Eastern Bloc constituted one of the most extensive efforts to remake human psychophysiology in modern history. As Lev Trotsky wrote in 1923, the socialist revolution would herald the advent of 'a higher social-biologic type, or if you please, a superman', whose ideal physical and mental state would be brought about through the harnessing of medical and scientific knowledge and the transformation of the social environment.[1] While Trotsky's statement captures the boundless ambition of the revolutionary moment, this was no fleeting goal; the desire to shape the minds and bodies of citizens persisted until the last days of the socialist experiment, as evidenced in the official belief that military service in the Soviet-Afghan War would forge young soldiers into 'a new (and presumably better) generation of men'.[2] Through institutional, social and individual practices, in scientific theories and in artistic production, the goal to create idealized human beings remained central to the frameworks and experience of state socialism.

The revolutionary desire to transform the mind and body was very much a product of its twentieth-century moment, when the rapidly expanding capacity of science and technology to perfect the human led the mind and body to emerge as sites of scientific investigation, medical intervention and technological innovation across Europe and beyond. Yet its particular contours in the Soviet and socialist context also reflected the institutional, social and ideological frameworks of Marxism and state socialism. The totalizing ambitions of the new revolutionary state to bring all aspects of public and private life under its control – however partial and incomplete the results – created new horizons of possibility. Soviet and other state socialist leaders spoke openly of their ambitions to shape the body and 'engineer the soul' in the service of building a bright future in communism. As Maksim Gorky, the Soviet writer, commented in 1928, 'Man was created to go forwards and upwards.'[3]

This volume examines attempts to reshape minds and bodies across the Soviet Union and the Eastern Bloc, from the early days of the revolution to the collapse of state socialism. In doing so it brings the history of human 'remaking' and the history of Soviet and Eastern Bloc socialism into conversation with each other. The chapters in the volume, many of which emerged from the international symposium of the same name at the University of Nottingham on 17–18 May 2019, are united by a shared focus on the multifaceted techniques developed in the socialist world in order to transform and revolutionize the human. They consider the ways in which science, culture and medicine overlapped with a mode of government that sought to manage, cultivate and regulate all aspects of human life in the service of an ideological goal. They trace the role of scientists, medical professionals, educational specialists and cultural producers in articulating new ideas about the body, health and human perfectibility. Finally, they explore some of the individual stories of those who transformed themselves, or who sought to transform others, as part of the wider Soviet 'project'.

This volume's exploration of 'technologies' of mind-body transformation seeks to offer a fresh perspective on the transformation of self and society in the Soviet Union and the Eastern Bloc. Derived from the Greek *techne* (art or craft) and *logos* (study of), 'technology' embodies a variety of different meanings. Science and technology studies scholars have drawn attention to three key 'layers of meaning' encompassed by the word 'technology': human knowledge (both in the sense of the 'know-how' pertaining to technological 'things' and specialized expertise); human activities, practices and processes; and finally, sets of physical objects or artefacts, such as cars or computers.[4] Indeed, the expansiveness of the term has allowed theorists like Michel Foucault to highlight the multiplicity of forces that have shaped understandings of what it is to be human – from technologies of production and sign systems that allow the manipulation of objects and representations, to technologies of power that shape human behaviour and technologies of self that permit individuals to transform 'their own bodies, souls, thoughts, conduct, and way of being'.[5] It is also notable that scholars have used the term to characterize the operation of complex and impersonal large-scale systems – Foucault's use of 'technology' to define relations of power presenting one vivid example – but also to describe individual craft and skills, strategies of self-development and 'techniques of the body'.[6] The lens of 'technology' similarly allows this volume to explore grand political visions of human remaking and the scientifically informed practices and techniques through which human conduct was transformed, without losing sight of the variety of ways in which individuals and collectives engaged with – or resisted – the transformative imperatives of the Soviet experiment. Thinking about mind-body transformation as a 'technology' also has the added benefit of allowing the coercive and repressive elements of this enterprise to be considered alongside its more 'positive' and productive aspects.[7]

The volume offers a broad interdisciplinary scope, bringing history into dialogue with cultural studies, the history of science and medicine, film studies, and science and technology studies. By engaging with current debates in these diverse fields – ranging from theories of biopolitics, to the haptic and the more-than-human – the volume re-interrogates the questions that have been raised in recent works on socialist remaking. Existing studies on individual and societal transformation in the Soviet Union and Eastern Europe (which will be outlined in greater detail below) have raised lingering questions. What was 'revolutionary' about Soviet techniques of 'reforging' individuals and populations? How did Soviet practices of population management differ from those deployed by other modern states? To what extent did the Russian Revolution mark a rupture with previous techniques of government? As Sergei Prozorov has recently noted in *The Biopolitics of Stalinism*, the search for an answer to such questions would benefit from an engagement with broader debates in contemporary social and critical theory.[8]

The volume examines the distinctive ways in which body-mind transformation was approached across the Soviet sphere of influence. The contributions cover not only the republics of the Soviet Union (including Soviet Russia, Ukraine and Latvia), but also the 'People's Democracies' of Bulgaria, Czechoslovakia and East Germany. Drawing attention to the unique experiences of state socialism in the countries of Eastern Europe, historians have increasingly questioned the tendency to assume that policies 'originated in Moscow and spread outwards'.[9] Through its geographical scope, *Technologies of Mind and Body* seeks to investigate the extent to which psychophysiological transformation should be seen as a common project across the Soviet Union and the Eastern Bloc. Is it fitting, our contributors ask, to consider the Soviet Union and Eastern Bloc as a common, if internally variegated, political, ideological and technological space?[10]

Existing studies on Soviet visions of human transformation have largely focused on the early Soviet and Stalinist periods.[11] By contrast, *Technologies of Mind and Body* seeks to explore the evolution of the project of psychophysiological remaking across the entire period of state socialism in Russia and Eastern Europe. The tendency of existing studies to focus on the early Soviet period is understandable given the predominance of utopian visions of bodily transformation during this time – from proposals for 'physiological passports' that were to be renewed when 'essential physiological changes have occurred in the human organism', to theories on the cessation of menstruation under Communism and research on rejuvenation.[12] The post-Stalin period, however, also gave rise to its fair share of radical transformative schemes. Seeking to better understand the fate of mind-body transformation under late socialism, our contributors explore how the urge for social and human engineering evolved in light of important post-war developments such as Cold War competition with the West, new technological advances and the waning of older models of heroism. The volume's contributors are particularly attentive to the role of the 'psy' disciplines in the Soviet Union and the Eastern Bloc, shedding light on the distinct approaches to questions of mental health and healing articulated in the Soviet sphere of influence. When Sarah Marks and Mat Savelli published their important volume *Psychiatry in Communist Europe* in 2015, they noted the reticence on behalf of historians to engage with the topic. '[P]sychiatry and mental illness rarely figured', they noted, in debates over 'the extent to which the countries of Eastern Europe underwent shared or unique experiences of Communism'.[13] The multiple essays on questions of mental health care and 'technologies of the mind' in this volume are a testament to the growth of scholarly interest in this previously under-researched topic over the last decade.

The chapters in *Technologies of Mind and Body* are divided into three sections, each of which addresses one of the 'layers of meaning' inherent in the concept of technology: knowledges, practices and artefacts. Separating out these layers of meaning enables the volume's authors to uncover the complexity of a project that stands at the intersection of political ambition, scientific enquiry and aesthetic and technological experiment, and that evolved over time. Yet the chapters – and this introduction – are also attentive to the myriad ways in which these layers overlap and intersect. Indeed, historians of modern state practices have shown that the production of knowledge cannot be 'easily disentangled from the exercise of power'.[14] New ideas about the mind and body facilitated the articulation of new programmes of personal and social 'remaking'; new technologies both reflected and enabled the emergence of distinct understandings and approaches to the human. This technological nexus of specialized knowledges, political programmes of transformation and material artefacts is the focus of this book.

Knowledges

One of the defining features of modern states is their proclivity to conceive society as an entity that can be identified, studied and manipulated. Modern statecraft, as James Scott notes, is predicated on the transformation of a previously inscrutable 'social hieroglyph into a legible and administratively more convenient format'.[15] The modern era saw the rulers of states beginning to tackle social questions in a new way, and becoming reliant on experts to resolve problems such as crime, poverty and suicide.[16] For the governed state, a particular form of knowledge, 'concrete, precise and measured' to use Foucault's formulation, became necessary.[17] The belief that society could be prophylactically engineered was intricately linked to what Lutz Raphael has termed the 'scientization' of the social.[18] The late nineteenth century saw a boom in social scientific research and its practical deployment by governments. Modern states began to amass knowledge about their subjects through 'new technologies of classifying and enumerating' (surveys, censuses, tests), which, as Ian Hacking has shown, led to new conceptualizations of the human subject.[19] Indeed, it was not only society that became a field of objective knowledge in the modern era. The self was also rendered a scientific issue, with disciplines such as psychology and psychiatry becoming intimately involved in 'establishing governing norms of human consciousness, conduct, and identity'.[20] As Greg Eghigian, Andreas Killen and Christine Leuenberger have shown, early-twentieth-century politicians and scientific and medical experts overlapped extensively in their efforts 'to turn the self into a project'.[21]

A considerable number of scholars have begun to explore the distinctive ways in which the social and human sciences were mobilized in the Soviet Union and socialist Eastern Europe in projects of social and individual reform.[22] Characterizing the Soviet regime as a 'social science state', scholars like Kenneth Pinnow have cast light on the vast expansion of expert intervention into the social realm in the Soviet era.[23] Prizing 'scientific government', Soviet leaders called on experts of all stripes – from pedologists and psychotechnicians to ethnographers, forensic experts and sexologists – to obtain the information about the population that was required for the implementation of transformative agendas and disciplinary practices.[24] The revolutionary transformation of group and individual identities was effected not only by coercion, Francine Hirsch notes, but through expert-driven 'technologies of rule' such as the census and the map that articulated new categories of self-understanding.[25] *Technologies of Mind and Body* further shows the integral role of scientific, medical and technical experts in elaborating new ideas about the body, health and human perfectibility.

In its focus on the interactions between the mind and body, this volume also builds on recent somatic and sensory 'turns' in Russian and East European studies.[26] Viewing embodiment and sensory perception as historically contingent and varied across time and space has enabled scholars to consider the unique understandings of and approaches to the body engendered by socialism. Indeed, recent studies have challenged the notion of the socialist body as homogeneous and tightly regulated by 'totalitarian' governance, pointing instead to the sheer variety of transformative practices of the body under socialism, and the sometimes-unexpected bodily ideals that they put forward. From the promotion of disabled masculinity in Soviet literature, to the use of film and other technologies to produce new kinds of sensory experience, scholars have considered the ways in which the 'alternative modernity' of Soviet socialism produced new ways of thinking about and experiencing the body.[27]

This volume traces the ways in which ideals of the body shifted over the socialist period and sheds new light on the bodily and sensory by linking them to frameworks of behaviour and psychological processes. Early scholarship focused on the various ways in which Soviet socialism promoted visions of the body and mind in distinctly utopian terms.[28] While Trotsky's famous 'superman' formulation was multifaceted and uncertain, recognizing the possibility of horizons of experience not yet envisioned, over time a more concrete ideal – a 'New Soviet Person' – solidified within Soviet culture and politics: a strong, muscular figure, predominantly masculine, aesthetically pleasing, and in sync with the machines of the factory. This ideal was perhaps best represented in the figure of the Stakhanovite, the hero worker who, following in the footsteps of the record-breaking miner Aleksei Stakhanov, sought to beat all production quotas.[29] The physical imperatives of the ideal body had military as well as industrial overtones, as seen in the generations of athletes who paraded on Red Square.[30] In their physical perfection, these individuals were seen to reflect the strength of the Soviet Union and the triumph of strong-willed, socialist humans over the flabby, weak citizens of the capitalist world.

Yet the physical and mental experiences of citizens of the Soviet Union, and later the state socialist societies of the Eastern Bloc, were far more complex than this early scholarship suggested. The Russian Revolution had taken place in a predominantly peasant society that fell far short of the ideals put forward by revolutionaries. Bodies and minds broken by war and disease, emaciated by hunger, or damaged by the rigours (and poor safety records) of the factory, could not easily conform to the Soviet ideal, if at all.[31] Gender and racial difference also proved difficult to reconcile; early dreams of the elimination of such physical markers through blood sharing, for example, failed to bear fruit.[32] Women, in particular, caused considerable anxieties, with their hormones and 'maternal natures' seen to open the door to capitalist corruption and mental decay.[33] Following the establishment of socialist regimes in the aftermath of the Second World War, Eastern Bloc nations found Soviet ideals competing with existing practices and imaginaries, as well as material realities, of the body and mind. Socialist individuals lived, breathed and often resisted the transformative imperatives imposed upon them.

This was not merely an issue of practical obstacle. The challenge posed by these problematic individuals was grounded in wider debates about the relationship between the mind and body, and about the competing influences of biology and society in shaping the human. In an atheist state, the materiality of the body – its muscles, bones, organs and cells – was central to understandings of not only physical but mental and social experiences. Yet while socialist specialists pledged allegiance to a monistic model of the human being throughout the Soviet period, understandings of mind-body interaction underwent considerable changes. The shift from the 'materialist' physiological explanations of human behaviour that rose to prominence after the revolution to a preoccupation with the question of 'consciousness' under Stalin has been particularly well documented.[34] Yet even as a new focus on the determining power of the will, intention and other mental factors over bodily processes took root, Soviet discourse often showed a remarkable sensitivity to the co-constitution and complex interaction of the psychic and the physiological. Insisting that phenomena like the emotions were not hardwired or 'instinctive', Stalinist psychology textbooks exalted the capacity of the human will to master physiological reactions but still affirmed that the 'brain cortex' was the 'substrate' of all psychical processes.[35]

In addition, while the monist attitudes of Soviet theorists saw consciousness as located at the level of the material brain or the cells (something that we might now refer to as the 'mindful body'), Soviet theorists of human nature were influenced by Marx's dictum that the social context, not biology, created the conditions that shaped human bodies and minds.[36] As Marx famously claimed, 'it is not the consciousness of men that determines their existence, but their social existence that determines their consciousness'.[37] The influence of this tradition is exemplified by the assertion of the early Soviet neurologist Aron Zalkind that different social environments cultivated 'a distinctive stock of reflexes'.[38] The belief in a plastic human nature that could be shaped (or 'forged', to use the industrial language of the early Soviet period) into new and ever more perfect forms underpinned much of the discussion of the body at this point. The tension between these two frameworks has been traced in a variety of socialist scientific contexts, from Soviet forensic medicine to the science of genetics and heredity.[39] In the latter, Darwinism was challenged by new theories, such as those put forward by the biologist Trofim Lysenko, suggesting that organisms could acquire new 'habits' and behaviours from their social surroundings that would then be handed down to future generations.[40] In the Soviet Union, Lysenko insisted, 'people are not born' but 'made'.[41]

While conversations around the mechanisms influencing the development of the human still predominantly focused on normative or idealized models of the body and mind, this shift from the paradigm of the 'strongest and fittest' to what Serguei Oushakine has termed the 'flexible and the pliant' made room for a multiplicity of approaches to human transformation, and for a variety of bodily states and experiences within the frameworks of the New Soviet Person[42]: from the valorization of disabled masculinity to the insistence that the myriad racial and ethnic minorities of the former Russian empire could become 'national in form, socialist in content'.[43] As many of the chapters in this volume show, however, the flexibility of the Soviet body and mind was not without limits, and the ideal of a perfect human (and the fear of an imperfect one) remained. How else to explain, for example, the persistent fears over women's physiological 'backwardness', or the desire for disabled people to 'overcome' their impairments and be 'rehabilitated' through prosthetic and other devices?[44] The drive to 'reforge' imperfect individuals reached its pinnacle in the practices of forced labour in the Gulag, which combined an imperative to transform the socially marginal through labour and discipline, with a more long-standing desire to quarantine the imperfect body from the 'healthy' body politic.[45] As Eric Naiman has argued, while early Soviet society looked to a utopian future of bodily perfection, it was often framed in the language of the gothic, haunted by imperfect bodies that contained within them problematic remnants of the past.[46] Such tendencies persisted throughout the Soviet period.[47] The contributors to this volume show that even the most pioneering technologies did not enable the 'overcoming' of physical impairments and the reintegration of problematic bodies into the Soviet body politic. Often, the imperfection of the body and the imperfection the mind were elided, with the body being scrutinized for clues as to the deviancy within.

The chapters in this section explore evolving understandings of the complex entanglement of mind and body across the socialist era. Anna Toropova's chapter on the thorny debates over the theory and practice of hypnosis in the early Soviet period shows the lingering influence of the work of nineteenth-century European specialists who had used hypnosis as technology for better understanding the recesses of the unconscious mind. She demonstrates that while the 1920s saw the emergence of seminal attempts to uncover the physiological mechanisms of hypnotic phenomena in the Soviet Union, many Soviet specialists continued to understand the hypnotic trance as the manifestation of a consciousness inaccessible to the waking self. Jakub Střelec's chapter on psychiatric knowledge and the management of crime in post-war Czechoslovakia examines the role of the psy-disciplines in developing new concepts of criminal behaviour and accountability. Pointing to an increased propensity of specialists to understand criminals as 'psychopathic' personalities rather than victims of psychosis, the chapter explores how psychiatric paradigms responded to social and political imperatives, such as tackling the growing problem of juvenile recidivism.

Siobhán Hearne's chapter explores the complex co-entanglement of mass media technologies, expert knowledge and political objectives in the articulation and dissemination of ideas about sexual health and morality in the Latvian Soviet Socialist Republic. The author examines how the late Soviet 'media boom' allowed medical advice to assume an unprecedented scope and reach, with venereologists tasked with preparing sex education lectures for dissemination via films, and radio and television broadcasts. Showcasing the Soviet state's reliance on expert opinion, Hearne connects sex education campaigns to sociological and demographic studies that laid bare alarming trends in the sphere of marriage and the family. Hearne's chapter reminds us of the degree to which expert knowledge in the Soviet Union was politically charged, with population statistics being subject to strict censorship and the battle against venereal disease conceptualized as the moral duty of every citizen. Similarly, the last contribution in this part, Jan Arend's chapter on late socialist popular health literature, explores the enlistment of health experts in the battle against the bodily and psychological 'consequences of advanced modernity' in Czechoslovakia and the German Democratic Republic. Arend traces how new post-war medical concerns about 'stress', 'health-related risk', and 'lifestyle diseases' travelled from the domain of the doctor's office and the research laboratory to the wider population via self-help literature, impacting everyday language as well as workplace practices. His chapter calls for a better appreciation of the extent to which socialist specialists' understandings of the mind and body were situated within international networks of knowledge transfer, and were thereby considerably influenced by research developed on the other side of the Iron Curtain.

The contributions on expert knowledge in this volume, many of which focus on the post-war decades, show that scientifically grounded techniques of state intervention by no means ran out of steam in the post-Stalin era, but in fact underwent important changes. The Soviet regime's reliance on experts to solve the problems of society continued apace, with a variety of professionals being called to tackle social issues and concerns that ranged from recidivism, to dwindling life expectancy, rising abortion rates, and mental overexertion. In this light, the contributions seem to provide little evidence of the post-war curtailment of the social engineering impulse pointed to by some scholars. For Amir Weiner, the post-war period was marked by a growing 'reluctance to accept without challenge the costs of radically transformative drives' and the emergence of 'softer gardening policies'.[48] By contrast, our contributors present the late socialist citizen as an individual targeted by a variety of prevention campaigns, bombarded with medical advice and instruction, and subjected to intrusive technologies of knowledge acquisition, such as health-monitoring programmes and contact tracing. Nevertheless, our authors acknowledge that the post-war period witnessed important developments such as the increased accessibility of therapy and counselling, as well as the growing public visibility of mental health problems, such as 'stress'. Moreover, for Hearne, the persistent framing of the battle for sexual health as a wider societal and political struggle is indicative of the Soviet state's attempts to counter waning faith in the promises of the socialist experiment. Arend, meanwhile, situates the growth of late socialist self-help literature, couched in a new language of 'kindness to oneself', in the context of the lessening hold of older discourses of socialist heroism and self-sacrifice.

Like other scholars exploring expert knowledge in the Eastern Bloc, our contributors show that the integration of scientific and medical expertise into the techniques of government did not necessarily mean that scientific disciplines were simply 'a hostage of the state'.[49] In his chapter, Střelec notes that the 'Sovietization' of Czechoslovak psychiatry was a much more complex process than often assumed. While psychiatrists increasingly read mental and somatic processes through the lens of Pavlov's teachings, the influence of medical paradigms and practices that were inherited from the Austro-Hungarian Empire remained strong. The fusion of Soviet models and native psychiatric traditions, Střelec shows, gave rise to a novel approach to mental health. Similarly, Toropova's chapter on the different scientific understandings of hypnosis in the early Soviet period demonstrates that Pavlovian paradigms did not have a complete monopoly over scientific and medical knowledge. Throughout the 1920s and early 1930s, physiological explanations of hypnosis as a process of brain inhibition were forced to contend with a highly influential tradition of understanding hypnotic phenomena as manifestations of the unconscious mind. Even in the mid to late 1930s, Toropova shows, specialists continued to resist the push for a single scientific explanation of the hypnotic state. Julian Chehirian's chapter elsewhere in this volume also reveals that the decisions implemented at the notorious Pavlov session of 1950 led to a pronounced 'somatic emphasis' in Bulgarian psychiatry, yet did not stop the Soviet approach to work therapy being subject to 'vernacular adaptations'.

Střelec, Arend, Hearne and Toropova not only showcase the expansion of the jurisdiction and authority of various fields of scientific and medical expertise, but also consider the limits of 'power-knowledge'. Střelec's chapter reminds us that there was often a gap between experts' strivings for influence over state policy and the actual implementation of scientific guidance. Psychiatrists and psychologists played a key role in the battle against religious belief and superstitions in post-war Czechoslovakia, and contributed to the articulation of models of socialist conduct and selfhood. Yet Střelec shows that even as psychiatrists made the case for the greater use of their expertise in assessing defendants undergoing criminal trials, their influence over the communist criminal-justice system remained limited. At least until the 1960s, judiciaries proved more inclined to explain criminal behaviour through the framework of class than through medical paradigms. Similarly, Toropova's chapter shows that the public uptake of scientific explanations lagged behind the aspirations of medical specialists. Despite doctors' efforts to present hypnosis as a scientifically justified and routine medical method, portrayals of hypnosis as an enigmatic and irrational phenomenon that was open to mis-use continued to proliferate in public culture. Hearne's chapter shows that despite considerable state investment in extending the public reach of medical sexual health advice in the late Soviet period, citizens' exposure to sex education was likely sparse outside of the urban centres where access to mass media was less consistent. Soviet authorities also remained frustrated by the under-deployment of new technologies of investigating the health of the social body, such as contact tracing. Moreover, Hearne highlights the presence of a disjunction between the models of dutiful deference to medical authority articulated in Soviet mass media and Latvian citizens' continued reluctance to seek out treatment for VD within the state healthcare system.

Practices

The Soviet state's attempt to cultivate a new type of human personality has remained an enduring topic of historical enquiry. In recent years, a growing number of historians have studied efforts to inculcate new behavioural norms, moral values and models of bodily discipline in the Soviet population through campaigns to improve public health and hygiene and interventions into spheres such as leisure, reproduction, sexuality and child rearing.[50]

The vast range of techniques of behaviour transformation explored by scholars include the campaigns targeting remnants of the 'old life' – from illiteracy, religion and traditional customs to sexual immorality – as well as health enlightenment propaganda and advice literature propagating new 'cultured' values.[51] Scholars have cast light on work-place strategies of forging model labourers, practices of 'productive rest', including vacation travel and stays at rest homes and health spas, and the new bodily regimes cultivated through physical culture.[52] The ways in which cities and living spaces functioned as 'training grounds' for 'model citizens' have received growing scholarly attention, as have the attempts to bring into being new ways of seeing through cinema, visual culture and cartographic practices.[53] Scholarship on Soviet subjectivity has also used a technological conception of power to foreground the disciplinary strategies of self-perfection and self-development through which New Men and Women made themselves into subjects.[54] As Jochen Hellbeck notes, subjectivizing practices such as diary-keeping served as 'both records and tools of psycho-physiological training', permitting their authors to scrutinize mental and bodily processes with a view to 'perfecting' them.[55]

Explorations of practices of self-development and population management have made clear the Soviet state's steadfast dedication to the 'sculpting', 'landscaping' and 'reworking' of human 'material'.[56] To paraphrase Peter Holquist's influential argument, the Bolsheviks viewed the socio-political body as an 'artefact' that could be operated upon and moulded to their liking.[57] Recent work on Soviet technologies of government and subjectivizing practices has been pivotal in helping to situate the Soviet case within a broader history of modern state intervention.[58] As Holquist notes, the 'technique' of population management became 'a value and an aesthetic goal' across Europe in the early twentieth century.[59] Not only were the Soviet regime's aspirations to mould new individuals shared by other modern governments, but the Bolsheviks' 'repertoire of practices' grew out of the methods deployed by the Imperial Russian state during the First World War. As many historians now recognize, the drive to remould society and individuals was not so much a marker of Soviet exceptionalism as a ubiquitous feature of the modern state, whose urge to 'landscape the human garden' was 'restrained by and accountable to no one'.[60]

Examinations of the procedures and methods employed by socialist states to regulate human bodies and behaviours have expanded scholarly understanding of the 'technologies of bio-power' through which human life is cultivated and managed. Theories of biopolitics – the exploration of a rationality of power that places human life at the centre of government, manifesting in procedures that centre on the '*anatomo-politics of the human body*', as well as those focused on 'the species body' or population – have been vital to elucidating the transformation of modern techniques of government.[61] While there has been much debate as to the applicability of biopolitics to the 'illiberal modernity' of Soviet and East European socialism, recent works have sought to challenge the tendency of scholarship to focus on the fascist and liberal incarnations of biopolitics and have begun to consider the specificity of a 'socialist governmentality of life'.[62]

Similarly, the socialist pathway of mental health care, characterized by the rejection of psychoanalytic psychotherapy in favour of a Pavlovian behaviourist model, has long been set in stark relief from that of the West.[63] In recent years, however, the focus on the repression of therapeutic practices that diverged from the tenets of 'Scientific Marxism' in Communist Eastern Europe has given way to attempts to trace the survival of a variety of psychotherapeutic modalities in the Eastern Bloc.[64] Uncovering psychotherapists' persisting interest in the unconscious aspects of the mind in Czechoslovakia and the German Democratic Republic and highlighting the flourishing of psychoanalytic psychotherapy in socialist Yugoslavia, this scholarship has helped to integrate developments in socialist science and medicine into a broader history of the psy-disciplines.[65] While much of this research has focused on the post-war period, the work of Benjamin Zajicek has shown that even under Stalin,

'Soviet psychiatrists were able to develop a sometimes surprisingly diverse range of approaches to the mind'.[66] Scholars have also begun to show that the vast growth of the psy-disciplines in the West in the post-war period, and the ensuing 'psychologisation of human subjectivity' was not only specific to Western liberal democracies.[67]

Further revealing the role of psychiatric and psychological professionals in 'defining standards and shaping perceptions of the individual subject', the contributors in this section explore the unique characteristics of therapeutic intervention under state socialism.[68] Julian Chehirian's chapter examining the role of psychotherapy in the political project of building communism in Bulgaria shows how closely the aims of therapeutic rehabilitation became intertwined with the economic objectives of the state. The growing psychotherapeutic emphasis placed on 'meaningful, purposeful and joyful work' reflected the influence of ideas about social usefulness as well as a steadfast dedication to the cultivation of a 'New Bulgarian Man'. Yet through the examination of the life and art of Nikola Kazakov, a psychiatric patient and brother to the better-known Bulgarian artist, Dimitar Kazakov, Chehirian reveals the complex and contested vision of the mind and body that this model produced. Aleksandra Brokman's chapter on Soviet psychotherapeutic methods and practices in the post-war period reads psychotherapy as not only a method of treatment but a technique for human transformation. The author shows how the purview of psychotherapy expanded beyond the clinical setting in the post-war decades, with psychotherapeutic methods targeting the optimization of human performance in spheres such as work and sport. As well as battling neurosis and mental disorders, psychotherapists turned to helping athletes cultivate specific skills and sporting abilities, boosting patients' self-confidence and promoting new attitudes and emotional outlooks. Brokman shows that the spoken word was seen as the central means of psychophysiological influence over the individual, assuming pride of place in practices of autogenic training, hypnosis and suggestion. Such techniques, Brokman argues, were used by Soviet psychotherapists to cultivate the resilience, self-assurance and strength of will that were ascribed to the 'New Soviet Person'.

Tricia Starks's chapter on the smoking cessation therapies deployed by Soviet medical specialists between 1920 and 1970 showcases the 'unique answers to tobacco danger' developed in the Soviet Union and the Eastern Bloc. Starks demonstrates how Soviet social medicine gave rise not only to the world's first cessation clinics but also to innovative chemical therapeutics. The development of the cytisine-based drug Tabex – a chemical replacement for nicotine – emerged as the link between nicotine and chemical dependency became better recognized in the post-war period. Despite these late Soviet breakthroughs, Starks sees a great deal of continuity in Soviet approaches to smoking cessation over the period. Ivan Pavlov's concept of the conditioned reflex remained fundamental to the methods of Soviet medical authorities. Through the lens of reflexology, smoking was perceived to be a cultivated habit that was reinforced by 'social and cultural cues'. Quitting smoking, Starks shows, was thereby largely framed as a process that depended on the training and strengthening of the will. Both Starks and Brokman see the pronounced emphasis placed on the will (and its 'training') in Soviet therapy as a crucial point of divergence with Western therapeutic practices. As Brokman notes, the will was conceptualized as the 'motor' of human activity. The overwhelming power attributed to this agency of self-perfection was evident in Soviet psychotherapists' view that willpower could conquer over both psychological and physiological processes.[69]

The case of socialist Eastern Europe presents particularly rich material for the analysis of the overlap between physicians' aspirations for health improvement and political ambitions to reform the social body.[70] Examining the turn to medical explanations in domains such as criminology, work and sexual morality, our contributors shed further light on the distinct manifestation of 'medicopolitics' that operated in the Soviet Union and the Eastern Bloc.[71] As a number of scholars have observed, the Soviet period saw the reach of medical jurisdiction expand 'beyond the traditional boundaries of clinical practice and into other domains of social and professional life'.[72] In this context, not only 'health' but 'development' fell into the purview of medical expertise and notions such as 'pathology' took on broader and more encompassing meanings.[73] Vividly illustrating the blurred lines between therapeutic practice and pedagogy, Brokman notes that the Soviet psychotherapist was not only a clinician but a 'teacher of life' who was to serve as an educator and a guide for his patients. Starks brings to light the unique therapeutic and political context that inclined Soviet cessationists to view smoking as less an addiction than a form of behaviour that could be modified through the training of the will and the influence of the collective. In her chapter in the previous section, Hearne similarly observes how closely 'discourses of health' became entangled with 'discourses of morality', with Soviet venereologists advocating measures to battle with VD that emphasized compliance to strict behavioural norms over the use of barrier contraceptives (in short supply throughout the Soviet period).

While showcasing the unique 'melding of the medical with the utopian and the political' in socialist Eastern Europe, the contributions nevertheless compel us to question narratives of 'exceptionalism'.[74] Starks acknowledges, for example, that the emphasis on peer support, group meetings and psychological influence in Soviet therapeutics could also be observed in many other countries tackling 'tobacco danger'. Brokman also recognizes that Soviet psychotherapists were not necessarily unique in targeting the self-perfection of the patient, with a broad array of psychotherapeutic methods elsewhere similarly directing clients towards the path of the 'good life'. Indeed, the contributions on post-war socialist medicine and psychotherapy in this volume all point out that Soviet specialists, much like their Western counterparts, were increasingly concerned about the stresses and tensions of modern life. As Arend also shows, East German and Czechoslovak self-help literature espoused the 'buzzwords' that became current across the modern world from the 1960s and 1970s, when experts in different countries turned their attention to the 'physical and mental health-related consequences of an industrial society perceived as fast-moving and performance-focused'. In this respect, the Soviet Union and its satellite states also saw key aspects of the 'therapeutic culture' that historians have long attributed to post-war Western societies, albeit without the attendant decline of the planned welfare state usually associated with 'therapeutisation'.[75]

Ideologies of human transformation were not limited to social and scientific fields, but also characterized Soviet and socialist approaches to culture. These concepts supplied a powerful imaginary that proved fruitful to writers, filmmakers and other artists. Indeed, the Soviet period was characterized by the slippage between science in the laboratory and on the page and screen. Recent studies have illustrated the extent to which cultural initiatives and developments in Russia and Eastern Europe were indebted to psychophysiological research and ideas. Whether exploring avant-garde theatre, dance and performance or socialist realist cinema, a growing number of scholars have turned their focus onto the terrain of scientific research that shaped Soviet cultural producers' engagement with the mind and body.[76] The creation of a socialist subject may have been a common objective that brought together 'seemingly incompatible scientific and artistic methods', but psychophysiological ideas about embodiment, affect and aesthetic reception were still appropriated in a plurality of ways.[77] As Ana Hedberg Olenina notes in her recent book *Psychomotor Aesthetics*, the 'incursion of neurophysiology into the arts' manifested in cultural initiatives that attempted to standardize and organize human behaviour, but also in projects that valorized open-ended experiment.[78]

The contributions in this volume explore how art, popular culture and mass media technologies translated the language of the human sciences into vernacular forms as well as spotlight the often-fruitful collaborations between scientists and cultural figures. As Chehirian's chapter shows, human reforging could take several alternate paths, from art to labour therapy and psychiatric intervention. To be sure, cultural practices and technologies also figure in this volume as important means of transmitting state-approved visions of 'health' and 'disease'. Films, radio and television broadcasts and newspaper articles disseminating sex education in Soviet Latvia, Hearne shows, starkly opposed 'normal' and 'perverted' sexual behaviour and reinforced traditional gender roles through their focus on men's behaviour. In this way, her chapter accords with Oksana Sarkisova's analysis of *kulturfilms* featuring Soviet national minorities, which has brought attention to the role of 'normative representations of health and illness' in sustaining a 'cultural hierarchy' of ethnicity and reinforcing binary oppositions of the 'primitive' and the 'modern'.[79]

Yet as Chehirian's exploration of art and therapy in socialist Bulgaria vividly demonstrates, artistic practice could give expression to states of consciousness that fell outside the accepted parameters of 'socialist subjectivity'. In the absence of a written record of Nikola Kazakov's experiences, his canvases and sculptures – 'effigies hand-carved from knobby, knotted tree branches' – present 'visceral archives and documents' of his psychic distress and social dislocation. As the chapters by Lilya Kaganovsky and Anna Toropova elsewhere in this volume similarly show, film and popular culture could facilitate new ways of experiencing the physical world, or register new mental and somatic states that posed a challenge to dominant scientific and ideological narratives within the socialist space.

Artefacts

The fascination of revolutionary socialism with science and technology's capacity to radically transform human nature remains an enduring focus of scholarly attention. The recent works of scholars such as Nikolai Krementsov have demonstrated the extent to which scientific research captured the imaginations of Bolshevik party leaders, fiction writers and the reading public.[80] From the early dreams of 'iron messiahs' and the fusing of human and machine parts, to the late Soviet fascination with cryotherapy and forms of 'grafting' of the human body, scholars have traced the ways in which the development of scientific devices and processes have shaped socialist understandings of, and attitudes to, the human.[81] Indeed, as Anya Bernstein has argued, the Soviet transformational project was steeped in understandings of 'technofuturism', which promised bodily perfection and even immortality.[82]

The centrality of science and technology to the Soviet socialist worldview was intimately entwined with the ideology of Marxism-Leninism, understood itself, as Ethan Pollock has argued, to be a 'science inextricably tied to the methodology and laws of the natural sciences'.[83] The sciences – from biology and physics to genetics and linguistics – were thus pressed into the service of the revolution. Science was seen as a tool both to understand the natural world and ultimately to transform it. As such, the role of science was not simply to bend to the whims of Marxist-Leninist ideology, but to provide new horizons of possibility for the revolutionary state.[84] As Krementsov suggests, science and technology 'supplied the ideas, ideals and techniques' that made cultural and political dreams "'real'" and "'living'".[85] The technical instrumentality so enthusiastically endorsed by the Soviet state – epitomising the subordination of technology to human interests that Martin Heidegger famously decries in his *Question Concerning Technology* – was not, however, the only approach to technology elaborated during the period, with avant-garde cultural producers imagining technologies that had 'exploratory' rather than 'exploitative' aims.[86]

While science and technology were ideologically central, their tenets were far from consistent. Fierce scientific debates characterized the entirety of the Soviet period, with some questions becoming more settled over time (occasionally by intervention from the 'coryphaeus' of Stalin or other Soviet leaders), and others becoming unsettled again by ideological shifts or the significant scientific developments that emerged within the socialist bloc or transcended the Iron Curtain.[87] The twentieth century was characterized by vast transformations in scientific and technological knowledge, from electrification to the nuclear bomb, microchips and the sequencing of DNA. These shifts mapped onto and interacted with developments inside the Soviet Union and the socialist bloc, such as the rhythms of the Five-Year Plans, the 'relaunch' of the Soviet project following the death of Stalin, or the economic issues that characterized the era of 'Stagnation'. Following the Second World War, they also became part of the wider crucible of the Cold War, as Naomi Oreskes has suggested, leading scholars to consider how 'the Cold War context either enabled or disabled certain kinds of investigations and intellectual achievements'.[88] Crucially, as contributions to this volume attest, technological transfer across the Iron Curtain was far from one-way: significant innovation could, and did, emerge from the socialist sphere.

Science and technology were therefore integral to revolutionary dreams of the mind and body, but their contours and imperatives shifted over time. In the early Soviet period, theorists focused particularly on the interaction between humans and their social context, and between external objects and the human mind-body nexus, to establish how best to facilitate the emergence of 'New People'. Scholars have identified biomechanics and the 'machine man' as central to this early vision, although as Johanna Conterio has revealed, there were alternative environmental models at play.[89] The notion of the human as part of a wider 'machine' or ecosystem characterized this period. The picture shifted in the 1930s, with the need for industrialization pushing a model of the human – and of nature more widely – that prioritized the strength of the will over the natural world and the desire to transcend all material limits, a phenomenon recognized by scholars as 'Soviet Prometheanism'.[90] While the capacities of science, as a manifestation of the human will to transform the world, were increasingly perceived to be limitless, its contours and scope were increasingly limited by the rigid ideological frameworks of Stalinism, and the exhortation that 'cadres decide everything' moved the focus decidedly from the primacy of technology onto the human.[91]

The Cold War and Khrushchev's Thaw prompted a return to science and technology as a source of innovative models and frameworks for the New Person; a moment that coincided with considerable developments in both the hard and applied sciences. The creation of new cities of science, and the development of technological competition with the United States, drove research that shaped new ways of thinking.[92] As Slava Gerovitch has shown, new scientific frameworks such as cybernetics took ideas of the human in new directions, using analogies of the computer to understand the 'feedback loops' that shaped the way people thought and behaved.[93] Similarly, the discovery of new technologies, such as electronics and electromagnetic radiation, created scope for new ways to graft and transform the human body and senses, imagining new relationships between bodies and objects: no longer 'machine men' but rather 'drilled humans', as Diana Kurkovsky-West argues.[94]

The chapters in this part trace the interplay of technological devices and the human body, and the ways in which technology was used to transform and perfect the human under socialism. Johanna Conterio's chapter focuses on the use of sun lamps in Soviet public health practices. She considers the shifting use of the lamp in the interwar period, from a means to treat the individual body, to a technology capable of transforming the environment (and by extension the people within it). As such, her chapter examines the ways in which the use of sun lamp technology tapped into wider Soviet theories of the nature of the human body, the aetiology of disease and the relationship of the environment to human health. Lilya Kaganovsky examines the body-technology relationship through the medium of women's cinema of the Soviet avant-garde, looking particularly at Lilya Brik's *Glass Eye* (*Stekliannyi glaz*, 1929) and Esfir Shub's *Today* (*Segodnia*, 1930). She focuses in particular on 'the haptic, material nature of the world as captured by the film camera' and traces the ways in which the filmmakers' practice – the hands-on engagement with the practice of film-making – creates new relationships between the body of the filmmaker and the body of the film itself. By doing so, she argues, these women filmmakers made a powerful case for cinema 'as an embodied technology that fragments and rearranges the world'.

Frances Bernstein's chapter examines the 'Russia Arm', the world's first functioning bionic arm, which dazzled audiences at the 1958 Brussels Expo. As she traces, the Russia Arm had several different 'lives': understood in the USSR as a technological marvel that would enable disabled veterans to return to normalcy, the arm's ability to be controlled by nerve impulses was understood by the Americans as an extension of the totalitarian 'brainwashing' that characterized the socialist world, and thus something to be feared. Bernstein also traces the arm as a commodity, marketed abroad to victims of the Thalidomide scandal to make money for the USSR, a process that belied its limited domestic use. Finally, Claire Shaw considers the Soviet discipline of 'deaf technology' in the 1960s and 1970s, tracing the ways in which the development of transistors and the emergence of microchips enabled the translation of sound waves into visual and tactile stimuli. She explores these innovations as an example of the utopian thinking of the late Soviet period, when types of technological synaesthesia promised to offer new and alternative ways of being in the world, but also considers how these types of sensory futurism were shaped and confined by long-standing Soviet ideologies of technology, the self and the senses.

In this respect, the chapters in this section engage with the recent 'material turn' in Soviet studies, which foregrounds material objects as a central aspect of socialist everyday life. At a recent conference in Cambridge, scholars from a variety of disciplines gathered to 'consider material and objects, their journeys through time and space, their processes of making and re-making, and [explore] how those perspectives might uncover alternative modernisms, defamiliarise Sovietness, and explore the diversity of Soviet experiences and identities'.[95] Alexei Golubev, in his influential work on materialism in late Soviet society and culture, has noted the particular power of 'elemental materialism' – 'a culturally rooted recognition of the power of matter and things to shape human bodies and selves' – in the socialist context.[96] He traces the ability of objects, such as bodybuilding equipment or steel frames for shattered bones, not only to enable transformations of the body, but to tap into powerful imaginaries that framed bodies and minds under socialism, such as the ubiquitous focus on 'iron' muscles and will. In a similar manner, the chapters in this section are each alive to the agency of objects, not only to shape the physical state and abilities of bodies, but to provoke new ways of thinking about the self and society. This focus on the 'tuning' of the human being to the material world, as Emma Widdis argues, was central to the revolutionary project from its very beginning: 'Soviet man or woman would feel the world differently, reborn into a revitalized sensory apprehension of the material.'[97]

Indeed, as the authors in this section show, the relationship between the body and the material world reveals both the body's own materiality, and the bodily nature of the material. As Rolf Hellebust has argued, Soviet and socialist literature abounds with conceptions of the body as a material, or technological, artefact: flesh becomes metal, nerves are electrical impulses and thoughts can be tangibly located in the brain.[98] These ways of thinking about the body are fundamental to the technological devices explored here; understanding the senses as electrical stimuli makes it possible to transform them using microchips; viewing thoughts as tangible impulses enables their conversion into bionic structures. As Kaganovsky shows, this parallel could (and often was) reversed: 'cinema is a technology that not only captures the human body [...], or relies on the human body for its production' but 'is itself a *body*, with "skin," "musculature," and "viscera"'. This blurring of the lines between body and technology is most evident in the field of prosthetic technology, but these imaginative frameworks, Kaganovsky shows, work even for those technologies that neither touch the body nor ape its processes.

The chapters in this volume also show how Soviet explorations of the body-technology interface play with certain binaries that we often consider to be fixed. Looking at the materiality of these objects and the processes of design and making reveals a complex set of practices that elide the fixed categories of the 'scientific' (formal, laboratory-based design processes) and the 'amateur' (the *ad hoc* or the handmade). As Bernstein and Shaw show, the Soviet Union actively encouraged the engagement of amateur inventors in the production of limb or sensory prosthetics, calling on the public to create their own technological solutions to problems of the body. Kaganovsky also demonstrates the ways in which women's cinema of the avant-garde elided the boundaries between masculine 'technology' and feminine 'faktura', or between seriousness and play in the creation of cinematic artefacts.

At the same time, considering the interplay of technologies and bodies also brings this volume into conversation with recent scholarship on the 'posthuman' under socialism. As Colleen McQuillen and Julia Vaingurt argue, the 'enmeshment of the human body with various forms of technology' was understood in unique ways in the Soviet period, from the decidedly humanist, rational approaches of Aleksei Gastev to the philosophical imaginaries of Russian Cosmism.[99] As such, the attention to posthumanism, which foregrounds the ways in which objects can enable bodies to 'transcend their physiological limits', enables scholars to ask new and probing questions about Soviet and socialist society. To date, these questions have been most extensively explored in the realm of culture (particularly in Anindita Banerjee and Elana Gomel's work on the body in Science Fiction), but these cultural imaginaries reflected, and sometimes even provoked, practical experimentation in using technology to extend and graft the body and mind.[100] Indeed, the very real technological artefacts explored in this section – the sun ray lamp, the Morse Code telephone, the cinema strip or the myoelectric arm – provoked new ways of thinking about the extension of human capacities under socialism, from the idea of 'mind control' of inanimate objects to forms of sensory augmentation and swapping.

In this way, several of the chapters in this volume engage with Donna Haraway's famous exploration of the cyborg, a 'theorised and fabricated hybrid of machine and organism'.[101] There is some debate within the literature about the applicability of cyborgs to state socialism: Elana Gomel notes that the utopian humanism of the New Soviet Man is very different from the postmodern hybridity that Haraway champions, but Slava Gerovitch, while he acknowledges that even the scientists involved in the space programme 'did not resort to cyborglike modifications of the human body', recognizes that the term was 'contemplated by Soviet physicians'.[102] In their engagement with very different socialist technologies, Bernstein, Kaganovsky and Shaw all engage with the slippery distinction between the prosthetic – an addition to the human body that replaces a missing or impaired function – and the cyborg, in which a productive melding of human and machine enables new forms of ability and selfhood to emerge.[103] Similarly, Conterio shows the ways in which the boundaries between human and environment, and human and machine, were blurred – both practically and imaginatively – by Soviet scientists' fascination with 'rays' and 'mechanical energy'.

The belief in the capacity of science and technology to transform the human and pave the way for a new future was characteristic of the socialist space until its collapse. In that respect, it complicates arguments made by scholars such as Leo Marx that a form of 'technological pessimism' set in after the Second World War: 'As the visible effects of technology became more dubious, modernism lost its verve and people found the romance less and less appealing.'[104] In the Soviet space, the 'verve' of technology continued to persist, even as its limitations became more evident. As Shaw shows in her chapter, the 1960s and 1970s were defined by a form of 'deaf futurism', characterized by an overriding belief that technology could create new forms of being in the world that would overcome bodily flaws. Similarly, Fran Bernstein considers the technological ambition encapsulated in the world's first myoelectric arm, while acknowledging at the same time that money, rather than ideology, was a driving factor, and that technologies often had lives, and were put to uses, that their inventors may not have intended.

Conclusion

In its examination of the various and multifaceted technologies of human remaking under socialism, *Technologies of Mind and Body* reveals the ideologies and understandings that underpinned social and scientific practices, and uncovers the competing agencies inherent in socialist approaches to the human. The desire to reshape the human population was not unique to socialism; in its engagement with wider discourses of science, technology and medicine, it reflects broader, modern practices of population management, social engineering and human remaking. Yet as this volume shows, the Soviet and Eastern Bloc example – both in its ambition and its practical, everyday realities – was indeed historically contingent and, in many ways, unique. In their attempts, not only to fix the various problems of the human body and mind, but to create 'a higher social-biologic type', Soviet and socialist scientists, doctors, engineers and policymakers created new ways of thinking about the interactions between the body, mind and society, and framed new, embodied ways of being in the world. While the utopia dreamed of by Trotsky was never realized, the legacy of these historical ideas of the future mind-body continues to persist, both in the former socialist world and elsewhere.

Notes

1   Leon (Lev) Trotsky, *Literature and Revolution*, ed. William Keach and trans. Rose Strunsky (Chicago, IL: Haymarket Books, 2005), 207.

2   Karen Petrone, 'Coming Home Soviet Style: The Reintegration of Afghan Veterans into Soviet Everyday Life', in Choi Chatterjee, David L. Ransel, Mary Cavender, Karen Petrone and Sheila Fitzpatrick, eds., *Everyday Life in Russia: Past and Present* (Bloomington, IN: Indiana University Press, 2015), 358. On Afghan veterans as 'new Soviet men', see also Aleksei Golubev, *The Things of Life: Materiality in Late Soviet Culture* (Ithaca, NY: Cornell University Press, 2020), 5.

3   Maksim Gor'kii, 'Rech' na torzhestvennom zasedanii plenuma Bakinskogo Soveta' [1928], in Akademiia nauk SSSR Institut mirovoi literatury im. A. M. Gor'kogo, *Sobranie sochinenii v tridtsati tomakh*, vol. 24 (Moscow: Goslitizdat, 1949), 392.
4   Donald Mackenzie and Judy Wajcman, 'Introductory Essay: The Social Shaping of Technology', in Donald Mackenzie and Judy Wajcman, eds., *The Social Shaping of Technology: How the Refrigerator Got Its Hum* (Milton Keynes: Open University Press, 1985), 2–25, here 3–4; Wiebe E. Bijker, 'Why and How Technology Matters', in Robert E. Goodin and Charles Tilly, eds., *The Oxford Handbook of Contextual Political Analysis* (Oxford: Oxford University Press, 2006), 681–706, 682. See also Sheila Jasanoff, 'Technology as a Site and Object of Politics', in Goodin and Tilly, eds., *The Oxford Handbook of Contextual Political Analysis*, 746–64. As scholars like Leo Marx have shown, the meaning of the word 'technology' has also undergone very significant shifts in recent history. It came to assume its modern connotations from about 1900 (in response to the advances of industrial society), previously being used to refer to a field of study – a 'branch of learning concerned with the mechanic arts'. See Leo Marx, 'Technology: The Emergence of a Hazardous Concept', *Social Research*, 51.3 (2010): 561–77.
5   Michel Foucault, 'Technologies of the Self', in Luther H. Martin, Huck Gutman and Patrick Hutton, eds., *Technologies of the Self: A Seminar with Michel Foucault* (Amherst: University of Massachusetts Press, 1988), 16–49, here 17–18.
6   As Leo Marx astutely notes, the word 'technology' in contemporary usage conjures images of '[w]hite male technicians in control booths watching dials, instrument panels, or computer monitors', while its origins lie in 'the mundane world of work, physicality, and practicality […] humdrum handicrafts and artisanal skills'. See Marx, 'Technology: The Emergence of a Hazardous Concept', 574. On Foucault's use of 'technology' and 'technique', see Michael C. Behrent, 'Foucault and Technology', *History and Technology*, 29.1 (2013): 54–104. Marcel Maus's analysis of the bodily techniques specific to each society focuses on 'culturally acquired skills'. See Marcel Maus, 'Techniques of the Body', *Economy and Society*, 2.1 (1973): 70–88.
7   As Michael Behrent notes, the term 'technology' has appealed to theorists of power relations like Foucault due to its 'neutral' and even 'potentially positive' connotations. See his 'Foucault and Technology', p. 56.
8   Sergei Prozorov, *The Biopolitics of Stalinism: Ideology and Life in Soviet Socialism* (Edinburgh: Edinburgh University Press, 2016), 39.
9   Sarah Marks and Mat Savelli, 'Communist Europe and Transnational Psychiatry', in Mat Savelli and Sarah Marks, eds., *Psychiatry in Communist Europe* (Basingstoke: Palgrave Macmillan, 2015), 1–26.
10 We are grateful to one of our anonymous reviewers for suggesting this point.
11 See, for example, Nikolai L. Krementsov and Yvonne Howell, eds., *The Art and Science of Making the New Man in Early 20th-century Russia* (London: Bloomsbury, 2021).
12 On Emmanuil Enchmen's proposal for physiological passports, and the ideological function of menstruation, see Eric Naiman, *Sex in Public: The Incarnation of Early Soviet Ideology* (Princeton: Princeton University Press, 1997), 76, 208–49. On rejuvenation, see Nikolai Krementsov, *Revolutionary Experiments: The Quest for Immortality in Bolshevik Science and Fiction* (Oxford: Oxford University Press, 2014).
13 Marks and Savelli, 'Communist Europe and Transnational Psychiatry', 1.
14 Francine Hirsch, *Empire of Nations: Ethnographic Knowledge and the Making of the Soviet Union* (Ithaca, NY: Cornell University Press, 2005), 11.

15 James C. Scott, *Seeing Like a State: How Certain Schemes to Improve the Human Condition Have Failed* (New Haven, CT: Yale University Press, 1998), 3.
16 David Horn, *Social Bodies: Science, Reproduction, and Italian Modernity* (Princeton, NJ: Princeton University Press, 1994); Lutz Raphael, 'Embedding the Human and Social Sciences in Western Societies, 1880–1980: Reflections on Trends and Methods of Current Research', in Kerstin Brückweh et al., eds., *Engineering Society: The Role of the Human and Social Sciences in Modern Societies, 1880–1980* (Basingstoke: Palgrave Macmillan, 2012), 41–56.
17 Michel Foucault, 'The Political Technology of Individuals', in Martin, Gutman and Hutton, eds., *Technologies of the Self*, 145–62, 151.
18 Raphael, 'Embedding the Human and Social Sciences', 41. See also Benjamin Ziemann et al., 'Introduction: The Scientization of the Social in Comparative Perspective', in Brückweh et al. eds., *Engineering Society*, 1–40.
19 Ian Hacking, *The Taming of Chance* (Cambridge: Cambridge University Press, 1990), 2–3; See also his 'The Invention of Split Personalities', in Alan Donagan, Anthony Perovich and Michael Wedin, eds., *Human Nature and Natural Knowledge: Essays Presented to Marjorie Grene on the Occasion of Her Seventy-Fifth Birthday* (Dordrecht: D. Reidel, 1986), 63–85.
20 Greg Eghigian, Andreas Killen and Christine Leuenberger, 'Introduction: The Self as Project: Politics and the Human Sciences in the Twentieth Century', *Osiris*, 22.1 (2007): 1–25, 3.
21 Ibid., 4.
22 Daniel Beer, *Renovating Russia: The Human Sciences and the Fate of Liberal Modernity, 1811–1930* (Ithaca, NY: Cornell University Press, 2008); Greg Eghigian, 'The Psychologization of the Socialist Self: East German Forensic Psychology and Its Deviants, 1945–1975', *German History*, 22.2 (2004): 181–205; Kateřina Lišková, *Sexual Liberation, Socialist Style: Communist Czechoslovakia and the Science of Desire, 1945–1989* (New York, NY: Cambridge University Press, 2018); Agnieszka Kościańska, *Gender, Pleasure, and Violence: The Construction of Expert Knowledge of Sexuality in Poland*, trans. by Marta Rozmysłowicz (Bloomington, IN: Indiana University Press, 2020); Frank Henschel, 'The Embodiment of Deviance: The Biopolitics of the "Difficult Child" in Socialist Czechoslovakia', *East European Politics and Societies*, 34.4 (2020): 837–57.
23 Kenneth Pinnow, *Lost to the Collective: Suicide and the Promise of Soviet Socialism, 1921–1929* (Ithaca, NY: Cornell University Press, 2010), 10–15.
24 Andy Byford, *Science of the Child in Late Imperial and Early Soviet Russia* (Oxford: Oxford University Press, 2020); Lewis H. Siegelbaum, '*Okhrana Truda*: Industrial Hygiene, Psychotechnics, and Industrialization in the USSR', in Susan Gross Solomon and John F. Hutchinson, eds., *Health and Society in Revolutionary Russia* (Bloomington, IN: Indiana University Press,1990), 224–45; Hirsch, *Empire of Nations*, 60; Dan Healey, *Bolshevik Sexual Forensics: Diagnosing Disorder in the Clinic and Courtroom, 1917–1939* (DeKalb, IL: Northern Illinois University Press, 2009); Susan Gross Solomon, 'Soviet Social Hygienists and Sexology after the Revolution: Dynamics of "Capture" at Home and Abroad', *Ab Imperio*, 4 (2014): 107–35.
25 Hirsch, *Empire of Nations*, 101–3.
26 Matthew Romaniello and Tricia Starks, eds., *Russian History through the Senses: From 1700 to the Present* (London: Bloomsbury, 2016).
27 Lilya Kaganovsky, *How the Soviet Man Was Unmade: Cultural Fantasy and Male Subjectivity under Stalin* (Pittsburg, PA: University of Pittsburgh Press, 2008); Emma Widdis, *Socialist Senses: Film, Feeling, and the Soviet Subject, 1917–1940*

(Bloomington, IN: Indiana University Press, 2017); Lilya Kaganovsky, *The Voice of Technology: Soviet Cinema's Transition to Sound, 1928-1935* (Bloomington, IN: Indiana University Press, 2018).

28 Toby Clark, 'The New Man's Body: A Motif in Early Soviet Culture', in Matthew Cullerne Bown and Brandon Taylor, eds., *Art of the Soviets: Painting, Sculpture and Architecture in a One-Party State* (Manchester: Manchester University Press, 1993), 33-50; Richard Stites, *Revolutionary Dreams: Utopian Vision and Experimental Life in the Russian Revolution* (New York, NY: Oxford University Press, 1989); David Hoffmann, *Cultivating the Masses: Modern State Practices and Soviet Socialism, 1914-1939* (Ithaca, NY: Cornell University Press, 2011).

29 Lewis Siegelbaum, *Stakhanovism and the Politics of Productivity in the USSR, 1935-41* (Cambridge: Cambridge University Press, 1988).

30 Susan Grant, *Physical Culture and Sport in Soviet Society: Propaganda, Acculturation and Transformation in the 1920s and 1930s* (New York, NY: Routledge, 2013).

31 Tricia Starks, *The Body Soviet: Propaganda, Hygiene and the Revolutionary State* (Madison, WI: University of Wisconsin Press, 2008).

32 Anindita Banerjee, *We Modern People: Science Fiction and the Making of Russian Modernity* (Middletown, CT: Wesleyan University Press, 2012), 141-51.

33 Naiman, *Sex in Public*.

34 The classic account of this shift is provided by Raymond Bauer, *The New Man in Soviet Psychology* (Cambridge, MA: Harvard University Press, 1952). For more recent explorations, see Igal Halfin, *Terror in My Soul: Communist Autobiographies on Trial* (Cambridge, MA: Harvard University Press, 2003), especially chapter 4.

35 K. N. Kornilov, A. A. Smirnov and B. M. Teplov, eds., *Psikhologiia* (Moscow: Gos. uchebno-pedagogicheskoe izd-vo Ministerstva prosveshcheniia RSFSR, 1948), 299.

36 On the 'mindful body', see Monique Scheer, 'Are Emotions a Kind of Practice (And Is That What Makes Them Have a History)? A Bourdieuian Approach to Understanding Emotion', *History and Theory*, 51.2 (2012): 193-220.

37 Karl Marx, *A Contribution to the Critique of Political Economy*, trans. S. W. Ryazanskaia and ed. Maurice Dobb (London: Lawrence & Wishart, 1971), 21.

38 A. B. Zalkind, *Zizhn' organizma i vnushenie* (Moscow and Leningrad: Gos. izd-vo, 1927), 123.

39 Pinnow, *Lost to the Collective*; Nikolai Krementsov, 'From "Beastly Philosophy" to Medical Genetics: Eugenics in Russia and the Soviet Union', *Annals of Science*, 68.1 (2011): 61-92.

40 Ethan Pollock, *Stalin and the Soviet Science Wars* (Princeton, NJ: Princeton University Press, 2006).

41 Trofim Lysenko, quoted in Evgeny Dobrenko, *Political Economy of Socialist Realism*, trans. by Jesse M. Savage (New Haven, CT: Yale University Press, 2007), 75.

42 Serguei Alex Oushakine, 'The Flexible and the Pliant: Disturbed Organisms of Soviet Modernity', *Cultural Anthropology*, 19.3 (2004): 392-428.

43 Kaganovsky, *How the Soviet Man was Unmade*; Brigid O'Keeffe, *New Soviet Gypsies: Nationality, Performance, and Selfhood in the Early Soviet Union* (Toronto: University of Toronto Press, 2013); Claire Shaw, *Deaf in the USSR: Marginality, Community and Soviet Identity, 1917-1991* (Ithaca, NY: Cornell University Press, 2017).

44 On women, see Naiman, *Sex in Public*; Sharon Kowalsky, *Deviant Women: Female Crime and Criminology in Revolutionary Russia, 1880-1930* (DeKalb, IL: Northern Illinois University Press, 2009). On disability, see Frances Bernstein, 'Prosthetic Manhood in the Soviet Union at the End of WWII', *Osiris*, 30.1 (2015): 113-33;

Claire McCallum, 'Scorched by the Fire of War: Masculinity, War Wounds and Disability in Soviet Visual Culture, 1941–65', *The Slavonic and East European Review*, 93.3 (April 2015): 251–85.

45 Peter Holquist, 'Violence as Technique: The Logic of Violence in Soviet Totalitarianism', in Amir Weiner, ed., *Landscaping the Human Garden: Twentieth-century Population Management in a Comparative Framework* (Stanford, CA: Stanford University Press, 2003), 19–45.

46 Naiman, *Sex in Public*, 151.

47 See, for example, Miriam Dobson's discussion of attitudes to the tattooed bodies of Gulag returnees in *Khrushchev's Cold Summer: Gulag Returnees, Crime, and the Fate of Reform after Stalin* (Ithaca, NY: Cornell University Press, 2009), 113–15.

48 Amir Weiner, 'Introduction: Landscaping the Human Garden', in Weiner, ed., *Landscaping the Human Garden*, 1–18, 17.

49 Lišková, *Sexual Liberation*, 9.

50 David Hoffmann, *Stalinist Values: The Cultural Norms of Soviet Modernity, 1917–1941* (Ithaca and London: Cornell University Press, 2003); Hoffmann, *Cultivating the Masses*; Stephen Kotkin, 'Modern Times: The Soviet Union and the Interwar Conjuncture', *Kritika*, 2.1 (2001): 111–64; Starks, *The Body Soviet*.

51 Michael David-Fox, 'What Is Cultural Revolution?', *The Russian Review*, 58.2 (1999): 181–201; Daniel Peris, *Storming the Heavens: The Soviet League of the Militant Godless* (Ithaca, NY: Cornell University Press, 1998); Matthias Neumann, *The Communist Youth League and the Transformation of the Soviet Union, 1917–1932* (London: Routledge, 2011); Frances Lee Bernstein, *The Dictatorship of Sex: Lifestyle Advice for the Soviet Masses* (DeKalb, IL: Northern Illinois University Press, 2007); Kate Transchel, *Under the Influence: Working-class Drinking, Temperance and Cultural Revolution in Russia, 1895–1932* (Pittsburg, PA: Pittsburgh University Press, 2006); Tricia Starks, 'A Revolutionary Attack on Tobacco: Bolshevik Antismoking Campaigns in the 1920s', *American Journal of Public Health*, 107.1 (2017): 1711–17; Catriona Kelly, 'The New Soviet Man and Woman', in Simon Dixon, ed., *The Oxford Handbook of Modern Russian History* (Oxford: Oxford University Press, 2013); Catriona Kelly and Vadim Volkov, 'Directed Desires: *Kul'turnost'* and Consumption', in Catriona Kelly and David Shepherd, eds., *Constructing Russian Culture in the Age of Revolution: 1881–1940* (Oxford: Oxford University Press, 1998), 291–313. As a number of historians have pointed out, these campaigns were often targeted at national and ethnic minorities. See, for example, Marianne Kamp, *The New Woman in Uzbekistan: Islam, Modernity, and Unveiling under Communism* (Seattle: Washington University Press, 2006) and Paula A. Michaels, *Curative Powers: Medicine and Empire in Stalin's Central Asia* (Pittsburgh: University of Pittsburgh Press, 2003).

52 Siegelbaum, *Stakhanovism and the Politics of Productivity*; Stephen Kotkin, *Magnetic Mountain: Stalinism as a Civilization* (Berkeley, CA: University of California Press, 1995); Diane Koenker, *Club Red: Vacation Travel and the Soviet Dream* (Ithaca, NY: Cornell University Press, 2013); Grant, *Physical Culture and Sport*; David Hoffmann, 'Bodies of Knowledge: Physical Culture and the New Soviet Man', in Igal Halfin, ed., *Language and Revolution: The Making of Modern Political Identities* (London: F. Cass, 2002), 228–42; Ben Krupp, 'How to Make a Soviet Body: Exercise as a Practice of Biopolitics', *Technologies of Mind and Body in the Soviet Union and the Eastern Bloc International Symposium*, 17 May 2019, University of Nottingham.

53 Stephen Kotkin, 'The Search for the Socialist City', *Russian History*, 23.1–4 (1996): 230–47. See also Victor Buchli, *An Archaeology of Socialism* (Oxford: Berg, 1999); Steven Harris, *Communism on Tomorrow Street: Mass Housing and Everyday*

Life after Stalin (Washington, DC: Woodrow Wilson Center Press, 2013); Andy Willimott, *Living the Revolution: Urban Communes & Soviet Socialism, 1917–1932* (Oxford: Oxford University Press, 2019); Christine Varga-Harris, *Stories of House and Home: Soviet Apartment Life during the Khrushchev Years* (Ithaca, NY: Cornell University Press, 2015); Heather DeHaan, *Stalinist City Planning: Professionals, Performance, and Power* (Toronto: Toronto University Press, 2013); Katherine Lebow, *Unfinished Utopia: Nowa Huta, Stalinism, and Polish Society, 1949–56* (Ithaca, NY: Cornell University Press, 2016). Recent scholarship on new practices of seeing includes Oksana Sarkisova, *Screening Soviet Nationalities: Kulturfilms from the Far North to Central Asia* (London: I.B. Tauris, 2017); Oksana Sarkisova, 'From *The Blind* to New Vision: Sergei Tretiakov and Soviet Ethnographic Optics', *Technologies of Mind and Body in the Soviet Union and the Eastern Bloc International Symposium*, 18 May 2019, University of Nottingham; Nick Baron, 'Mapping the Soviet: Cartographic Culture and Political Power from Lenin to Stalin', in *Language, Culture, and Society in Russian/English Studies: The Proceedings* (London: Senate House, University of London, 2013), 12–25; Nick Baron, 'Transforming Vision: Maps and Technologies of Seeing in the Soviet 1930s', *Technologies of Mind and Body in the Soviet Union and the Eastern Bloc International Symposium*, 18 May 2019, University of Nottingham; Galina Orlova, '"Karty dlia slepykh": Politika i politizatsiia zreniia v stalinskuiu epokhu', in E. R. Iarskaia-Smirnova and P. V. Romanov, eds., *Vizual'naia antropologiia: Rezhimy vidimosti pri sotsializme* (Moscow: OOO 'Variant', TsSPGI, 2009), 57–104.

54 Jochen Hellbeck, *Revolution on My Mind: Writing a Diary under Stalin* (Cambridge, MA: Harvard University Press, 2006); Oleg Kharkhordin, *The Collective and the Individual in Russia: A Study of Practices* (Berkeley, CA: University of California Press, 1999); Igal Halfin, *From Darkness to Light: Class, Consciousness, and Salvation in Revolutionary Russia* (Pittsburgh, PA: University of Pittsburgh Press, 2000); Anatoly Pinsky, ed., *Posle Stalina: pozdnesovetskaia sub"ektivnost'* (1953–1985) (St. Petersburg: Izdatel'stvo Evropeiskogo universiteta v Sankt-Peterburge, 2018); Anatoly Pinsky, 'Subjectivity after Stalin', *Russian Studies in History*, 58.2-3 (2019): 79–88.

55 Jochen Hellbeck, 'Working, Struggling, Becoming: Stalin-Era Autobiographical Texts', *The Russian Review*, 60.3 (2001): 340–59, 351.

56 Weiner, 'Introduction: Landscaping the Human Garden'; Holquist, 'Violence as Technique'; Oushakine, 'The Flexible and the Pliant'.

57 Holquist, 'Violence as Technique'.

58 See, for example, Yanni Kotsonis and David L. Hoffmann, eds., *Russian Modernity: Politics, Knowledge, Practices* (Basingstoke: Macmillan, 2000).

59 Holquist, 'Violence as Technique', 20.

60 Weiner, 'Introduction: Landscaping the Human Garden', 20.

61 Michel Foucault, *The History of Sexuality, Volume 1: Introduction*, trans. by Robert Hurley (New York, NY: Pantheon Books, 1978), 139.

62 Prozorov, *The Biopolitics of Stalinism*, 8. See also Magdalena Lopez, 'Socialist Biopolitics: Flesh and Animality in Cuba and Venezuela', *Latin American Research Review*, 56.2 (2021): 417–36. For a discussion of the applicability of the biopolitical paradigm to Soviet socialism, see Laura Engelstein, 'Combined Underdevelopment: Discipline and the Law in Imperial and Soviet Russia', *American Historical Review*, 98.2 (1993): 338–53; Stephen Kotkin, *Magnetic Mountain: Stalinism as a Civilisation* (Berkeley, CA: University of California Press, 1995).

63 Greg Eghigian, 'Was There a Communist Psychiatry?: Politics and East German Psychiatric Care, 1945–1989', *Harvard Review of Psychiatry*, 10.6 (2002): 364–8; Savelli and Marks, eds., *Psychiatry in Communist Europe*; Mat Savelli, 'Beyond Ideological Platitudes: Socialism and Psychiatry in Eastern Europe', *Palgrave Communications*, 4.1 (2018).
64 Christine Leuenberger, 'Socialist Psychotherapy and Its Dissidents', *Journal of the History of the Behavioural Sciences*, 37.3 (2001): 267–373; Melinda Kovai, 'The History of the Hungarian Institute of Psychiatry and Neurology between 1945 and 1968', in Savelli and Marks, eds., *Psychiatry in Communist Europe*, 117–33; Sarah Marks, 'From Experimental Psychosis to Resolving Traumatic Pasts: Psychedelic Research in Communist Czechoslovakia, 1954–1974', *Cahiers du Monde Russe*, 56.1 (2015): 53–76; Sarah Marks, 'Suggestion, Persuasion and Work: Psychotherapies in Communist Europe', *European Journal of Psychotherapy & Counselling*, 20.1 (2018): 10–24; Aleksandra Brokman, 'The Healing Power of Words: Psychotherapy in the USSR, 1956–1985', PhD Thesis (University of East Anglia, 2018).
65 Leuenberger, 'Socialist Psychotherapy'; Roy Decarvalho and Ivo Cermak, 'History of Humanistic Psychology in Czechoslovakia', *The Journal of Humanistic Psychology* 37.1 (1997): 110–30; Mat Savelli, 'The Peculiar Prosperity of Psychoanalysis in Socialist Yugoslavia', *The Slavonic and East European Review*, 91.2 (2013): 262–88; Ana Antic, 'Raising a True Socialist Individual: Yugoslav Psychoanalysis and the Creation of Democratic Marxist Citizens', *Social History*, 44.1 (2019): 86–115. The polarized picture of Eastern and Western psychological medicine has also been contested by studies highlighting the post-war appeal of Pavlovian paradigms to British and American doctors disillusioned with Freudian theories. See Kate Davison, 'Cold War Pavlov: Homosexual Aversion Therapy in the 1960s', *History of the Human Sciences*, 34.1 (2021): 89–119.
66 Benjamin Zajicek, 'Scientific Psychiatry in Stalin's Soviet Union: The Politics of Modern Medicine and the Struggle to Define "Pavlovian" Psychiatry, 1939–1953', PhD dissertation (University of Chicago, 2009), 234.
67 Eghigian, 'The Psychologization of the Socialist Self'.
68 Ibid., 182.
69 Scholars such as Agnieszka Kościańska have also pointed to the uniqueness of the 'schools of thought and therapy' developed in the Eastern Bloc, emphasizing that socialist experts offered 'solutions fundamentally different from those of their Western counterparts'. See her *Gender, Pleasure, and Violence*, 3.
70 Frances L. Bernstein, Christopher Burton and Dan Healey, eds., *Soviet Medicine: Culture, Practice and Science* (DeKalb, IL: Northern Illinois University Press, 2010).
71 Kenneth Pinnow has argued that the Soviet period gave rise to 'a particular form of medicopolitics that sought to control ideological, rather than infectious, disease'. See his *Lost to the Collective*, 190.
72 Byford, *Science of the Child*, 14. As Frances L. Bernstein, Christopher Burton and Dan Healey also note, the Soviet period saw the intensification of the process of medicalization that saw state leaders 'turn to medicine to regulate questions with a moral or aesthetic component'. See their 'Introduction: Experts, Expertise, and New Histories of Soviet Medicine', in Bernstein, Burton and Healey, eds., *Soviet Medicine*, 8.
73 Byford, *Science of the Child*, 15.
74 Bernstein, Burton and Healey, 'Introduction', 8.
75 Lutz Raphael links the rise of 'an all-embracing "therapeutic culture"' to the 'end of planning and a growing political dispute about the welfare state and its cost'. See his 'Embedding the Human and Social Sciences', 53.

76 Pivotal works include: Margarete Vohringer, *Avangard i psikhotekhnika: Nauka, iskusstvo i metodiki eksperimentov nad vospriiatiem v poslerevoliutsionnoi Rossii* (Moscow: Novoe literaturnoe obozrenie, 2019); Irina Sirotkina, *Svobodnoe dvizhenie i plasticheskii tanets v Rossii* (Moscow: Novoe literaturnoe obozrenie, 2011); Irina Sirotkina and Roger Smith, *The Sixth Sense of the Avant-garde: Dance, Kinaesthesia and the Arts in Revolutionary Russia* (London: Bloomsbury Methuen Drama, 2017); Ana Hedberg Olenina, *Psychomotor Aesthetics: Movement and Affect in Modern Literature and Film* (New York, NY: Oxford University Press, 2020); Widdis, *Socialist Senses*; Anna Toropova, *Feeling Revolution: Cinema, Genre, and the Politics of Affect under Stalin* (Oxford: Oxford University Press, 2020).
77 Vohringer, *Avangard i psikhotekhnika*, 289.
78 Olenina, *Psychomotor Aesthetics*, xv.
79 Sarkisova, *Screening Soviet Nationalities*, 114–37.
80 Nikolai Krementsov, *Revolutionary Experiments: The Quest for Immortality in Bolshevik Science and Fiction* (Oxford: Oxford University Press, 2014); Nikolai Krementsov, 'New Sciences, New Worlds, and "New Men"', in Kremenstsov and Howell, eds., *The Art and Science of Making the New Man*, 85–104.
81 Richard Stites, *Revolutionary Dreams: Utopian Vision and Experimental Life in the Russian Revolution* (New York, NY: Oxford University Press, 1989); Rolf Hellebust, *Flesh to Metal: Soviet Literature and the Alchemy of Revolution* (Ithaca, NY: Cornell University Press, 2003). See also the Annual Interdisciplinary Graduate Student Conference 'Grafting the Self' (Princeton, 19–21 October 2017).
82 Anya Bernstein, *The Future of Immortality: Remaking Life and Death in Contemporary Russia* (Princeton, NJ: Princeton University Press, 2019), 7.
83 Pollock, *Stalin and the Soviet Science Wars*, 3.
84 On Soviet science, see Nikolai Krementsov, *Stalinist Science* (Princeton, NJ: Princeton University Press, 2007); Loren Graham, ed., *Science and the Soviet Social Order* (Cambridge, MA: Harvard University Press, 1990); Hiroshi Ichikawa, *Soviet Science and Technology in the Shadow of the Cold War* (Abingdon and New York: Routledge, 2018).
85 Nikolai Krementsov, 'Introduction: On Words and Meanings', in Kremenstsov and Howell, eds., *The Art and Science of Making the New Man*, 1–23, 3.
86 Julia Vaingurt, *Wonderlands of the Avant-Garde: Technology and the Arts in Russia of the 1920s* (Evanston, IL: North-western University Press, 2013), 13; Martin Heidegger, *The Question Concerning Technology, and Other Essays* (New York, NY: Harper & Row, 1977), 3–35.
87 Pollock, *Stalin and the Soviet Science Wars*, 1.
88 Naomi Oreskes, 'Introduction', in *Science and Technology in the Global Cold War*, eds. Naomi Oreskes and John Krige (Boston, MA: Massachusetts Institute of Technology, 2014), 3. On Cold War science on the other side of the Iron Curtain, see Audra J. Wolfe, *Competing with the Soviets: Science, Technology, and the State in Cold War America* (Baltimore, MD: Johns Hopkins University Press, 2013).
89 Johanna Conterio, 'Curative Nature: Medical Foundations of Soviet Nature Protection, 1917–1941', *Slavic Review*, 78.1 (2019): 23–49.
90 Ibid., 24. See also Paul R. Josephson, *Would Trotsky Wear a Bluetooth: Technological Utopianism under Socialism* (Baltimore, MD: Johns Hopkins University Press, 2010); Colleen McQuillen and Julia Vaingurt, eds., *The Human Reimagined: Posthumanism in Russia* (Boston, MA: Academic Studies Press, 2018).
91 On the competing paradigms of 'technology decides everything' and 'cadres decide everything', see Slava Gerovitch, '"New Soviet Man" Inside Machine: Human

Engineering, Spacecraft Design, and the Construction of Communism', *Osiris*, 22.1 (2007): 135–57, 140.

92 On the city of science, see Paul Josephson, *New Atlantis Revisited: Akademgorodok, the Siberian City of Science* (Princeton, NJ: Princeton University Press, 1997). On Cold War competition, see Susan Reid, 'Who Will Beat Whom?: Soviet Popular Reception of the American National Exhibition in Moscow, 1959', *Kritika: Explorations in Russian and Eurasian History*, 9.4 (2008): 855–904.

93 See Slava Gerovitch, *From Newspeak to Cyberspeak: A History of Soviet Cybernetics* (Cambridge, MA: MIT Press, 2002).

94 Diana Kurkovsky-West, '"Drilled Humans" or Automated Systems?: Reconsidering Human-Machine Integration in Late Soviet Socialism', in McQuillen and Vaingurt, eds., *The Human Reimagined*, 114–35. On late Soviet imaginaries of 'grafting' the human body, see Ekaterina Vikulina, 'Media, Science and the Body in the Soviet Photography of the 1960s', *Technologies of Mind and Body in the Soviet Union and the Eastern Bloc International Symposium*, 18 May 2019, University of Nottingham.

95 *Soviet Materialisms*, 11–12 April 2022, Jesus College, Cambridge: https://www.sovietmaterialities.org. Works on aspects of materiality under socialism include: Susan Reid and David Crowley, *Pleasures in Socialism: Leisure and Luxury in the Eastern Bloc* (Evanston, IL: North-western University Press, 2010); Eli Rubin, *Synthetic Socialism: Plastics and Dictatorship in the German Democratic Republic* (Chapel Hill, NC: University of North Carolina Press, 2008); Natalia Chernyshova, *Soviet Consumer Culture in the Brezhnev Era* (London: Routledge, 2013); Graham H. Roberts, ed., *Material Culture in Russia and the USSR: Things, Values, Identities* (London: Bloomsbury Academic, 2017).

96 Golubev, *The Things of Life*, 5.

97 Widdis, *Socialist Senses*, 2.

98 Rolf Hellebust, *Flesh to Metal: Soviet Literature and the Alchemy of Revolution* (Ithaca, NY: Cornell University Press, 2003). See also Keith A. Livers, *Constructing the Stalinist Body: Fictional Representations of Corporeality in the Stalinist 1930s* (Lanham, MD: Lexington Books, 2004).

99 Colleen McQuillen and Julia Vaingurt, 'Introduction', in *The Human Reimagined*, 1–36.

100 Banerjee, *We Modern People*; Elana Gomel, *Science Fiction, Alien Encounters, and the Ethics of Posthumanism: Beyond the Golden Rule* (London: Palgrave Macmillan, 2014).

101 Donna Haraway, 'A Manifesto for Cyborgs: Science, Technology and Socialist Feminism in the 1980s', in *The Haraway Reader* (New York, NY: Routledge, 2004), 8.

102 Elana Gomel, 'Gods like Men: Soviet Science Fiction and the Utopian Self', *Science Fiction Studies*, 31.3 (2004): 358; Gerovitch, '"New Soviet Man"'.

103 On the cyborg and Soviet posthumanism, see also McQuillen and Vaingurt, 'Introduction', 50–2.

104 Leo Marx, 'The Idea of "Technology" and Postmodern Pessimism', in Yaron Ezrahi, Everett Mendelsohn and Howard Segal, eds., *Technology, Pessimism, and Postmodernism* (Amherst, MA: University of Massachusetts Press, 1994), 237–57, 253.

Part One

Knowledges

1

'Rest for the brain' or 'technology of the unconscious?': Hypnosis in early Soviet medicine and culture

Anna Toropova

The early Soviet period witnessed an intense scientific and medical interest in hypnosis and suggestion. Soviet doctors and scientists sought to reclaim a therapeutic method long tarnished by its association with stage performers, occult practices and theories of animal magnetism.[1] At the heart of efforts to demystify hypnosis and fully exploit its 'healing powers' were the studies on hypnotic phenomena conducted by the followers of Ivan Pavlov and Vladimir Bekhterev in the 1920s. Uncovering the physiological mechanisms of hypnosis, this research reinterpreted the hypnotic state as a process of internal 'inhibition' that did not fundamentally differ from the normal state of sleep.[2] Even as physiologists proclaimed their explanation as a definitive scientific 'unmasking' of the 'enigma' of hypnosis, many aspects of the hypnotic state continued to be debated and discussed. In consonance with a late-nineteenth-century tradition of research that placed hypnosis at the heart of a 'new experimental science of the unconscious mind', many Soviet specialists continued to read the hypnotic trance as the manifestation of a consciousness inaccessible to the waking self.[3] The understanding of hypnosis as a 'technology of the unconscious' exerted a lingering influence not only on Soviet medical and scientific specialists, but filmmakers, writers and literary theorists.

The debate over the meaning of hypnosis was ostensibly settled by the mid-1930s, with the reflexological reading of hypnosis carving out a clear dominance in the scientific and medical sphere. In the context of growing attacks on psychoanalysis, the Pavlovian paradigm of 'inhibition' offered a convenient way of setting hypnosis in sharp relief from 'discredited' Freudian theories and practices.[4] The tendency to stress the divergence of hypnosis and psychoanalysis has largely prevailed in scholarly accounts, with the unabated popularity of hypnosis in the Soviet Union having been linked to the triumph of authoritarianism.[5] The persisting framing of hypnosis as 'a technology for unlocking unconscious forces' in popular culture as well as in scientific scholarship, however, suggests that the ascendancy of Pavlovian paradigms in the Soviet psy-disciplines did not necessarily spell the end of all discussion of the unconscious aspects of the psyche.[6] In defiance of the physiological reading of hypnosis as a state of mental 'inhibition' and inactivity, a wide variety of medical experts as well as cultural producers continued to conceptualize this phenomenon as a gateway into the unconscious mechanisms of the mind.

As Julia Mannherz has shown, in the decade after the October Revolution doctors came a long way in stamping their authority over hypnosis and turning it into a legitimate form of medical therapy.[7] Eminent neurologists and psychotherapists such as Vladimir Bekhterev emerged as vocal champions of suggestion and hypnosis in the treatment of so-called 'functional' disorders, psychological illnesses with no determinate physical origin.[8] The 'psycho-neuroses' – including pathological fears and invasive thoughts, hysteria, mania and depression – were all thought to be highly treatable by hypnosis and suggestion.[9] In addition, Soviet doctors vouched for the success of hypnosis in treating a wide variety of unhealthy habits and addictions, especially alcoholism, tobacco use, morphinism and other forms of drug addiction.[10] As Tricia Starks's contribution to this volume shows, hypnosis and suggestion were key therapeutic methods within the network of narcological clinics (or 'narcodispensaries') established in the 1920s.[11] These specialist clinics allowed the wider implementation of the modes of group hypnotherapy and suggestion therapy that Bekhterev and his associates had first developed in the late Imperial period.[12] Hypnosis and suggestion were also advanced as valuable tools in the task of 're-education' targeting anti-social behaviour and moral defects.[13] These methods were also thought to bring hope of curing the sexual 'perversions' and dysfunctions (including homosexuality, masturbation and impotence) that had proven resistant to other treatments.[14]

It was not only in the treatment of neuroses, addictions and unhealthy habits that Soviet doctors turned to hypnosis. Enthused by the possibilities of achieving anaesthesia and analgesia under hypnosis, specialists boasted of their success in using hypnosis as a means of pain relief during labour, dentistry, minor operations and even major surgery.[15] So enchanted were Soviet doctors with the healing powers of hypnosis that they frequently advocated its use as a treatment for a range of ailments and afflictions, from morning sickness to migraines and skin conditions such as eczema.[16] Indeed, hypnosis became a 'cure-all', to be used in any case 'where the restoration of a good appetite, sleep, a cheerful mood and faith in the efficacy of treatment were needed'.[17]

Demystifying hypnosis

Attempts to rid hypnosis of the notoriety it had gained through association with the Viennese doctor Franz Anton Mesmer had begun long before the October Revolution. At the same time as the famous late-nineteenth-century enquiries into hypnotic phenomena were being undertaken by Jean-Martin Charcot in Paris and Hippolyte Bernheim in Nancy, Russian scientists also strove to disprove Mesmer's claims that hypnosis was a force premised on 'animal magnetism'. Having observed Charcot's work at the Salpêtrière first hand, Bekhterev and his associates (including A. Pevnitskii and A. F. Lazurskii) undertook a series of laboratory investigations into the effects of hypnosis that were published in the 1890s and 1900s.[18] Through showcasing the physiological changes to a hypnotised patient's pulse, breathing rate and cardiovascular system, Bekhterev and his collaborators were able to demonstrate the objective reality of hypnotic phenomena like hallucinations, blindness and analgesia.[19]

The attempt to understand the 'objective' mechanisms of hypnosis continued in the early Soviet period as Bekhterev and his students, as well as the laboratory of Ivan Pavlov, turned to understand hypnosis and suggestion through the lens of their research on conditioned (or, in Bekhterev's case, 'associative') reflexes.[20] Bekhterev's student, the Kharkiv doctor Konstantin Platonov, embarked upon extensive experimental research that could serve as 'proof of the changes in the organism provoked by verbal suggestion'.[21] Platonov's findings, published in his influential 1930 monograph, *The Word as a Physiological and Therapeutic Factor*, showed the concrete psycho-physiological effects of suggestion. Framing the words of the psychotherapist as associative, conditioned stimuli, Platonov unravelled their influence on the sensory organs, the nervous system and on the emotions.[22] The attempt to strip hypnosis of its mystique using 'purely objective' methods was also carried out at Pavlov's laboratory.[23] Experiments conducted by Boris Birman showcased how alert dogs could be put into a state of 'experimental sleep' using a number of different stimuli that took on 'hypnotic' properties through their association with the conditioned reflex of sleep.[24]

The reconceptualization of hypnosis as 'experimental sleep' (Birman) or 'reflexological sleep' (Platonov) demonstrated a central tenet of the physiological re-assessment of hypnotic phenomena – the idea that hypnosis was not fundamentally different from the normal state of sleep.[25] As early as 1893, Bekhterev, following Bernheim, had insisted that hypnosis was closely linked to the state of sleep.[26] Hypnosis, Bekhterev asserted, was nothing other than the 'modification' of normal sleep. The similarity between hypnosis and sleep was reinforced by Pavlov's theories on 'internal inhibition'. Characterizing the activity of the nervous system as a perpetual balancing act between 'excitation' and 'inhibition', Pavlov posited that sleep ensued when a brain cell became exhausted due to prolonged stimulation. The exhausted cell fell into a state of inactivity – 'inhibition' – which, due to the 'law of irradiation', then spread further to eventually take hold of all the cells in the cortex and the lower parts of the brain.[27] According to Pavlov, 'inhibition and sleep' were 'one and the same process'.[28] Reinterpreted as 'experimental'/'reflexological sleep', hypnosis was presented as a perfectly ordinary biological process, a natural defensive mechanism designed to prevent the over-exhaustion of the brain.[29] Soviet physiologists saw their experimental studies on hypnotic suggestion as providing irrefutable scientific 'proof' of the position upheld by the proponents of the 'Nancy school' of hypnosis founded by Hippolyte Bernheim and Ambroise-Auguste Liébeault.[30] Bernheim had famously challenged Jean-Martin Charcot's interpretation of hypnosis as a pathological phenomenon, a form of artificially induced hysteria, by contending that hypnosis was a normal, sleep-like process rooted in a naturally occurring characteristic of the human mind – suggestibility.[31]

The physiological demystification of hypnosis was hailed as nothing less than a landmark achievement of Russian and Soviet science. Soviet specialists boasted that the theory of conditioned reflexes, founded on 'purely objective experimental methods', had finally provided the 'key' to unlocking the 'mystery' that had long seemed inaccessible to science.³² The advances in knowledge generated by Soviet physiological research on hypnosis were thought vastly superior to the efforts of Western European scientists, who were deemed profoundly hindered by an allegiance to a 'subjective-psychological' understanding of hypnosis.³³ Until Western authors grasped the superiority of the 'physiology of Pavlov and the reflexology of Bekhterev', Platonov noted, they would continue to languish behind Soviet scholars.³⁴

The pinning of hypnotherapy's legitimacy on reflexological explanations is vividly demonstrated in the 1929 health enlightenment film, *To Your Health* (*Za vashe zdorov'e*, Dubrovskii). Aleksandr Dubrovskii's film sought to normalize the medical use of hypnosis by portraying hypnotherapeutic treatment as one of a number of therapies available for alcoholics at a narcodispensary. The young male specialist administering the treatment, identified on screen as Dr Ia. G. Livshits, is pictured in a white doctor's coat worn over a smart suit. As an article publicising *To Your Health* was keen to emphasize, the young and dynamic doctor depicted on screen was a stark departure from the stock figure of the mysterious 'magnetiser' and his infamous 'gestures' and 'manipulations'.³⁵ The traditional resort to 'passes' and shiny objects to impel hypnosis was eschewed by the doctor for an authoritative look at his patient and a firm command to 'sleep'. The intertitles explained Dr Livshits's delivery of suggestions about quitting the bottle to a patient under hypnosis as a process of 'forming' 'a new REFLEX of aversion to alcohol'.

The theory of 'inhibition' was illustrated in *To Your Health* through the trope of hypnotic catalepsy. The demonstration of a session of individual hypnosis with a male alcoholic identified on screen as A. P. Chistiakovich captured the patient's rigid pose as he continued to hold his arms upright long after the doctor placed them in this position (Figure 1.1). The phenomenon of hypnotic catalepsy was frequently invoked in physiological accounts as a testament to the 'paralysis' of consciousness that occurred under hypnosis.³⁶ Indeed, a large part of the beneficial effect of hypnosis was seen to reside in the capacity of hypnosis to 'inhibit' brain activity. It was argued that the partial or complete paralysis of activity in specific parts of the brain during hypnosis, much like in normal sleep, preserved vital energy and provided essential rest and recuperation.³⁷ The phenomenon of hypnotic catalepsy also allowed hypnosis to be framed as a phenomenon analogous to passive defensive states in animals.³⁸

In line with the characterization of hypnosis as a form of mental and somatic 'inhibition' in physiological accounts, the hypnotherapy sequence in *To Your Health* culminated in a startling demonstration of suggested anaesthesia and analgesia. To show the suppression of the perception of pain under hypnosis, the film captures Livshits's assistant inserting a long needle through the skin of a hypnotized patient's forearm. The unsuspecting subject chosen for the experiment continues to sit obliviously as his pierced arm is moved from side to side in front of the camera to make sure the 'miracle' is captured from every angle (Figure 1.2). After the removal of the needle, another extreme close-up hones attention on the lack of blood produced by the experiment. The sequence was likely inspired by a similarly sensationalist display of the capacity of hypnosis to 'switch off feelings of pain' in Curt Thomalla's 'kulturfilm' *A Look into the Depth of the Soul: A Film about the Unconscious* (*Ein Blick in die Tiefen der Seele. Der Film vom Unbewussten*, 1923), which was imported to the Soviet Union in the 1920s.

Technology of the Unconscious 33

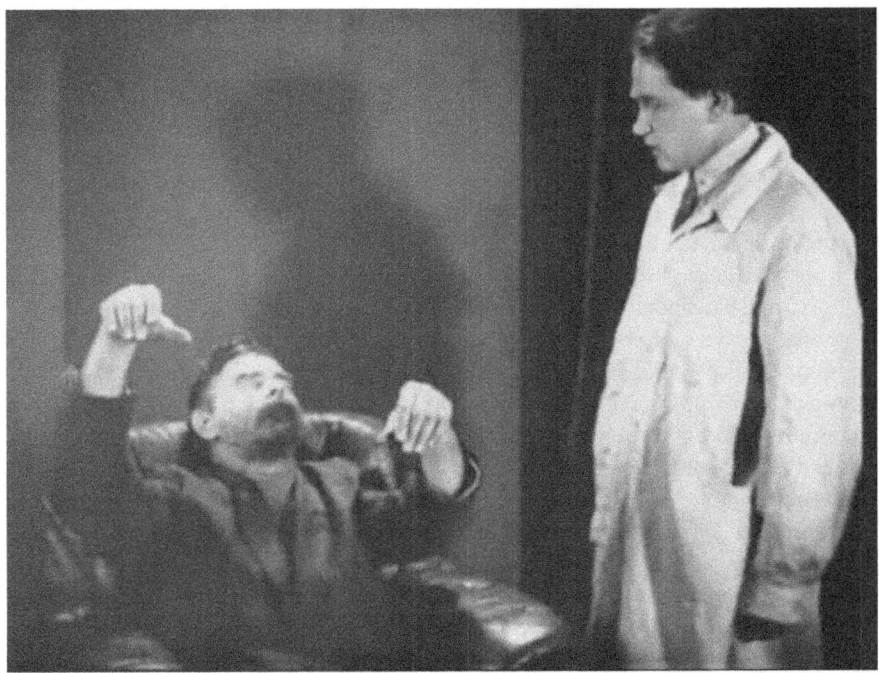

Figure 1.1 Hypnosis on screen: Film still from *To Your Health* (*Za vashe zdorov'e*, dir. Aleksandr Dubrovskii, 1929).

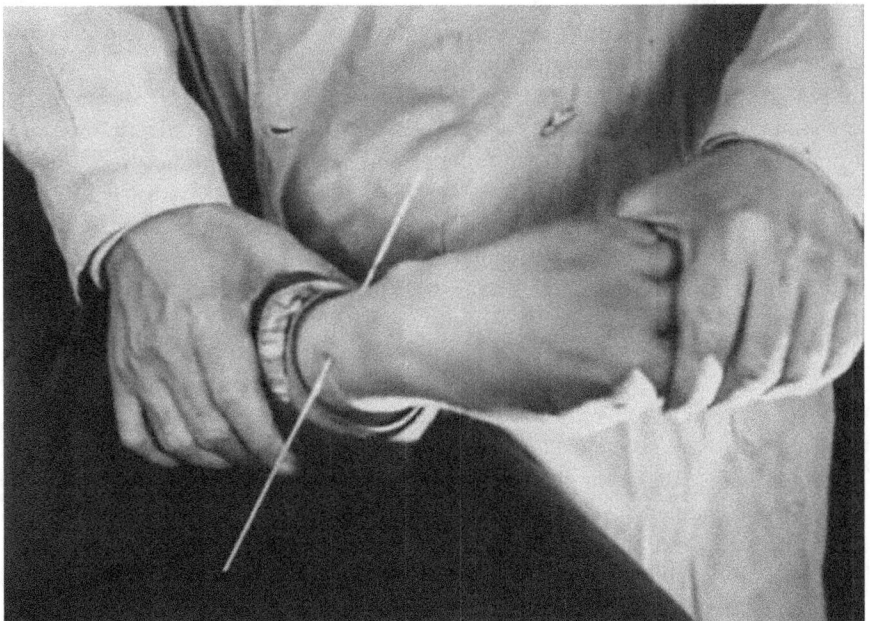

Figure 1.2 Paralysed consciousness: Film still from *To Your Health* (*Za vashe zdorov'e*, dir. Aleksandr Dubrovskii, 1929).

The completeness of the mental 'switch off' experienced by patients undergoing hypnotherapy was also emphatically stressed in the published account of the filming of *To Your Health*.[39] The *Soviet Screen* reporter witnessing the shoot marvelled in awe at the spectacle of oblivious alcoholics, contorted in different poses of sleep, being transported like waxworks across the set without stirring. So deep was the sleep that enveloped the patients, the reporter related in amazement, that when a piece of burning coal fell out from one of the overhead lights during filming onto the legs of a hypnotized patient, he continued to doze peacefully.[40]

Even as *To Your Health* marvelled at the obliteration of the hypnotized subject's sensory and perceptive capacities, however, the film was also fascinated with the hypnotist's powers of control over the patient. Indeed, the film's demonstration of hypnotic catalepsy ultimately gave way to the portrayal of the hypnotist's ability to manipulate the movements of the somnambulist. Chistiakovich's rigid pose is shown to instantly relax in response to the hypnotist's instructions. The film's showcase of a group hypnotherapy session, in which an entire room of alcoholic patients is pictured sinking into a deep, uninterruptible slumber under Dr Livshits's command, similarly culminates in an awe-striking display of bodily manipulation. The somnambulists who are first shown to be dull to the doctor's prods and enquiries respond instantaneously to his suggestion to lift up their left arms, lowering them only when instructed to do so.

The radical psycho-physiological pliability effected by hypnosis was an endless source of fascination in physiological accounts. Bekhterev asserted that the hypnotized patient became 'a machine in the literal meaning of the word, with the ignition key lying in the hands of the hypnotist'.[41] The physiologist Vasilii Danilevskii was similarly struck by the malleability of the subject under hypnosis. A 'blank space opens up', he noted, 'a psychical emptiness which can be effortlessly filled with whatever content that is desired'.[42] Illustrating the 'wax-like plasticity' of the body during hypnosis, Danilevskii's and Platonov's works on hypnosis featured image after image of bodies that had compliantly assumed the position desired by the hypnotist[43] (Figure 1.3).

For many medical experts, the 'wax-like pliability' of the hypnotized mind-body was synonymous with the dawn of new scientific and medical horizons, as well as bodily capacities. The suppression of the patient's will, Danilevskii noted, radically increased the physician's powers of healing by surrendering the patient's mind and body to the 'the full disposal' of the doctor.[44] Granting the physician with unprecedented access to the depths of a person's mind, Danilevskii continued, hypnosis made possible the performance of 'a mental vivisection'.[45] Reflexologists like Platonov and V. V. Sreznevskii contended that the inhibition of brain processes under hypnosis significantly increased the ease of breaking existing reflexological chains and of establishing 'new conditioned associations' through suggestions.[46] The inhibition of parts of the brain, Platonov noted, removed the conscious opposition that could hinder the education of new habits and ways of thinking. The possibilities of therapeutic re-education opened up by hypnosis looked to be truly endless; a thief, Platonov insisted, could be transformed into an honest person.[47] Seemingly anticipating the post-war psychotherapeutic applications that Aleksandra Brokman explores in her chapter in this volume, early Soviet experts also contemplated the 'performance enhancing' potential of hypnotic suggestion. Studies on the effect of hypnosis on the 'higher nervous functions' conducted by

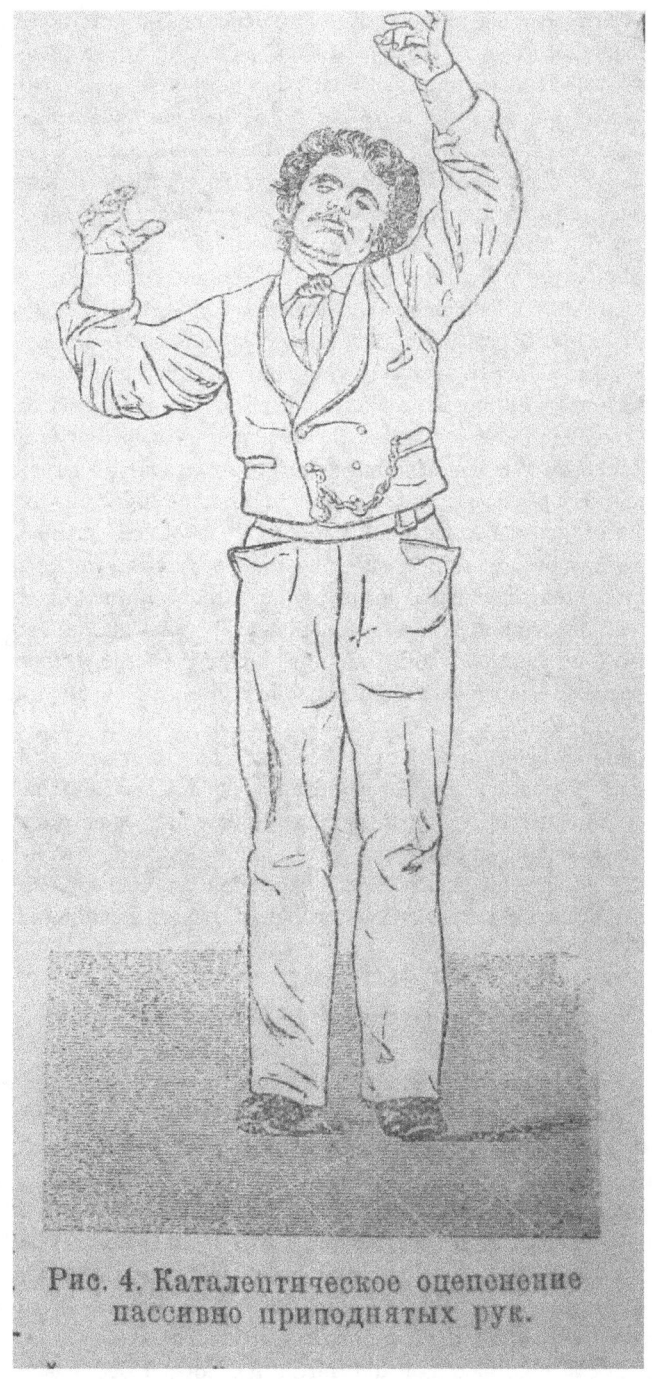

Figure 1.3 'Wax-like plasticity': Illustration of Hypnotic Catalepsy in V. Ia. Danilevskii, *Gipnotizm* (Kharkiv: Put' prosveshcheniia, 1924), 43.

Platonov's research team had found a positive influence on concentration, memory and associative mental processes.[48] The experiments carried out by physiologists studying labour in the 1930s similarly indicated that subjects who had been instructed under hypnosis to perceive their labour tasks as easy required less oxygen during the work and recovery process, had a slower pulse rate and accomplished more at a faster pace.[49]

Even as it stirred fantasies of unbridled scientific reach and unfettered medical power, the spectre of the hypnotized subject's suggestibility and malleability raised difficult questions for the inhibition theory of hypnosis. Simply put, if hypnosis was a state of brain inactivity that provided beneficial rest and recuperation for the brain, how was the hypnotist able to compel the patient to comply with his suggestions? The well-publicized capacity of the hypnotist to effect spectacular 'transformations of the personality' – compelling test subjects to act out suggested emotions or to assume childhood personas – did not appear readily explicable by the theory of inhibition.[50] As Platonov pondered after observing the heightening of memory capacity under hypnosis, '[b]ut why is it that such an activation (*ozhivlenie*) of large quantities of organic traces takes place much more readily in a state of artificially induced, sleep-like inhibition of the brain cortex?'[51] While Pavlov's laboratory attempted to answer such conundrums by conceding that some limited parts of the brain (so-called 'guarding points') remained active during hypnosis and permitted the establishment of a rapport with the hypnotist, the exact relationship between alertness and inhibition remained ill-defined in physiological accounts of hypnosis.[52] The profound ambiguity of the hypnotic state – in which, as Jonathan Crary notes, 'the paradoxical qualities of heightened mental alertness and a loss of conscious agency are united' – continued to pose a profound challenge to Soviet physiologists, who visibly struggled to place the diverse facets of hypnotic phenomena under the explanatory rubric of 'rest for the brain'. Indeed, the attempt to account for phenomena such as enhanced perceptual capabilities, vivid hallucinations and access to memories that were off-limits to the waking subject led some medical hypnotists like Platonov to conceptualize hypnosis as both a process of rest and inactivity *and* 'the highest stage of wakefulness'.[53]

Hypnosis and the unconscious

The inconsistencies found in Platonov's characterization of hypnotic phenomena are perhaps unsurprising given that, like several other Soviet physiologists, he endorsed the 'inhibition theory' while remaining sympathetic to another tradition of understanding hypnosis. From the nineteenth century, prominent medical hypnotists including Hippolyte Bernheim, Albert Moll and August Forel had characterized hypnosis as an intervention into the unconscious mechanisms of the mind. Contesting the association of hypnosis with the '"depressing of cortical activity", a kind of experimental imbecility', these doctors were united in insisting that the consciousness of the hypnotized subject continued to remain active during hypnotic sleep, much as it did during the normal sleep state.[54] '[N]atural sleep does not necessitate the abolition of thought and consciousness, any more than artificial sleep does', Bernheim noted, 'we are self-conscious during sleep, we think, we dream, we work'.[55] The notion that suggestion could take place in the hypnotic state 'without consciousness' was simply 'inconceivable', Moll asserted.[56] Rather than contending that the psychical faculties were 'destroyed' during 'active somnambulism', these scholars argued that the consciousness of the hypnotized patient was 'modified'.[57] This altered state of consciousness, often likened to 'dream-consciousness', was thought to be the bedrock of a better scientific understanding of the mind.

Hypnotic experiments had played a central role in demonstrating that the life of the human mind was not limited to the activity of the waking consciousness. As Moll noted, hypnotic phenomena could only be 'comprehensible if, besides the primary consciousness, a secondary consciousness works intelligently in us'.[58] For many specialists, hypnosis provided incontestable proof of the co-existence of this 'secondary consciousness' (or 'hypoconscious', 'dream-consciousness', 'unconceived' or 'unconscious' realm, as it was variously identified) with the consciousness that was fully known and accessible to the individual in the waking state.[59] Nineteenth-century neurologists and psychologists, from Charcot to Forel and Max Dessoir, saw immense value in hypnotism's capacity to render unconscious phenomena reproducible and scientifically observable. With the help of hypnosis, a part of the mind that was usually inaccessible in waking life could be subjected to scientific scrutiny.[60] Indeed, the 'father' of psychoanalysis, Sigmund Freud, began his therapeutic practice by using hypnotic techniques to gain access to the unconscious life of his patients. While famously turning his back on hypnosis later in his career, Freud nevertheless acknowledged that the 'science of the unconscious' had emerged out of the bedrock of hypnotism.[61]

The understanding of hypnosis as a state that activated unconscious mental activity had a lasting legacy in the Soviet Union. Works by foreign doctors who saw hypnosis as a means of facilitating access to the sphere of the unconscious circulated widely in the Soviet Union in the decade following the October Revolution. The 1920s saw the publication of the Russian translation of the twelfth edition of Forel's *Der Hypnotismus* (1924), a pivotal work that attributed the revelation of the co-existence of waking cognition (described by Forel as the 'superconsciousness') and 'other forms of consciousness' to hypnosis. Works by the German physicians Leopold Löwenfeld and Arthur Kronfeld, which presented hypnosis as a technique of unearthing 'deeply hidden psychic mechanisms', also appeared in translation.[62] To be sure, these translations were typically accompanied by a 'preface' by leading Soviet physiologists who spelled out the 'correct' interpretation of hypnosis to readers. Sreznevskii used his preface to Forel's monograph to reiterate that hypnosis was an 'inhibitory process' akin to catalepsy in animals, while Platonov's preface to Löwenfeld's *Hypnotismus und Medizin* (1922) cautioned readers that the book reflected the view-point of 'subjective psychology' all too common amongst Western authors.[63] During the 1920s, however, these foreign works of scholarship were still presented as 'authoritative' statements that had 'shaped the understanding of hypnosis and suggestion not only in the West, but also in Russia'.[64]

In addition to foreign literature, imported films also served to popularize the reading of hypnosis as a technology of the unconscious. In the summer of 1924, Mezhrabpomfil'm acquired *A Look into the Depth of the Soul*, a 1923 German film on 'the problem of consciousness and the unconscious, hypnosis and suggestion' (which had been produced in consultation with Arthur Kronfeld) for screening in Soviet cinemas under the title *Hypnosis and Suggestion*.[65] Presenting waking consciousness as but a fraction of the vast depths of the mind, the film framed hypnosis as a vital means of influencing the unconscious. The close intertwinement of the 'higher' and 'lower' consciousness was illustrated through the images of a sea that juxtaposed the calmness of its surface with the hidden life teeming underneath. The subsequent depiction of a storm at sea demonstrated the power of the 'lower consciousness' over human actions. The film proceeded to showcase the 'pivotal' role that the unconscious played in human life through the examples of mental illness, artistic inspiration and dreams. The access to the unconscious facilitated by hypnosis was depicted in a diagram that pictured the human mind as a house composed of an upper floor and a basement. The hypnotist's influence was represented through the act of dimming the lights on the upper floor (switching off the waking consciousness) while shining a spotlight onto the lower depths (igniting the 'lower consciousness'). A sensational sequence of hypnotic acts – featuring hypnotized subjects taking imaginary infants and dogs into their arms or being made to pour water over their interlocutors – demonstrated the hypnotist's seemingly limitless power of surreptitious influence.

To be sure, certain Soviet physiologists warned against understanding hypnosis as a manifestation of unconscious psychic processes. 'Theories that explained hypnosis as the manifestation of the unconscious "I" or the "lower consciousness"', Birman asserted, whilst of interest 'from a philosophical point of view', had 'no scientific value'.[66] Nevertheless, many Soviet specialists, even those who firmly identified as physiologists, continued to understand hypnosis as a 'window' onto the workings of the unconscious mind. Indeed, in the early 1920s, physiologists often saw no contradiction between championing a reflexological understanding of hypnosis, and connecting the hypnotic state to unconscious psychical activity. The year before Konstantin Platonov published his pivotal attempt to read hypnosis through the lens of reflexology, *Hypnosis and Suggestion in Practical Medicine* (1925), he wrote a foreword to a book titled *The Psychoanalysis of Communism* by Georgii Malis. Drawing attention to the common ground between reflexology and psychoanalysis and acknowledging the 'invaluable contribution' made by Freudian psychoanalysis to the 'understanding of nervous processes', the foreword asserted that hypnosis had proved the existence of unconscious phenomena beyond all doubt.[67] Platonov's own experiments with re-activating the unconscious thoughts and feelings of hypnotized patients had convinced him of hypnotism's serviceability in uncovering the sources of neurotic symptoms.[68]

Platonov was not alone in recognizing the promise of hypnosis in helping to recover the 'conditioned stimuli' that had generated pathological 'conditioned reflexes'. Another former associate of Bekhterev, V. V. Sreznevskii, experimented with using hypnosis to retrieve the thoughts and feelings which were no longer accessible to consciousness. Corroborating the thesis advanced by the Austrian psychiatrist, Richard Kraft-Ebbing, Sreznevskii cited the case of a twenty-five-year-old patient called 'Ania', whose recovery of childhood experiences long expelled from memory he had facilitated using hypnosis. Asserting that he was

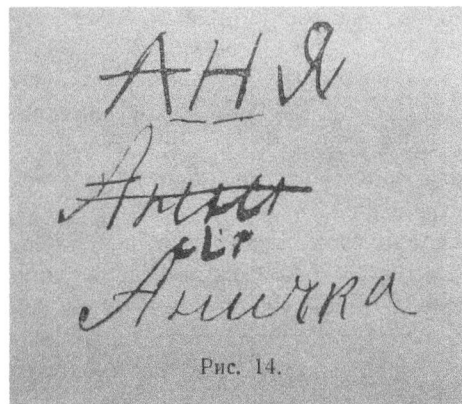

Figure 1.4 From 'Ania' to 'Anichka': Illustration of age regression under hypnosis in V. V. Sreznevskii, *Gipnoz i vnushenie* (Petrograd: Akademicheskoe izd-vo, 1923), 31.

able to 'return' Ania to the ages of six and nine under deep hypnosis, Sreznevskii illustrated the authenticity of the psychical regression through handwriting samples[69] (Figure 1.4).

The attempts of researchers like Sreznevskii to merge hypnosis with the investigation of the unconscious mind crystallized in the foundation of a new therapeutic method – 'hypnoanalysis'. Envisaged as a means of reconstructing the facts of distant childhood events, hypnoanalysis enabled the patient to 'relive' and process repressed infantile trauma.[70] The head of the Moscow Hypnological Society, S. Ia. Lifshits, emerged as one of the leading proponents of this synthesis of hypnosis and psychoanalysis. While acknowledging Freud's critique of hypnosis, Lifshits insisted that hypnosis was fully compatible with the aims of psychoanalytic investigation and the recovery of repressed memories. 'The foremost achievement of hypnology', Lifshits argued, was its discovery of a means of switching off the higher consciousness and its 'censorship' and 'penetrating the activity of the lower, dream consciousness and analysing it'.[71] The emphasis on the shared ground between psychoanalysis and hypnosis was common amongst the enthusiasts of hypnoanalysis. Calling attention to Freud and Josef Breuer's initial reliance on hypnosis in psychotherapeutic treatment, hypnologists like A. P. Nikolaev noted that no method was as effective as hypnosis at attaining 'limitless truthfulness' and re-activating repressed psychical traces.[72]

Probing the unconscious: Experiment and control

It was not only Soviet psychotherapists who saw hypnosis as a valuable tool of probing the unconscious, prominent psychologists like Alexander Luria also harnessed hypnosis in the service of 'experimental psychoanalysis'.[73] As part of his seven-year study into the impact of acute affective states on 'systems of psychological function', published in English in 1932 as *The Nature of Human Conflicts*, Luria called on hypnosis to create artificial conflict situations that gave rise to affective disorganization. Luria's research team put test subjects into a deep hypnotic state and suggested a variety of situations that conflicted with the subjects' normal behaviour and beliefs – the theft of a wallet from a friend, the performance of an illegal abortion, the beating of a small child. Having been instructed to forget the 'traumatic situation' suggested to them under hypnosis upon awaking, test subjects were analysed through free association and word association tests (which included 'triggering' word-stimuli) in order to explore the correlation between subjects' verbal responses and their motor reactions. Variations in reaction times and motor disturbances recorded during the post-hypnotic experiments indicated that while the artificially induced psychological trauma was ostensibly removed from consciousness, it still remained active.[74] Luria conceptualized the technique as a means of creating an 'experimental unconscious'; hypnosis allowed the experimenter to 'insert' specific feeling states into the hypnotized subject's psyche and to bring into being 'complexes' or 'affect traces' that continued to shape the test subject's behaviour without their conscious awareness.[75]

Cultural sources such as Ivan Prutkov's 1928 one-act play *Hypnosis* (*Gipnoz*), submitted to the main literary censorship body, Glavlit, in March 1928, testify to the potency of the association between hypnosis and the revelation of unconscious psychic material.[76] Prutkov's play enacts a hypnotic experiment at a social gathering hosted by one of the 'former people' displaced by the revolution, Nikolai Pritykin.[77] One of the invited guests, a doctor who happens to be a specialist in hypnosis, is called to provide some after-dinner entertainment by demonstrating his craft on Pritykin. The guests gathered together at Pritykin's flat marvel at the spectacle of their hypnotized host being made to re-live his actions from an ordinary day in the winter of 1919. The experiment in 'journeying into the past' brings only embarrassment to Pritykin; his guests witness their host spend his day during the 'heroic period' of the Civil War grumbling about food shortages and attempting to keep his wife's valuables hidden from the Red Guards. The depiction of hypnosis as means of unearthing the secrets of a person's soul in Prutkov's play echoed hypnologists' framing of their practice as a technique of 'limitless truthfulness'.

Many other early Soviet cultural producers found inspiration in scientific research that demonstrated hypnotism's capacity to open access to the hidden life of the mind. The leading director of the Soviet film avant-garde, Sergei Eisenstein, who began to actively engage with Luria's work from the mid-1920s, asked the psychologist to conduct a number of special hypnotic experiments as a means to test out his ideas about 'one of the fundamental laws' underlying expressive movement – 'recoil'.[78] In experiments conducted in December 1928 to study how 'a movement in any specific direction' was preceded by 'a somewhat smaller, preliminary movement in the opposite direction', Luria and Eisenstein suggested conflict situations to subjects under hypnosis.[79] In the first two experiments, test subjects were asked to walk clockwise in a circle as if they were taking a stroll in a park. They were to notice a column standing in the middle of the room bearing a desired object, which took the shape of an appetizing pear in the first experiment and an attractive bunch of flowers in the second.[80] Once the test subjects were within grasp of their desired object, an awareness of an obstacle was suggested to them – a wasp buzzing around the pear, and a hissing snake in the midst of the bouquet of flowers, respectively. While the hypnotist's suggestions were to compel the first test subject to conquer their fear of wasps and to grab hold of the pear, the second subject was to remain overwhelmed by feelings of fear.[81] The third experiment conducted by Luria allowed Eisenstein to observe the actions of a hypnotized subject who was instructed to experience a burning desire to stand up and articulate their feelings at the same time as finding themselves unable to communicate verbally.[82] The experiments, which produced graphs of movement that took the shape of spirals and zigzags, affirmed Eisenstein's theory that a particular goal was achieved through 'denial' and 'false movements'. For both Luria and Eisenstein, hypnosis provided an expedient means of studying motivations and impulses that were usually repressed. Eisenstein's hypnotic experiments probed the 'conflict between different strata of consciousness' – the 'atavistic' and the 'progressive', the emotional and the rational.[83]

Eisenstein was not the only cultural producer who saw great promise in hypnosis and suggestion as techniques of exploring different layers of the psyche. In 1925–6, the Psycho-Physiological Section at the State Academy of Artistic Sciences (GAKhN) saw the establishment of two commissions dedicated to the study of hypnosis and suggestion. The 'Commission for the Study of Aesthetic Production and Reception under the Influence of Hypnosis' was headed by the literary and aesthetic theorists A. V. Bakushinskii and P. N. Kapterev.[84] The 'Commission for the Study of the Suggestive Effects of the Word' was organized under the leadership of the psychiatrist, P. I. Karpov.[85] Bakushinskii and Kapterev's commission conducted a series of experiments to explore the drawings produced by adult subjects who had been transposed to childhood stages under hypnosis.[86] Examining the techniques used by orators from antiquity to the present day, Karpov's commission sought to establish the 'laws' and principles underlying the suggestive effects of oral communication.[87] The concept of the unconscious was pivotal to both research groups' understanding of hypnosis and suggestion. While the first commission framed hypnosis as a form of 'psychical regression', Karpov's team explicitly characterized suggestibility as a property of the 'unconscious "I"'.[88] Moreover, Karpov made clear that his commission's research into the laws of suggestion aimed to facilitate 'the penetration into the depths of unconscious functions and the casting light on the darkness that was unconscious mental activity' – a task which stood at the forefront of contemporary critical enquiry in Europe, Karpov insisted.[89]

While Bakushinskii and Kapterev's research on hypnosis and artistic production appeared to be chiefly driven by the goal of expanding creative capabilities, the objectives of the 'Commission for the Study of the Suggestive Effects of the Word' were focused on practical and political implications. The chief aim of the commission's investigations into suggestibility was the discovery of the techniques and strategies through which the process of suggestion could be rendered 'easier' and 'more effective'.[90] Hypnosis and suggestion, in the eyes of Karpov's researchers, presented techniques of influence and control that were indispensable not only to doctors, teachers, lawyers, and judiciaries, but also to political activists.[91] A skilful politician or public servant was tellingly framed by the commission as a master manipulator of the unconscious. Just as a lawyer adept at finding a way to sway jurors or a doctor skilled in influencing the behaviour of his patient, the political orator was to be well versed in the art of 'opening up access to the sphere of the unconscious', Karpov reasoned.[92]

The tradition of understanding hypnosis as a technology of the unconscious mind not only informed the work of researchers who were enthused by the possibilities opened up by hypnosis, but by those who were highly critical of the practice. Concerns about the dangers of hypnotism voiced during the early Soviet period frequently equated hypnotic suggestion to a process of surreptitious influence facilitated by the diminishment of the 'conscious' and 'rational' aspects of the mind. Staunch opponents of hypnosis like the neurologist Aron Zalkind, for example, were horrified by what the wide implementation of hypnosis and suggestion could mean for 'the field of active critical control'.[93] For Zalkind, hypnosis was a therapeutic practice based on surreptitious suggestion and fundamentally at odds with the qualities of active resistance and independence of thought required for the class struggle. Suggestibility, Zalkind argued, was a pernicious corrupting force – an 'infection' – that had to be fought and resisted with all of one's might rather than cultivated in medical treatment.[94] This 'opiate' that 'put patients to sleep, stupefied them, and weakened their reason' could, like other narcotics, be resorted to as a 'necessary evil' in some circumstances, Zalkind noted, but was dangerous to deploy on a mass scale.[95]

The association of hypnosis and suggestion with unconscious control and the disablement of the critical faculties proved pervasive in public culture. At the same time as Soviet physiologists asserted the medical benefits of the sleep-like state of hypnosis, images of hypnotists who exploited their power over the unconscious minds of their victims abounded in the cultural sphere. The period of the New Economic Policy saw the wide distribution of imported foreign films like *The Cabinet of Dr Caligari* (*Das Cabinet des Dr Caligari*, Wiene, 1920). A tale of a medical specialist who instructs a somnambulist under his command to conduct a series of crimes, Robert Wiene's film reflected the revival of medical interest in the question of post-hypnotic suggestion and hypnotic crime.[96] In 1924, another film on the abuse of hypnotic influence, Fritz Lang's *Dr Mabuse, the Gambler* (*Dr Mabuse, der Spieler*, 1922), appeared on Soviet screens.[97] The criminal protagonist of Lang's film, the mastermind of an underground criminal gang, was shown to be both a skilled hypnotist and an expert in psychoanalysis.[98] Lavishly advertised and extensively discussed on the pages of the Soviet film press, *The Cabinet of Dr Caligari* and *Dr Mabuse* were key reference points for the depiction of hypnosis in one of the highest grossing Soviet films of the 1920s, the detective thriller, *Miss Mend* (Otsep and Barnet, 1926).[99] The clandestine anti-Bolshevik 'Organization' depicted in *Miss Mend* is headed by the evil scientist 'Chiche' (played by Sergei Komarov), a striking amalgam of Caligari and Mabuse. Like Caligari, he uses hypnosis to keep his victim, the millionaire Gordon Stern, in a passive somnambulist trance. Using only the power of his gaze, Chiche is able to force Stone to sign a will surrendering his vast fortune. In a clear nod to *Dr Mabuse*, Chiche is a master of disguise and a manipulator of women's affections, holding Stone's widow Elisabeth under his spell.[100]

The misuse of hypnotic influence was also imagined in literary works like Mikhail Zoshchenko's 1926 satirical short story, 'Hypnosis', in which a worker who undergoes hypnosis to help him to quit smoking suspects that he has overpaid the hypnotist under the influence of suggestion.[101] Such cultural portrayals not only indicate that scientific efforts to dispel the lingering public distrust of hypnosis had some way to go, but also suggest that the 'inhibition' paradigm had little currency in the popular imagination. Figuring hypnosis as an inroad to the mysterious recesses of the mind, portrayals such as Zoshchenko's short story invoked the trope of post-hypnotic suggestion, the phenomenon cited by Freud as one of the most vivid illustrations of the existence of the unconscious.[102]

To be sure, not all cultural representations of the hypnotic rapport invoked the prospect of nefarious unconscious influence. A satirical 1927 play by L. Miliugin and Vladimir Ivanov titled *Woe from Hypnosis* (*Gore ot gipnoza*) associated the medical hypnotist's power with socially beneficial re-education.[103] Echoing Platonov's heady fantasies of the radical social conditioning that could be effected with the aid of suggestion, the play presents a series of experiments with the 'method of transforming inveterate criminals into honest people'.[104] One session of hypnosis converts a folk healer who specialises in backstreet abortions and a recidivist hooligan into model Soviet citizens for the duration of one week. On the day after being hypnotized, the folk healer develops pangs of conscience and is no longer able to trade in charlatanism. Van'ka the street hooligan similarly begins to experience the stirrings of 'proletarian virtue' in his soul and 'red worker-peasant blood' pumping through his veins, coming to denounce hooliganism as the most 'evil of evils'.[105] The man who previously itched to live out fantasies of violence now declares his intent to battle social disorder arm in arm with his former arch enemy – the Soviet policeman. Even cultural representations that entertained the socially beneficial possibilities of hypnosis, however, still portrayed the practice as a technique of unconscious control. Despite the hypnotist telling the folk healer and Van'ka that they are free at the end of their session, the influence of post-hypnotic suggestion overpowers the will of both subjects. On the stroke of 4 o'clock, the folk healer is compelled to reveal the truth about her 'treatments' to her customers and Van'ka, who is poised to land a blow against a local policeman, abandons the attack and unfurls his fist into a handshake.

Conclusion

The repression of psychoanalysis as a theory and practice in the Soviet Union in the early 1930s ensured that the conception of hypnosis as a 'technology of the unconscious', which co-existed alongside the physiological interpretation of hypnotic phenomena for much of the 1920s, was largely effaced from scientific discourse. From the late 1920s, medical films and books that explicated hypnosis with recourse to theories of the unconscious were subjected to sustained criticism. The critical reception of Curt Thomalla's *Hypnosis and Suggestion* is a vivid example. By the end of the 1920s, the film that explicitly framed hypnosis as a means of exploring the unconscious life of the mind was attacked for failing to advance a 'biological' explanation of hypnosis 'from the point of view of the inhibition of the brain cortex'.[106] The growing intolerance of the psychological paradigm was similarly illustrated by the heavy-handed editing of foreign works on hypnosis. The 1929 edition of the Russian translation of Kronfeld's *Hypnosis and Suggestion*, edited by Aron Zalkind, abounded with editorial footnotes that sought to translate Kronfeld's 'metaphysical constructions' into the language of objective reflexology.[107] By the mid-1930s, psychotherapists who had previously seen the merits of both the physiological and the psychological accounts of hypnosis, such as Konstantin Platonov, insisted on the need to cement a single definition.[108] The basis of this 'unified' interpretation, Platonov insisted, could only be Pavlov's 'materialist' teaching on 'inhibition'.[109]

While the portrayal of hypnosis as a technology that opened up access to the unconscious mind was increasingly rendered off limits in official scientific and medical discourse, the cultural sphere betrayed the lingering influence of this paradigm. In the same year as Platonov's article was featured in a leading psychiatric journal, the writer Leonid Lench published a short story titled 'A Hypnotist's Séance' ('*Seans gipnotizera*', 1935).[110] The satirical tale, set at a public hypnosis demonstration, framed hypnosis as the 'breaking through of repression' that allowed the abuses of power perpetuated by the director of a local poultry trust office (comrade Verepetuev) to publicly unravel.[111] Indeed, efforts to instate the Pavlovian inhibition paradigm as the definitive explanation of hypnosis continued to be resisted. Even in the mid-1930s, some doctors continued to assert that hypnosis facilitated the physician's access to 'the unconscious sphere of psychobiological mechanisms', and questioned whether hypnosis could be solely explained through Pavlov's theories.[112] Insisting that hypnosis was a state in which the 'qualities of inhibition and activation, sleep and wakefulness' co-existed, the prominent psychotherapist Iurii Kannabikh noted that the state of 'physiological sleep' induced in dogs at Pavlov's laboratories should not be characterized as hypnosis.[113] 'Hypnosis', another doctor not fully satisfied with the physiological explanation noted in 1937, 'is a phenomenon far more complex than we had previously assumed.'[114]

Notes

1   On conceptions of hypnosis in late Imperial Russia, see Julia Mannherz, *Modern Occultism in Late Imperial Russia* (Ithaca: Cornell University Press, 2012), 87–110.
2   B. N. Birman, *Eksperimental'nyi son* (Leningrad: Gos. izd-vo, 1925); K. I. Platonov, *Slovo kak fiziologicheskii i lechebnyi faktor: k fiziologii psikhoterapii* (Kharkiv: Gos. izd-vo Ukrainy, 1930).
3   Andreas Mayer explores the emergence of hypnosis as a prime technique in the 'experimentalization of the unconscious mind'. See his *Sites of the Unconscious: Hypnosis and the Emergence of the Psychoanalytic Setting* (Chicago: University of Chicago Press, 2013), 1–2.
4   On the rise and fall of psychoanalysis in the Soviet Union see Martin A. Miller, *Freud and the Bolsheviks: Psychoanalysis in Imperial Russia and the Soviet Union* (New Haven, CT: Yale University Press, 1998) and Alexander Etkind, *Eros of the Impossible: The History of Psychoanalysis in Russia*, trans. by Noah and Maria Rubins (Oxford: Westview Press, 1997).
5   Alexander Etkind has asserted that 'the authoritarian mentality, with its primitivism, its abrogation of responsibility, and its magical expectations, has something in common with hypnosis'. See his 'How Psychoanalysis Was Received in Russia, 1906–1936', *Journal of Analytical Psychology* 39.2 (1994): 191–202, 194.

6   Pasi Väliaho describes hypnotism's deployment for this purpose by nineteenth-century neurologists and psychologists. See his *Mapping the Moving Image: Gesture, Thought and Cinema circa 1900* (Amsterdam: Amsterdam University Press, 2010), 69.
7   Julia Mannherz, 'Hypnosis in Russian Popular Culture during the Era of War and Revolution', in Boris Kolonitskii, Steven Marks and Melissa Stockdale, eds., *Russian Culture in War and Revolution, 1914–22*, book 1 (Bloomington, IN: Slavica, 2014), 101–17.
8   V. M. Bekhterev, 'O lechenii gipnozom', *Vestnik znaniia*, 2 (1926): 85–96.
9   E. I. Dubnikov, 'Gipnoterapiia v praktike', *Sovetskii vrachebnyi zhurnal*, 2 (1939): 109–20; K. I. Platonov, 'K ucheniiu o prirode gipnoza i gipnosuggestivnoi terapii, kak lechebnom faktore', *Sovremennaia psikhonevrologiia*, 3.3 (1926): 132–40.
10 Bekhterev, 'O lechenii gipnozom'; A. P. Nikolaev, *Teoriia i praktika gipnoza v fiziologicheskom osveshchenii* (Kyiv, 1927), 56; B. A. Tokarskii, 'Psikhoterapiia alkogolizma', *Sovremennaia psikhonevrologiia*, 5.11 (1927): 393–6; F. B. Tseikinskaia and N. L. Utevskii, 'K ambulatornomu lecheniiu alkogolikov', in K. I. Platonov, ed., *Psikhoterapiia: Sbornik statei* (Kharkiv: Gos. izd-vo Ukrainy, 1930), 267–83; P. I. Istomin, 'K probleme morfinizma: opyt ambulatornogo gipnosuggestivnogo lecheniia', in Platonov, ed., *Psikhoterapiia*, 251–65.
11 As well as Tricia Starks's chapter in this volume, see also her 'A Revolutionary Attack on Tobacco: Bolshevik Antismoking Campaigns in the 1920s', *AJPH*, 107.11 (2017): 1711–17, 1716.
12 Nikolaev, *Teoriia i praktika gipnoza*, 57; See also V. Bekhterev and V. Sreznevskii, 'Novyi metod kollektivnogo lecheniia bol'nykh khronicheskim alkogolizmom', 1-oi Vsesoiuznyi s"ezd psikhiatrov i nevropatologov, *Sovremennaia psikhonevrologiia*, 6.1 (1928): 103–4.
13 V. Ia. Danilevskii, *Gipnotizm* (Kharkiv: Put' prosveshcheniia, 1924), 209.
14 I. M. Apter, *Seksual'nye nevrozy i ikh terapiia* (Kharkiv: Nauchnaia mysl', 1929); Bekhterev, 'O lechenii gipnozom', 93.
15 Nikolaev and Platonov reported their success in achieving full anaesthesia during gynaecological, surgical, dental and optical operations. See Nikolaev, *Teoriia i praktika gipnoza*, 45–6 and K. I. Platonov and M. V. Shestopal, *Vnushenie i gipnoz v akusherstve i ginekologii* (Kharkiv: Gos. izd-vo Ukrainy, 1925).
16 The use of hypnosis and suggestion in the sphere of dermatology attracted particular attention in the early Soviet period. See A. I. Kartamyshev, *Gipnoz v dermatologii* (Tashkent: Gos. izdat. UzSSR, 1936).
17 Nikolaev, *Teoriia i praktika gipnoza*, 57. See also I. M. Protopopov, 'Primenenie gipnoza v sanitarnykh usloviiakh', *Vrachebnoe delo*, 9 (1928): 733–4.
18 A. F. Lazurskii, 'O vliianii vnushennykh v gipnoze chuvstvovanii na pul's i dykhanie', *Izvestiia Imperatorskoi Voenno-Meditsinskoi Akademii*, 4 (1900): 329–50; V. M. Bekhterev, 'Ob ob"ektivnykh priznakakh vnushenii, ispytyvaemykh v izuchenie ob"ektivnykh priznakov podeistvovavshego vnusheniia' [1905], in *Gipnoz. Vnushenie. Telepatiia* (Moscow: Mysl', 1994), 57–64.
19 V. M. Bekhterev and V. Narbut, 'Ob"ektivnye priznaki vnushennykh izmenenii chuvstvitel'nosti v gipnoze' [1902], in *Gipnoz. Vnushenie. Telepatiia*, 64–75.
20 V. M. Bekhterev and N. M. Shchelovanov, 'O vliianii gipnoza i vnusheniia na sochet. refleksy', in B. M. Bekhterev ed., *Novoe v refleksologii i fiziologii nervnoi sistemy* (Leningrad and Moscow: Gos. izd-vo, 1925), 179–204.
21 Platonov, *Slovo kak fiziologicheskii i lechebnyi faktor*, 10.

22 Ibid., 9–19.
23 Ibid.
24 Birman, *Eksperimental'nyi son*.
25 K. I. Platonov, *Gipnoz i vnushenie v prakticheskoi meditsine* (Kharkiv: Nauchnaia mysl', 1925), 22.
26 Bekhterev and Shchelovanov, 'O vliianii gipnoza', 181; V. M. Bekhterev, 'Gipnoz, vnushenie i psikhoterapiia i ikh lechebnoe znachenie' [1911], *Gipnoz. Vnushenie. Telepatiia*, 255.
27 Ivan Pavlov, *Lectures on Conditioned Reflexes: Conditioned Reflexes and Psychiatry*, Vol. 2 (London: Lawrence and Wishart Ltd, 1941), 39–43; Platonov, *Gipnoz i vnushenie*, 17–18.
28 Ivan Pavlov, *Lectures on Conditioned Reflexes: Twenty-Five Years of Objective Study of the Higher Nervous Activity (Behaviour) of Animals*, Vol. 1 (London: Martin Lawrence Limited), 307.
29 Platonov and Shestopal, *Vnushenie i gipnoz*, 58.
30 As K. I. Platonov noted, 'all of Bernheim's claims are scientifically being proven by the contemporary Russian physiological teaching on the higher functions of the nervous system (Bekhterev and Pavlov)'. See his 'Predislovie k russkomu izdaniiu', in L. Levenfel'd, *Gipnoz i ego tekhnika*, trans. by P. Ia. Gal'perin (Kharkiv: Kosmos, 1929), 5–11, 7.
31 Soviet scientists typically saw themselves as reconciling the two rival readings of hypnotic phenomena, backing the Nancy school's interpretation of hypnosis as psychological suggestion while also acknowledging that hypnosis could be impelled by physiological stimuli. See V. Bekhterev, 'Gipnoz' [1925], *Gipnoz. Vnushenie. Telepatiia*, 51.
32 Platonov, *Gipnoz i vnushenie v prakticheskoi meditsine*, 15, 17.
33 Ibid., 5–6.
34 Ibid., 7. See also Nikolaev, *Teoriia i praktika gipnoza*, 59.
35 Dal', 'Massovyi gipnoz v kino', *Sovetskii ekran*, 39 (1928): 19.
36 See, for example, Danilevskii, *Gipnotizm*, 43, 195–6.
37 Platonov, *Gipnoz i vnushenie*, 17–18.
38 Pavlov, *Conditioned Reflexes*, 411; Bekhterev, 'Gipnoz', 54; Danilevskii, *Gipnotizm*, 195–6; V. V. Sreznevskii, 'Predislovie k russkomu izdaniiu', in Avgust Forel', *Gipnotizm ili vnushenie i psikhoterapiia* (Leningrad: Obrazovanie, 1928), 3–8.
39 Dal', 'Massovyi gipnoz v kino'.
40 Ibid.
41 Bekhterev, 'O lechenii gipnozom', 88.
42 Danilevskii, *Gipnotizm*, 182.
43 Ibid., 43; Platonov, *Gipnoz i vnushenie*, 32–6.
44 Danilevskii, *Gipnotizm*, 249.
45 Ibid., 247.
46 Platonov, *Gipnoz i vnushenie v prakticheskoi meditsine*, 35. See also Platonov, 'Predislovie', L. Levenfel'd, *Gipnoz i ego tekhnika*, 9. Suggestion under hypnosis, Sreznevskii claimed, could be used to establish 'dominanty' (Uspenskii) that could shape behaviour in a specific direction. See his 'Predislovie' to Forel', *Gipnotizm*, 5.
47 Platonov, *Gipnoz i vnushenie*, 37.
48 K. I. Platonov and A. N. Matskevich, 'Gipnoz i alkogolizirovnnaia nervnaia sistema', in A. I. Geimanovich, ed., *Voprosy obshchei i sotsial'noi psikhonevrologii* (Kharkiv: Iuridicheskoe izd-vo Ukrainy, 1930), 93–106, 93.

49 V. M. Vasilevskii and E. M. Kagan, 'Vliianie gipno-suggestivnykh vozdeistvii na funktsii organizma v rabote i v restitutsii', *Fiziologicheskii zhurnal SSSR*, 29.1 (1935): 79–92.
50 K. I. Platonov and E. A. Prikhodivnyi, 'K ob"ektivnomu dokazatel'stvu eksperimental'nogo izmeneniia lichnosti', in Platonov, ed., *Psikhoterapiia*, 191–202.
51 Ibid., 200. Julia Vassilieva notes that early Soviet researchers also conducted studies that demonstrated the heightening of sensory sensitivity under hypnosis. See her 'Hypnosis, Psychotechnics and Magic of Art', in Ian Christie and Julia Vassilieva, eds., *The Eisenstein Universe* (London: Bloomsbury, 2021), 130–51, 137–8.
52 Birman, *Eksperimental'nyi son*, 62; Platonov and Prikhodivnyi, 'K ob"ektivnomu dokazatel'stvu', 201–2.
53 Platonov, *Gipnoz i vnushenie*, 17.
54 Sigmund Freud, 'Review of August Forel's Hypnotism' [1889], *The Standard Edition of the Complete Psychological Works*, ed. and trans. by James Strachey (London: Hogarth Press, 1966), Vol. 1, 89–102, 96.
55 H. Bernheim, *Hypnosis and Suggestion in Psychotherapy* [1886], trans. by Christian A. Herter (New York: University Books, 1965), 152.
56 Albert Moll, *Hypnotism* (London: Walter Scott, 1890), 267.
57 Bernheim, *Hypnosis and Suggestion*, 143–4, 148.
58 Moll, *Hypnotism*, 251.
59 See August Forel, *Hypnotism or Suggestion and Psychotherapy*, 5th edn., trans. by H. M. Armit (New York: Rebman Company, 1907), 1. As Adam Crabtree has shown, it was on the basis of hypnosis that psychologists like Max Dessoir posed the existence of a 'double-ego', a split in the human subject between the spheres of the conscious and the unconscious. See his *From Mesmer to Freud: Magnetic Sleep and Roots of Psychological Healing* (New Haven, CT: Yale University Press, 1993), 344–50.
60 Heather Wolffram, *The Stepchildren of Science: Psychical Research and Parapsychology in Germany, c. 1870–1939* (Amsterdam: Rodopi, 2009), 97; Mayer, *Sites of the Unconscious*.
61 'It is not easy to over-estimate the importance of the part played by hypnotism in the history of the origin of psychoanalysis,' Freud noted. See his 'A Short Account of Psychoanalysis', in *The Standard Edition*, Vol. 19, ed. and trans. by James Strachey (London: Hogarth Press, 1961), 191–209, 192.
62 Forel', *Gipnotizm ili vnushenie i psikhoterapiia*; Levenfel'd, *Gipnoz i ego tekhnika*; Artur Kronfel'd, *Gipnoz i vnushenie*, 2nd edn., trans. by S. Tsederbaum (Moscow: Gos. izd-vo, 1929).
63 Sreznevskii, 'Predislovie' to Forel', *Gipnotizm*, 5. Platonov also asserted that the Soviet physiological school was 'more valuable' since it was built on 'laboratory experiment'. See his 'Predislovie k russkomu izdaniiu', 7.
64 Platonov, 'Predislovie k russkomu izdaniiu', 5.
65 G. Sh., 'Gipnoz i vnushenie', *Pravda*, 19 August 1924, 8; V. E., 'Gipnoz i vnushenie', *Kino-gazeta*, 26 August 1924, 2. The 'shooting script' for the film was published in L. M. Sukharebskii, *Patokinografiia v psikhiatrii i nevropatologii* (Moscow: Biomedgiz, 1936), 65–9.
66 Birman, *Eksperimental'nyi son*, 14–15.
67 K. Platonov, 'Predislove', Georgii Malis, *Psikhoanaliz kommunizma* (Kharkiv: Kosmos, 1924), 6, 29.
68 Ibid., 10.
69 V. V. Sreznevskii, *Gipnoz i vnushenie* (Petrograd: Akademicheskoe izd-vo, 1923), 30–1.

70 S. Ia. Lifshits, *Gipnoanaliz infantil'nykh travm u isterikov* (Avtorizovannoe izdanie, 1927), 31–2.
71 Ibid., 8.
72 The expediency of hypnoanalysis as a psychotherapeutic method was clearly an appealing factor. Whereas Freudian psychoanalysis required a programme of treatment that could span anywhere from six months to two years, Nikolaev noted, hypnoanalysis could uncover deeply buried psychical trauma in as little as twenty sessions. See Nikolaev, *Teoriia i praktika gipnoza*, 44.
73 A. R. Luria, *The Nature of Human Conflicts or Emotion, Conflict and Will: An Objective Study of Disorganisation and Control of Human Behaviour*, trans. and ed. by W. Horsley Gantt (New York: Liveright, 1932), 150.
74 Ibid., 130–147.
75 Ibid., 130.
76 Letter from the head of Leningrad Oblastlit to Glavlit, 18 March 1928, Russian State Archive of Literature and Art (RGALI), f. 656, op. 1, d. 2401, l. 1.
77 'Iv. Prutkov, *Gipnoz: P'esa v 1 deistvii i v trekh godakh*', RGALI, f. 656, op. 1, d. 2401, ll. 2–8.
78 On Eisenstein's and Luria's shared interest in hypnosis, see Vassilieva, 'Hypnosis, Psychotechnics and Magic of Art'.
79 S. M. Eisenstein, 'Rhythm and Repetition: Recoil and Expressive Movement', in *The Primal Phenomenon: Art*, ed. by Oksana Bulgakowa, trans. by Dustin Condren (Berlin: Potemkin Press, 2017), 12. See also his 'The Montage of Film Attractions' [1924] in *Selected Works, Vol. 1: Writings, 1922–34*, ed. and trans. by Richard Taylor (London: BFI, 1988), 39–58.
80 'Protokol opyta', 13 December 1928, RGALI, f. 1923, op. 1, d. 2739, ll. 2–5. For an analysis of this experiment in relation to Eisenstein's conception of recoil and Luria's theories, see Oksana Bulgakova, 'From Expressive Movement to the "Basic Problem": The Vygotsky-Luria-Eisensteinian Theory of Art', in Anton Yasnitsky, Rene van der Veer and Michel Ferrari, eds., *The Cambridge Handbook of Cultural Historical Psychology* (Cambridge: Cambridge University Press, 2014), 423–48, 430; and Julia Vassilieva, 'The Eisenstein-Vygotsky-Luria Collaboration', *Projections*, 13.1 (2019): 23–44, 26, 33–4.
81 'Protokol opyta', ll. 3–4.
82 Ibid., l. 5.
83 Eisenstein, 'Rhythm and Repetition', 26–7; 'The Montage of Film Attractions', 52.
84 'Protokol no. 16', RGALI, f. 941, op. 12, d. 54, l. 32.
85 'Protokol no. 19', RGALI, f. 941, op. 12, d. 54, l. 37.
86 'Fiziko-Psikhologicheskoe otdelenie', *Biulleteni GAKhN*, 4–5 (1926), 26.
87 'Protokol no. 1: Zasedaniia komissii', 2 November 1925, RGALI, f. 941, op. 12, d. 20, l. 4; 'Godovoi otchet za 1925/26 g', RGALI, f. 941, op. 12, d. 20, l. 46.
88 'Protokol no. 1: Zasedaniia komissii', 2 November 1925, RGALI, f. 941, op. 12, d. 20, l. 4; 'Tezisy k dokladu P. I. Karpova, "Vnushenie kak kharakternaia osobennost' podsoznatel'noi deiatel'nosti"', RGALI, f. 941, op. 12, d. 20, l. 7.
89 'Plan rabot komissii', RGALI, f. 941, op. 12, d. 20, l. 35.
90 'Godovoi otchet za 1925/26 g', RGALI, f. 941, op. 12, d. 20, l. 46.
91 Ibid., l. 46.
92 'Tezisy doklada, "Psikhologicheskogo razbora rechi A. V. Lunacharskogo" N. N. Vinogradova', 15 November 1926, RGALI, f. 941, op. 12, d. 20, l. 33.

93   A. B. Zalkind, *Zhizn' organizma i vnushenie* (Moscow and Leningrad: Gos. izd-vo, 1927), 94.
94   Ibid.
95   Ibid., 124.
96   Stefan Andriopoulos, *Possessed: Hypnotic Crimes, Corporate Fiction, and the Invention of Cinema*, trans. by Peter Jansen and Stefan Andriopoulos (Chicago: University of Chicago Press, 2008), 97.
97   The film was re-edited for Soviet release by Esfir Shub and Sergei Eisenstein. See Vassilieva, 'Hypnosis, Psychotechnics and Magic of Art', 130.
98   As Andriopoulos notes, a disguised Mabuse is shown giving a lecture on 'Psychoanalysis as a Factor in Modern Therapeutics', which compares the relationship between the analyst and the patient to the rapport established in hypnosis. See Andriopoulos, *Possessed*, 104.
99   'Nasha tribuna o: "Kabinete doktora Kaligari"', *Kino: dvukhnedel'nik*, 1/5 (1923): 15–18. For an example of the advertising of these films, see *Kino-zhizn'*, 1 (1923): 8. I am grateful to Ana Hedberg Olenina for alerting me to the representation of hypnosis in *Miss Mend*.
100 Perhaps in a nod to the claims of some Soviet doctors that only the weak-willed and suggestible could be successfully hypnotised, *Miss Mend* showed its Soviet heroes as much less susceptible to Chiche's hypnotic influence: a comic episode showing one of the film's heroes (Hopkins) being able to snap out of Chiche's hypnotic trance, ultimately dismisses hypnosis as a 'dupe'. See Ana Hedberg Olenina's commentary on this film, 'Miss Mend: A Whirlwind Vision of an Imagined America', in *Miss Mend: An Adventure Serial in Three Parts*, DVD produced by Jeffery Masino and David Shepard (Flicker Alley, 2009).
101 M. Zoshchenko, *Nervnye liudi* (Kharkiv: Proletarii, 1927), 33–5.
102 'Even before the time of psychoanalysis, hypnotic experiments and especially post-hypnotic suggestion, had tangibly demonstrated the existence and mode of operation of the mental unconscious,' Freud noted. See his 'The Unconscious' [1915], *The Standard Edition*, Vol. 14, 168–9.
103 'L. Miliugin and Vl. Ivanov, *Gore ot gipnoza: obozrenie v 6-ti kartinakh*', RGALI, f. 656, op. 1, d. 1945.
104 Ibid., l. 2.
105 Ibid., l. 6ob.
106 L. M. Sukharebskii, *Obzor sanprosvetitel'nykh kinofil'm za 10 let proletarskoi revoliutsii, 1917–1927* (Moscow: Izd-vo Moszdravotdela, 1928), 14.
107 A. Zalkind, 'Predislovie redaktora', in Kronfel'd, *Gipnoz i vnushenie*, 7.
108 K. I. Platonov, 'K novomu obosnovaniiu psikhoterapii', *Nevropatologiia, psikhiatriia, psikhogigiena*, 4.11 (1935): 85–90.
109 Ibid., 86.
110 L. S. Lench, 'Seans gipnotizera' [1935], in *Trudnaia sluzhba: Satir. i iumorist. rasskazy* (Moscow: Khudozh. literatura, 1967), 15–19.
111 Stage hypnotist 'Fernando' invites the lowly watchman of a poultry farm onto the stage to be hypnotized in front of the trust director Verepetuev and his second in command who are seated in the audience. With his usual inhibitions having being removed by hypnosis, the watchman unleashes a flood of home truths about his superior whilst Verepetuev looks on in horror.

112 Kartamyshev, *Gipnoz v dermatologii*, 22; Iu. V. Kannabikh, 'Mesto gipnoza v sisteme sovetskoi psikhoterapii i psikhogigieny', *Sovetskaia nevropatologiia, psikhiatriia i psikhogigiena*, 3.9 (1934): 50–60.
113 Kannabikh, 'Mesto gipnoza', 52.
114 G. P. Amfiteatrov, 'Obezbolivanie rodov gipnozom', *Akusherstvo i ginekologiia*, 12 (1937): 17–23, 23.

2

From psychosis to psychopathy: Psychiatry and crime in communist Czechoslovakia (1948–70)

Jakub Střelec

Researchers have recently turned their attention to how the views of experts from various fields shaped people's everyday lives in post-war Europe – from the building of the welfare state to the planning of new cities and the provision of marriage counselling.[1] As the recent literature shows, the psy sciences (disciplines dealing with human behaviour and mental health, such as psychology, psychiatry and psychotherapy) played an essential role in shaping the modern 'self' of people in the workplace, in the family and in politics.[2] Over the last decade, much of the new work has focused on the role of the psy sciences in communist Europe and the Soviet Union.[3] Drawing inspiration from Foucauldian theories, the study of the history of the 'socialist psy sciences' is an evolving field of research dealing with varied topics, from the history of medical knowledge to the history of the transnational exchange of ideas and practices across the Iron Curtain. Despite the growing number of studies in the field, there is still little research into the role of the psy sciences in the criminal justice system and the anti-crime policies of communist regimes. While the political abuse of psychiatry in the Soviet Union has been well studied, the question of how the ideas and concepts of the psy sciences impacted the management of everyday crime in socialist societies has attracted less scholarly attention.[4] This chapter seeks to shed further light on this question by investigating the concept of 'insane' and 'deviant' criminal behaviour constructed in forensic psychiatric knowledge in communist Czechoslovakia. It examines the ideas and practices developed by psychiatrists to deal with criminal behaviour as well as the interaction between the communist criminal justice system and forensic experts.

Czechoslovakia between 1948 and 1970 offers an excellent case for studying the relationship between psychiatry and criminology. Psychiatrists and other psy experts in Czechoslovakia found themselves in an unusual position at the beginning of the

---

The study was supported by the Charles University through a project of the Grant Agency of the Charles University (GAUK), no. 164119. I would like to thank the editors for their careful reading of my manuscript and their insightful comments and suggestions.

Cold War. On the one hand, the adoption of official Soviet policies in the areas of health and social welfare was underway; on the other hand, psychiatry and other fields were still rooted in the medical knowledge and practices of German-speaking scientists that were inherited from the Austro-Hungarian Empire. This created a unique amalgam of knowledge, which manifested itself in a 'holistic' concept of mind and body developed by Czechoslovak psychiatrists, who perceived mental activity as the product of the whole body, rather than the brain alone.

A closer look at primary sources reveals a certain discrepancy between the propagation of the concept of the 'socialist self' in psychiatry textbooks and its actual influence on the governing praxis of the communist state. This discrepancy can be demonstrated by the role of psychiatrists in criminal trials. Especially in the 1950s, psychiatric opinion played a less influential role in the courts' decision-making process than other factors, such as the defendant's class origin, the subversive nature of the crime and the threat the crime posed to the people's democratic regime. This slowly began to change in the 1960s alongside a rise in juvenile recidivism, which became a major issue for socialist society and forensic experts. Psychiatrists and other experts started to engage in various research projects studying the causes of crime and consequently began to point to links between psychopathy, criminal behaviour and recidivism. Using new language borrowed from the social sciences and humanities, psychiatrists stressed that the roots of criminal psychopathy could be identified in 'dysfunctional family backgrounds' and 'disordered behavioural traits'. The 'rise of psychopathy' was related to broader changes in anti-crime policy in post-Stalinist Czechoslovakia. Twenty years after the communist coup in 1948, it was no longer possible to attribute crime to the class struggle because there was a whole new generation of recidivists who had been raised under socialism. Searching for a different cause of crime, psychiatrists and other experts grasped at a new theory that placed the blame for crime on psychopathy.

Between Kuffner and Pavlov: Mind and body in early communist Czechoslovak psychiatry and psychology

After the communist coup in 1948, Czechoslovak psychiatry was 'Sovietized'. Psychiatric care had to be reformed according to the Soviet model, which was characterized by centralization, nationalization and planning.[5] The infrastructure of psychiatric care in Czechoslovakia was inherited from the Austro-Hungarian Empire and most psychiatric hospitals and facilities were established at the turn of the twentieth century.[6] Therefore, in 1953 a new psychiatric reform was introduced that aimed to reorganize psychiatric care, propagate Pavlovian medicine and support psychiatric research.[7] The theoretical framework of Czechoslovak psychiatry was reoriented around the principle of 'dialectical materialism, the Leninist theory of reflection, the physiology of I.P. Pavlov, and the biology of Michurin'.[8] This mirrored the approach to mental health disorders presented in Soviet psychiatry textbooks. Based on the Pavlovian principle of unity between organism and environment, psychiatrists argued that mental disorders were a pathological reaction of an organism to negative external stimuli. Among such stimuli were infections, brain injuries, intoxication, emotional shocks and other external factors such as light or noise.[9] The authors of a 1953 psychiatry textbook, for example, argued that 'mental activity, the psyche, is a property of highly organized matter, in this case, the brain'.[10] Mental activity was understood to be the result of the long-term development of the human nervous system, which had adapted and responded to external conditions and the environment over time. Moreover, Pavlov's theory of higher nervous activity impacted other disciplines dealing with human behaviour such as pedagogy, psychology and penology. Experts began to stress the role of education instead of punishment, especially for correcting the behaviour of repeat offenders.[11] They contended that there was a certain 'plasticity' of higher nervous activity that would allow experts to shape the future development of 'deviant' and 'defective' individuals.[12]

The adoption of the Soviet model in Czechoslovak psychiatry was not a one-sided process, however. The concepts of Pavlovian medicine merged with the traditions of Czech psychiatry, which reached back to the end of the nineteenth century, when it was first established as an independent field. Czech psychiatric knowledge had stressed that mental illness manifests not only in deviant behaviour patterns but also in physical, bodily symptoms. The influence of this tradition is evident in a prominent psychiatry textbook written by Zdeněk Mysliveček, who was the head of the Prague psychiatric clinic between 1929 and 1957. Mysliveček contended that mental illnesses were disorders of the whole 'somatopsychic' unit.[13] It was 'necessary to look at the human being', Mysliveček argued, 'as a somatopsychic unit in which it is impossible to distinguish between bodily and mental symptoms because both are the expression of the entire organism and biological processes'.[14] He stressed that mental illness cannot be localized in particular parts of the brain, but instead manifests itself in the functions of the body and the mind together.[15] This 'holistic concept' of mind and body was already present in the texts of Karel Kuffner, who founded modern Czech psychiatry at the turn of the twentieth century and who was a teacher of Zdeněk Mysliveček. Kuffner emphasized a similar approach to mental disorders, and in particular the need to understand the person in his or her totality.[16] Because of the prominent role of Charles University in the Czech lands as the centre of research and education, the knowledge and practices produced at the Prague psychiatric clinic by Kuffner and Mysliveček influenced the development of psychiatry in the whole of Czechoslovakia. Moreover, the 'Kuffner school' retains authority in Czech psychiatry to this day. References to the works of Mysliveček can be found in contemporary textbooks.[17]

During the 1950s, forensic psychiatrists in Czechoslovakia were mainly involved with the criminal justice system in an advisory capacity. Forensic psychiatry was not considered an independent field of research but rather part of clinical psychiatry. There was no specialized research institute dealing with forensic psychiatry nor was there a postgraduate educational programme in this field. The main task of psychiatrists was to provide expert answers to a court's questions about whether the offender was responsible for their actions and to determine whether the offender suffered from a mental disorder at the time of the crime. Defendants could be determined 'insane' and therefore not responsible for their conduct if they were unable to recognize the danger of their actions or could not control them. To serve as a defence for criminal liability, the loss of cognitive and volitional ability had to be the result of a mental disorder and had to have occurred at the time of the crime.[18]

It is important to point out that the Czechoslovak concept of criminal responsibility differed from that in the West. In the United Kingdom, for example, the offender's sanity was tested against the so-called M'Naghten rules, which emphasized the offender's inability to recognize the 'nature and quality of the act' and to distinguish right from wrong.[19] In Czechoslovakia, an 'insanity defence' could be based not only on the disorder of reasoning and judgement but also on a disruption of volitional control. This meant that offenders could be found not liable for their behaviour if, despite being conscious of their actions, they were unable to control themselves. By contrast, the inability to control one's own behaviour due to mental disorder was not relevant under the M'Naghten rules. Czechoslovak psychiatrists contended that their concept of criminal liability, inspired as it was by Soviet medicine, was more progressive and modern. The M'Naghten rules were deemed proof of the 'backwardness' of Western psychiatry.[20]

Not only psychiatrists but also psychologists began to develop new concepts of mind and body in the post-war period. In 1952, a group of Czechoslovak psychologists published two volumes about the development of the personality under socialism.[21] In the introduction, the psychologists rejected 'idealist theories' which had 'overestimated' the role of the individual in history and were typical of 'bourgeois' philosophers.[22] According to the understanding of dialectical materialism and the theory of reflection, the authors noted, human nature was the outcome of social relations and the reflection of objective reality. The authors were convinced that the creation of a new communist society would create a new type of socialist personality that would demonstrate qualities such as 'collectivist spirit', 'socialist patriotism', 'socialist discipline', 'socialist will' and 'socialist character'. The authors emphasized that the new socialist personality would also have different interests, needs and feelings. Unlike the 'feelings of a bourgeois man', who was interested only in himself, the socialist man would empathize with the collective and working people. The psychologists believed that under socialism, the 'antagonism' between feelings for the individual and feelings for the collective would disappear. Moreover, the interests and needs of people living under socialism would evolve. Whereas under capitalism, people were driven solely by the logic of money and profit, their personal interests under socialism would be motivated by a desire to educate their fellow citizens.[23] The psychologists expected that the new socialist man would take an active interest in public affairs, in contrast with the political passivity of people under capitalism.[24]

Despite ambitious reform plans and the new concepts presented by psychologists and psychiatrists in the early 1950s, psychiatry was not a top priority of the new communist regime. On paper, psychiatric care was part of a robust and all-embracing system of mental health institutions focused on treatment and prevention. However, the reality of the post-war economy and the priority placed on the development of heavy industry often thwarted those intentions. Almost a decade after the first plans for reforming mental health institutions were put forward, Czechoslovak ministry officials had to admit that not all of them had been implemented.[25]

Identifying 'deviant' criminal behaviour in the 1950s: Class struggle, religious beliefs and psychosis

In the 1950s, psychiatrists occupied an ambiguous position in the communist criminal justice system. They actively participated in a variety of educational activities, primarily of a political nature, which aimed to 'liberate' the masses from 'irrational' beliefs and superstitions propagated by religion. Psychiatrist Ivan Horvai, who published two books examining religious beliefs from a psychiatric point of view, is a good example of a politically conscious psychiatrist.[26] Challenging the 'idealistic' interpretation of the human soul in his works, Horvai contended that the soul was exclusively the product of the body's higher nervous activity and the second signalling system.[27] Horvai came to this conclusion by examining some of the fundamental tenets of religious belief, especially those of the Catholic Church. Religious belief, Horvai asserted, shared some characteristics with psychopathologies. After all, religious miracles were 'faked' incidents arranged by priests to support faith in God among ordinary people.[28] Horvai further claimed that hysterical persons often experienced miracles and speculated that some saints must have suffered from schizophrenia. Similarly, Horvai saw epilepsy and hysteria as the root cause of the 'fanatical' behaviour of 'dogmatic' believers.[29]

Yet despite psychiatrists' key role in anti-religious and educational discourses and the stress on psychiatry's importance in building the new socialist society, psychiatry's actual position within the communist criminal justice system was limited. The limits of psychiatric authority are evident in the criminal cases of religious prosecution in Liberec and Ústí nad Labem in the 1950s.[30] Of thirteen such cases, where individuals were charged with crimes because of their beliefs or affiliation with Jehovah's Witnesses, only one contained a psychiatric assessment. In the case in question, the accused, M.R., was prosecuted for the crime of supporting fascism, an offence with a maximum sentence of ten years.[31] In 1958, M.R. sent letters with 'religious content' to different state offices and people to warn the addressees about the end of the world. Classed as a 'fanatical believer' by the prosecutor, M.R., was a woman who lived with her brother following her husband's death in a concentration camp. After the war, M.R. and her brother moved to the countryside, where they began to study the Bible. Her behaviour was described as 'highly dangerous for society'. The police inspector testified that both M.R. and her brother had avoided gainful employment for several years. In her testimony, M.R. stressed that God had commissioned her and her brother to spread His word and that she was only following in Moses' footsteps. The first psychiatric assessment concluded that M.R. was suffering from a rare mental disorder, *folie à deux*, combined with delusions of religious persecution, and that M.R. was not responsible for her acts.[32] However, the state prosecutor was not satisfied with this assessment. He argued that the report was 'unclear', 'based on assumptions' and did not reflect 'prevailing opinion in forensic psychiatry that religious madness is considered psychopathy without regard for the criminal liability of the accused person'.[33] Consequently, M.R. was sent to a psychiatric hospital in Prague for more extensive observation. In that second assessment, Prague psychiatrists pointed out that M.R. had 'megalomaniac delusions and hallucinations' and suffered from 'manic moods'.[34] Her severe delusions and other symptoms led psychiatrists to conclude that M.R. was suffering from 'paraphrenia with paranoid religious delusions' and that therefore she was not responsible for her acts.[35] They recommended that she be treated in a psychiatric hospital. Based on the second assessment, the court ultimately acquitted her of all charges and ordered her to undertake psychiatric treatment.

M.R.'s case shows that psychiatrists were gradually gaining authority in criminal trials. The state prosecutor challenged the psychiatrists' original opinion and a second evaluation was ordered. The prosecution argued that the conclusions of the first assessment were invalid and that the proceedings should go forward. Only following the second assessment, which was conducted by psychiatrists from Prague, was the court persuaded to acquit. It is also notable that psychiatrists did not use Pavlovian language to describe M.R.'s mental health in their assessments. Nor did they look for the cause of the offender's unusual behaviour. Rather, they merely described M.R.'s current condition, pointing out her 'delusional' state. In their evaluation they briefly mentioned her physical condition and her family history and specified whether she had suffered any serious injuries.

In other prosecutions of religious people in regional courts (mainly against Jehovah's Witnesses), the court's decisions were based on the political relevance of the criminal act and no psychiatrists were invited to the hearings at all. For example, in a trial from 1959, two persons were convicted of 'subverting the republic' with their religious activities as Jehovah's Witnesses and were sentenced to one year in prison.[36] They were accused of 'being hostile to the people's democratic establishment' and 'carrying out subversive activities'. Specifically, the allegations included efforts to 'undermine citizens' confidence in the stability of the state' and 'establish an illegal organization of Jehovah's Witnesses'.[37] At trial, several people testified that the accused had claimed that it was God's will to destroy humanity and leave only Jehovah's Witnesses remaining.[38] In their testimony, the defendants stated that they met regularly to study the Bible and other texts, and had tried to convince people from the neighbourhood about their beliefs. They were accused of undermining women's right to work and discouraging people from military service.[39] These were significant allegations since compulsory military service and the integration of women into the workforce were essential goals of the newly established regime. The defendants denied all the accusations. In the final verdict, it was pointed out that the accused were unable to establish a large organization and that their teaching had not resonated with the people. Their working-class family backgrounds were considered, but nevertheless they both were sentenced to one year in prison.

Generally, the defendant's class background tended to overrule any purported medical condition, as was made clear at another trial from 1958. J.S. was accused of distributing anonymous letters and leaflets with 'hostile content', which 'terrorized the supporters of the people's democratic establishment' and 'undermined the republic'.[40] J.S.'s partner sent a letter to the court asking that he receive a psychiatric examination because he was showing 'signs of a mental disorder'. It is unclear whether that was a strategy to help J.S. and reduce his sentence or if he really did have a mental disorder. Nevertheless, the request was rejected and J.S. was sentenced to two years in prison. Because of his class background as a *kulak* and his past criminal record, the court found no mitigating circumstances and even increased the final sentence from that demanded by the prosecution.

The cases examined, albeit limited in number, suggest that the political aspects of criminal acts (e.g. establishing 'illegal' organizations such as Jehovah's Witnesses) were more decisive than psychiatrists' attempts to medicalize defendants' religious beliefs. Criminologists pointed out that Czechoslovakia was in a 'transition' period from a capitalist to a socialist system. This 'transition' period was associated by criminologists with increased crime resulting from the survival of 'capitalist' habits and class consciousness among ordinary people.[41] Even though psychiatrists were attempting to make the case for the greater use of their forensic expertise in determining the presence or absence of mental illness, the communist judicial system still favoured the class-based explanation of crime. The role of psychiatrists in communist criminal proceedings began to slowly change in the 1960s with the emergence of new issues such as recidivism, which challenged the Stalinist belief that crime was a 'transitional' phenomenon.

Identifying 'deviant' criminal behaviour in the 1960s: Psychopathy and recidivism as a new danger to socialist society

In 1965, the Third International Criminalistics Conference took place in Prague. Delegations from the socialist countries of the Eastern Bloc were among the prominent guests. In the opening speech, Josef Kudrna, Czechoslovakia's Interior Minister, stated that the main task of forensic experts was to 'analyse the conditions and roots of crime committed by those born in the new socialist society'.[42] He continued, 'From this point of view, we consider criminal recidivism to be a profoundly serious problem, one which is certainly of interest to all socialist countries.'[43] Kudrna's concerns were also shared by police, criminologists and forensic experts who pointed out the growing proportion of recidivism in the total number of crimes. Whereas in 1957, repeat offenders had committed approximately 17 per cent of all crimes, in 1960 it was 20 per cent.[44] In some regions, the number was even higher. For example, in the Ostrava region, recidivists were responsible for 34 per cent of all crimes committed.[45] Juvenile recidivism was particularly disturbing for the communist criminal justice system. In a document prepared for the Public Security headquarters, the rise in juvenile recidivism was perceived as 'undesirable' in light of the political and economic situation in the country.[46] In a 1960 survey, it was discovered that of 269 recidivists, 190 were twenty-four years of age or younger. The report's authors highlighted that juvenile recidivism did not stem from 'social issues' but from 'improper educational methods', 'broken families', 'affiliation to gangs' or the 'desire for western morality'.[47]

The urgent need to deal with recidivism was an opportunity for psychiatrists and other psy experts to present new explanatory models of criminal behaviour that were based on their specialized knowledge of the human mind and body. Psychiatrists claimed that it was necessary to study the role of psychopaths in modern societies in order to fully understand recidivism. Psychopathy, a previously under-researched topic, received increasing scholarly attention in the 1960s. A 1968 Czechoslovak textbook on psychiatry framed psychopathy as a disharmony of the personality which led to a 'change in the system of values'.[48] Perceived as rooted in an imbalance between the biological and the social aspects of the human mind, psychopathy was recognized as a diagnosis akin to neurosis, psychosis and organic illness.[49] Czechoslovak psychiatry distinguished different types of psychopaths: 'restless', 'aggressive', 'hyperthymic', 'paranoid', 'chronic complainers', 'hysterical', 'schizoid' and 'cyclothymic'.[50] Characterizing psychopaths as individuals suffering from an 'abnormality of the value system', 'insufficient ethical and moral principles', 'agitation', 'inflexible behaviour' and 'impulsiveness',[51] Czechoslovak psychiatrists came to believe that any of these pathological behavioural traits could lead to criminal behaviour under certain circumstances. Psychopathy was henceforth understood to be the most common cause of violent crime.[52]

During the 1960s, psychiatric evaluations of offenders showed a new concern with questions of personality and family background. For instance, the psychiatric assessment of an unemployed man accused of breaking into a canteen and stealing one thousand crowns in 1969 devoted attention to the defendant's family background, heredity, childhood and 'adult' (i.e. sexual) life. The psychiatrist stressed that the defendant had grown up in a 'deficient' family environment as an extramarital child. Since his childhood, the defendant had been reclusive and his intellect was described as below average. The psychiatrist framed these personal traits as the principal cause of his criminality. He concluded that the defendant had a 'psychopathic personality with signs of neurotic depression and decreased intellectual function bordering on simple-mindedness'.[53]

In another case involving an accused who had been charged with theft, pilferage of socialist property, unlawful possession of a firearm and forgery, the psychiatrist reported that the accused suffered from 'emotional apathy', a distinctive feature of an 'asocial' personality.[54] The psychiatrist also emphasized that the offender had tried to 'block out' his 'antisocial' character traits, which only led to an 'inner conflict' within his personality that caused him anxiety and other neurological issues. He concluded that the accused was a 'psychopath with antisocial behavioural traits and neurotic syndrome'.[55] The accused had a lengthy criminal record, had spent three years in prison and had appeared in court five times between 1959 and 1965. He also had already been treated in a psychiatric hospital in Pilsen and at the Bohnice mental hospital in Prague in 1968. According to the criminal file, in 1968 the accused had stolen money from the state betting company, stolen a car and broken into a gun shop where he took eight pistols, two air guns and ammunition. He had also unsuccessfully attempted to steal jewellery. In addition, the accused broke into an art shop using a duplicated key and stole two jacks from a car repair shop in the summer of 1968. In the same year, he also stole the personal documents of a foreign citizen and assumed a false identity.

In both cases, psychiatrists focused on the psychology and social background of the offenders in order to explain their antisocial behaviour. In the first case, the psychiatrist stressed the role of the defendant's 'deficient' family environment as the main cause of his criminal behaviour. In the second case, the accused's internal psychological conflict was the main factor identified as motivation for recidivism. Both offenders were found to be responsible for their acts and were given prison terms. This was the result of the long-standing view in Czech psychiatry that psychopaths should be held accountable for their actions. Only in severe cases of delusion and paranoia were psychopaths deemed to be 'insane' and therefore not responsible for their crimes. Zdeněk Mysliveček, in his textbook from the 1930s, recommended that psychopathy not be considered an extenuating circumstance to avoid an increase in crime. Similarly, Ferdinand Knobloch and Jiřina Knoblochová, in their forensic psychiatric textbook published in 1965, stressed that psychopathy was a 'condition' of the personality shaped by social relations and the environment. Psychopaths were thereby deemed responsible for their crimes in most cases.[56] This view was also adopted by the criminal justice system.

The new focus on the social and psychological explanations of crime was an outcome of the cooperation between psychiatrists, forensic experts and the police. Psychiatrists started to conduct surveys to study the relationship between recidivism and psychopathy. In 1961, in cooperation with doctors and psychologists, police conducted the first nationwide survey on recidivism and mental disorders. A sample of 769 recidivists were examined by psychiatrists and psychologists, who concluded that 88 per cent had a mental disorder or personality defect. Only 12 per cent were without any mental health issues.[57] The examined recidivists were largely found to suffer from psychopathy, intellectual defects or alcoholism, and, often, a combination of all three. The authors also stressed that the highest number of those who were mentally ill was among the youngest recidivists. In a three-year study conducted between 1967 and 1970 using a sample of 244 criminal psychopaths that were classified according to 30 different socio-economic characteristics, the authors outlined four common factors among criminal psychopaths: alcoholism, a broken family background, an unfavourable position in the family hierarchy and a stint in an orphanage.[58] In another study published in a criminological journal, the authors examined a variety of factors such as school attendance and upbringing in order to explain the rise of recidivism in socialist Czechoslovakia. They found that the so-called 'cultural transfer' of bad family habits and behavioural traits played a vital role in causing recidivism.[59] With these studies, the picture of the 'criminal psychopath' was coming into clearer focus in Czechoslovakia. Perceived as the leading cause of violent crime, psychopathy gradually became a common diagnosis in psychiatric assessments in criminal trials because it covered such a wide variety of 'abnormal' behaviours.[60]

This shift reflected a broader transformation in the criminal justice system during de-Stalinization. Whereas in the 1950s, criminologists and criminalists emphasized the 'bourgeois' class background of the perpetrators, in the 1960s, the criminal justice system focused on fighting against various 'antisocial parasitic elements', 'violent criminals' and 'individuals violating the socialist order'.[61] This change in the state's criminal policy went hand in hand with the increasing role of psychiatrists and other experts in the criminal justice system, a shift reflecting the 'scientification' of socialist society.[62]

Conclusion

The communist takeover of Czechoslovakia in 1948 gave rise to a new form of conceptualizing the human mind and body, characterized by an emphasis on the theory of 'higher nervous activity' in the psy sciences and the ideal of the socialist personality introduced by Soviet psychologists. However, the newly introduced concepts of Pavlovian medicine did not completely dominate the thinking of Czechoslovak experts. Rather, Pavlovian concepts were integrated into the longer tradition of psychiatry in the Czech lands, which approached mental health as a holistic problem involving both mental and bodily processes. This tradition proved to be quite compatible with Pavlov's emphasis on the unity of the organism and the environment. From the state's perspective, the role of psychiatrists was not only to treat mental illnesses but also to actively engage in educating the masses. This can be illustrated by the participation of psychiatrists in the anti-religion campaigns of the 1950s. Psychiatrists were called upon to help 'liberate' the masses from superstition and 'unscientific' beliefs about the human mind and body. Yet their influence over courts' decisions in anti-religion trials was limited. Political factors, such as the class origin of the defendant, the level of danger posed by the crime to the state and the threat the crime posed to the people's democratic regime, carried more weight in the courts' decision-making.

The role of psychiatry in state criminal policy began to change with the advent of de-Stalinization and especially with the rise of juvenile recidivism. Juvenile recidivism became a major topic of discussion for forensic experts in the 1960s. The Stalinist theory of crime, which assured citizens that there would be no crime in the new utopian society after the 'transition' from capitalism to socialism, failed to explain the rise in juvenile recidivism. Accordingly, psychiatrists and other experts searched for a new theory of crime that would not undermine the legitimacy of communist ideology. Seizing the opportunity to actively shape the state's anti-crime policies, psychiatrists developed psychopathy into a broad, loosely defined diagnosis that could be applied to various behaviour patterns and could take the blame for the increase of criminal recidivism in Czechoslovakia's socialist society.

Notes

1   Lutz Raphael, 'Die Verwissenschaftlichung des Sozialen als methodische und konzeptionelle Herausforderung für eine Sozialgeschichte des 20. Jahrhunderts', *Geschichte und Gesellschaft*, 22 (1996): 165–93; Greg Eghigian, Andreas Killen and Christine Luenberger, eds., 'The Self as Project: Politics and the Human Sciences in the Twentieth Century', *Osiris*, 22 (2007): 1–25; Kerstin Brückweh, Dirk

Schumann, Richard F. Wetzell and Benjamin Ziemann, eds., *Engineering Society. The Role of the Human and Social Sciences in Modern Societies, 1880–1980* (London: Palgrave Macmillan, 2012); Frank Huisman and Harry Oosterhuis, eds., *Health and Citizenship: Political Cultures of Health in Modern Europe* (London and New York: Routledge, 2014); Janet Weston, *Medicine, the Penal System and Sexual Crimes in England, 1919 to 1960s: Diagnosing Deviance* (London: Bloomsbury Academic Publishing, 2017); Michal Kopeček, ed., *Architekti dlouhé změny. Expertní kořeny postsocialismu 1980–1995* (Prague: Argo, Ústav pro soudobé dějiny AV ČR, FF UK, 2019); Vítězslav Sommer et al., *Řídit socialismus jako stát. Technokratické vládnutí v Československu 1956–1989* (Prague: Ústav pro soudobé dějiny AV ČR, 2019); Łukasz Stanek, *Architecture in Global Socialism: Eastern Europe, West Africa, and the Middle East in the Cold War* (Princeton, NJ: Princeton University Press, 2020).

2 Michel Foucault, Luther H. Martin and Huck Gutman, eds., *Technologies of Self: A Seminar with Michel Foucault* (Amherst, MA: The University of Massachusetts Press, 1988); Nikolas Rose, 'Engineering the Human Soul: Analyzing Psychological Expertise', *Science in Context* 5 (1992): 351–99; Nikolas Rose, *Governing the Soul: The Shaping of the Private Self*, 2nd edn (London: Free Association Books, 1999).

3 Sarah Marks and Mat Savelli, eds., *Psychiatry in Communist Europe* (London: Palgrave Macmillan, 2016); Sarah Marks, 'Suggestion, Persuasion and Work: Psychotherapies in Communist Europe', *European Journal of Psychotherapy & Counselling* 20.1 (2018): 10–24; Mat Savelli, 'Peace and Happiness Await Us: Psychotherapy in Yugoslavia, 1945–85', *History of the Human Sciences* 31.4 (2018): 38–57; Ana Antic, 'Raising a True Socialist Individual: Yugoslav Psychoanalysis and the Creation of Democratic Marxist Citizens', *Social History* 44.1 (2019): 86–115; Adéla Gjuričová, 'Proměna socialistického člověka v liberální individuum? Psychoterapie v Československu po roce 1968', in *Architekti dlouhé změny. Expertní kořeny postsocialismu v Československu*, ed. Michal Kopeček (Prague: Argo – Ústav pro soudobé dějiny AV ČR – Univerzita Karlova, Filozofická fakulta, 2019): 185–221; Frank Henschel, 'Embodiment of Deviance: The Biopolitics of the "Difficult Child" in Socialist Czechoslovakia', *East European Politics and Societies* 34.4 (2020): 837–57; Kate Davison, 'Cold War Pavlov: Homosexual Aversion Therapy in the 1960s', *History of the Human Sciences* 34.1 (2021): 89–119.

4 On the abuse of psychiatry, see Stephen Faraone, 'Psychiatry and Political Repression in the Soviet Union', *American Psychologist* 37.10 (1982): 1105–12; Sidney Bloch and Peter Reddaway, *Soviet Psychiatric Abuse: The Shadow over World Psychiatry* (London and New York: Routledge, 1985); Theresa C. Smith and Thomas Oleszczuk, *No Asylum: State Psychiatric Repression in the Former USSR* (New York, NY: NYU Press, 1996); Sonja Süß, *Politisch mißbraucht? Psychiatrie und Staatssicherheit in der DDR* (Berlin: Ch. Links Verlag, 2000). Recent works on the psy sciences and the management of crime under socialism include Greg Eghigian's study of the forensic sciences and crime in East Germany between 1945 and 1975. Eghigian points out that psy experts influenced the state's crime policies by introducing the concept of 'socialist personality' into the penal system. See Greg Eghigian, 'The Psychologization of the Socialist Self: East German Forensic Psychology and Its Deviants, 1945–1975', *German History* 22 (2004): 181–204. See also Dan Healey, *Bolshevik Sexual Forensics: Diagnosing Disorder in the Clinic and Courtroom, 1917–1939* (DeKalb, IL: Northern Illinois University Press, 2009); Riccardo Nicolosi and Anne Hartmann, eds., *Born to be Criminal: The Discourse on Criminality and the Practice of Punishment in Late Imperial Russia and Early Soviet Union. Interdisciplinary Approaches*

(Bielefeld: Transcript, 2017); Sharon Kowalsky, *Deviant Women: Female Crime and Criminology in Revolutionary Russia, 1880–1930* (DeKalb, IL: Northern Illinois University Press, 2009); Siobhan Hearne, 'Sanitising Sex in the USSR: State Approaches to Sexual Health in the Brezhnev Era', *Europe-Asia Studies*, 74.1 (2022): 1793–1815; Christiane Brenner, 'Sex and Scientific-Observation: Research on Prostitution in Socialist Czechoslovakia', *Mitteilungen des Sonderforschungsbereichs 1369 'Vigilanzkulturen'*, no. 1 (2021): 11–17.

5 Jakub Rákosník and Igor Tomeš, *Sociální stát v Československu. Právně-institucionální vývoj v letech 1918–1992* (Prague: Auditorium, 2012), 304.

6 For instance, one of the most famous psychiatric hospitals in Prague was established in 1909 in the suburb of Bohnice; other big psychiatric hospitals were founded in Kosmonosy (1869), Dobřany (1881), Kroměříž (1909) and Horni Beřkovice (1891).

7 Ivan P. Pavlov received the Nobel Prize (1904) for research on classical conditioning and higher nervous activity. Pavlovian medicine became the basic scientific framework in the Soviet Union and was propagated at regularly organized conferences. See Benjamin Zajicek, 'Scientific Psychiatry in Stalin's Soviet Union: The Politics of Modern Medicine and the Struggle to Define Pavlovian Psychiatry, 1939–1953' PhD diss., (The University of Chicago, Chicago, IL 2009); Dušan Bílý, 'Plnění dokumentu strany a vlády', *Neurologie a psychiatrie československá* 17.4 (1954): 223–6.

8 Ibid., 1.

9 Josef Hádlík, *Speciální psychiatrie* (Prague: SPN, 1955), 10–11.

10 Josef Hádlík, *Repetitorium psychiatrie* (Prague: SPN, 1953), 3.

11 Ferdinand Knobloch and Jiřina Knoblochová, *Soudní psychiatrie pro právníky a lékaře* (Prague: Orbis, 1957), 93. See also Greg Eghigian, *The Corrigible and the Incorrigible: Science, Medicine, and the Convict in Twentieth-Century Germany* (Ann Arbor, MI: University of Michigan Press, 2015).

12 Miloš Sovák, 'Pojetí defektologie podle učení I.P. Pavlova', *Pedagogika* 4 (1953): 242. Cf. Frank Henschel, 'Defectology, the State, and Eugenic Biopolitics in Czechoslovakia 1938–1989', in Victoria Schmidt, ed., *The Politics of Disability in Interwar and Socialist Czechoslovakia: Segregating in the Name of the Nation* (Amsterdam: Amsterdam University Press, 2019), 109–44.

13 Zdeněk Mysliveček, *Repetitorium všeobecné psychiatrie a speciální psychiatrie* (Prague: SPN, 1952), 5.

14 Zdeněk Mysliveček, *Obecná psychiatrie*, 2nd edn (Prague: SZdN, 1959), 12.

15 Ibid., 17.

16 Ota Konrád, Rudolf Kučera, *Cesty z apokalypsy. Fyzické násilí v pádu a obnově střední Evropy 1914–1922* (Prague: Masarykův ústav a Archiv AV ČR, 2018), 81. Cf. Karel Kuffner, *Psychiatrie: pro studium i praktickou potřebu lékaře, Díl 1. Část povšechná* (Prague: Bursík & Kohout, 1897).

17 E.g. Pavel Pavlovský, *Soudní psychiatrie a psychologie* (Prague: Grada, 2009).

18 Knobloch and Knoblochová, *Soudní psychiatrie*, 15.

19 'To establish a defence on the ground of insanity it must be clearly proved that, at the time of committing the act, the party accused was labouring under such a defect of reason from disease of the mind, as not to know the nature and quality of the act he was doing, or if he did know it, that he did not know that what he was doing was wrong.' See Rebecca Jackson, *Learning Forensic Assessment: Research and Practice* (London and New York: Routledge, 2007), 110; Keith Rix, 'Towards a More Just Insanity Defence: Recovering Moral Wrongfulness in the M'Naghten Rules', *BJPsych Advances* 22.1 (2016): 45.

20 Knobloch and Knochlochová, *Soudní psychiatrie*, 17–18.
21 Josef Linhart et al., *Vývoj osobnosti a její rozvoj v socialismu. Díl I.* (Prague: SPN, 1952).
22 Ibid., 12.
23 Josef Linhart et al., *Vývoj osobnosti a její rozvoj v socialismu. Díl II.* (Prague: SPN, 1952), 354. For further reading on this topic, see Emma Widdis, 'Socialist Senses: Film and the Creation of Soviet Subjectivity', *Slavic Review*, 71 (2012): 590–618; Anna Toropova, *Feeling Revolution: Cinema, Genre and the Politics of Affect under Stalin* (Oxford: Oxford University Press, 2020).
24 Ibid., 355.
25 'Zpráva o psychiatrickém stavu v ČSSR a jejím rozvoji', in Ministerstvo zdravotnictví (1945–1968), Materiály pro schůzi vlády, file 5, no. LP/3-270-27.2.1962, The Czech National Archives (Prague).
26 Ivan Horvai, *Záhady duševního života* (Prague: Naše vojsko, 1957); Ivan Horvai, *Zázraky očima psychiatrie* (Prague: SNPL, 1959).
27 Horvai, *Záhady duševního života*, 40.
28 Ibid., 25. In this context, it is necessary to mention the so-called 'Číhošť miracle', an alleged miracle that happened in 1949 in the church in the village Číhošť. This event became the pretext for anti-religion repression in Czechoslovakia. Communist propaganda claimed that the miracle was a hoax arranged by the Catholic Church.
29 Horvai, *Zázraky očima psychiatrie*, 126.
30 To protect sensitive personal data of the actors, I do not provide all personal details of the accused persons.
31 Criminal Code 1950, §83/1,2.
32 'Lékařský nález a posudek, Mudr. Bohuslav Vitík', The State Regional Archive Litoměřice, Krajský soud Liberec, T 3/59.
33 'Krajská prokuratura v Liberci, dopis ze dne 18. června 1959', The State Regional Archive Litoměřice, Krajský soud Liberec, T 3/59, 1 kv 22/59-31.
34 'Posudek, 7. září 1959., J. Semotán, K. Hofmeister', The State Regional Archive Litoměřice, Krajský soud Liberec, T 3/59.
35 'Rozsudek, 29. září 1959', The State Regional Archive Litoměřice, Krajský soud Liberec, T 3/59.
36 Criminal Code 1950, §81.
37 'Rozsudek, 23. února 1959', in The State Regional Archive Litoměřice, Krajský soud Ústí nad Labem, T 1/59.
38 'Svědecká výpověď Miroslava Hakla', in The State Regional Archive Litoměřice, Krajský soud Ústí nad Labem, T 1/59, 8.
39 'Výpověď obžalované', in The State Regional Archive Litoměřice, Krajský soud Ústí nad Labem, T 1/59, 3.
40 'Rozsudek, 3. října 1958', in The State Regional Archive Litoměřice, Krajský soud Liberec, T 58/60.
41 *Základy kriminalistiky*, 21. See also Volker Zimmermann, 'Kriminalität und Kriminologie im Staatssozialismus', in Michal Pullmann and Volker Zimmermann, eds., *Ordnung und Sicherheit, Devianz und Kriminalität im Staatssozialismus Tschechoslowakei und DDR 1948/49–1989* (Munich: Vandenhoeck & Ruprecht, 2011): 57–81; David Shearer, 'Recidivism, Social Atavism, and State Security in Early Soviet Policing', in Nicolosi and Hartmann, eds., *Born to Be Criminal*, 119–48.
42 'III. Mezinárodní Kriminalistické Symposium', *Kriminalistický sborník* 9.14 (1965): 707.

43 Ibid.
44 'Zpráva o situaci na úseku kriminální recidivy', in Materiály z kriminalistické konference o recidivitě a recidivistech, konané ve dnech 29.-31.3.1961, Archivní fondy ministerstva vnitra České socialistické republiky, Hlavní správa VB, H 1-4 i.j. 493, The Security Service Archives (Prague), 2.
45 Ibid., 12.
46 Ibid., 2.
47 Ibid.
48 Ivan Horvai, *Psychopatie* (Prague: SZN, 1968), 234.
49 Ibid., 38, 68.
50 Ferdinand Knobloch and Jiřina Knoblochová, *Základy soudní psychiatrie pro právníky* (Prague: SPN, 1969), 28–37.
51 Horvai, *Psychopatie*, 217.
52 Vladimír Študent, *Soudní psychiatrie a trestní právo* (Prague: SPN, 1989), 56.
53 Knobloch and Knoblochová, *Základní soudní psychiatrie pro právníky*, 36.
54 Miroslav Dufek, *Soudně psychiatrická expertýza. Sbírka výtahů soudně psychiatrických expertýz* (Prague: SPN, 1978), 60.
55 Ibid., 62.
56 Knobloch and Knoblochová, *Základní soudní psychiatrie pro právníky*, 29.
57 Miroslav Dufek, *Soudní psychiatrie pro právníky a lékaře* (Prague: Orbis, 1978b), 226.
58 Ibid., 69.
59 Jiří Podleský, 'První poznatky z výzkumu kriminální recidivy', *Kriminalistický sborník* 9, no. 14 (1965): 333.
60 Študent, *Soudní psychiatrie a trestní právo*, 56.
61 *Československé trestní právo. 1. Obecná část* (Prague: Orbis, 1969), 6.
62 Raphael, 'Die Verwissenschaftlichung des Sozialen', 165–93; Susan Reid, 'The Khrushchev Kitchen: Domesticating the Scientific-Technological Revolution', *Journal of Contemporary History* 40.2 (2005): 289–316.

3

Broadcasting communist morality: Sex education in Soviet Latvia

Siobhán Hearne

Readers of the Soviet Latvian daily tabloid *Rīgas Balss* (*The Voice of Riga*) opened their newspapers on 6 October 1973 to find graphic descriptions of the rashes, lesions and secretions that they could expect to find if they were ever to become infected with syphilis. An article published that day, entitled 'I trusted him ...' and penned by Doctor V. Zhukov (chairman of the Latvian Republic's Scientific Society of Dermato-Venereologists), told the harrowing story of a young woman who caught syphilis after having sex with a man who promised to marry her.[1] After recounting the woman's story, Zhukov insisted that venereal diseases (VD) were exclusively spread by people who violated the 'norms of socialist morality' by drinking alcohol to excess and engaging in casual sex. In order to prevent the spread of VD, it was apparently necessary to use education, persuasion and coercion to fight against 'parasites, drunks, and people leading antisocial, immoral lifestyles'. Newspaper articles like this were not uncommon in the Latvian Soviet Socialist Republic (SSR) in the 1970s. Throughout the Brezhnev era, Soviet leadership looked to mass media to articulate ideas about sex that would directly serve the broader pronatalist goals of the state. Mass media was a technology with significant transformative potential. Radio, television and print media reached audiences of millions upon millions, and media consumption cut across generational, social, ethnic and gender lines. For Soviet leadership, technologies of mass media offered fruitful opportunities to mould sexual behaviour to fit the ideals of the state.

In sex education materials, adherence to specific standards of sexual morality was presented as an individual, societal and national responsibility of all Soviet citizens. Those who failed to heed the advice of medical professionals not only faced the painful, and sometimes life-altering, physical consequences of VD, but they also endangered the collective and future generations by jeopardizing their reproductive capacities. Taking the case study of the Latvian SSR, this chapter explores how state policies related to the dissemination of sexual knowledge played out at a republican level to examine the entanglement between sexual health and politics in the former Soviet Union.

Mass media had been an important technology of sexual enlightenment long before the Brezhnev era. In the 1920s, the Department of Sanitary Enlightenment produced and disseminated a large variety of sex education materials in an attempt to reach broad segments of the population, including films, posters, newspaper articles, travelling exhibitions, journals and brochures.[2] Early Soviet sexual enlightenment propaganda implored individuals to eradicate bad habits and overcome personal weaknesses in order to ensure good sexual health. Sex was categorized as a public health matter, as a healthy populace was deemed necessary for the construction of socialism. Soviet citizens were instructed to refrain from engaging in 'unhealthy' practices that were presumed to spread VD, such as sharing spoons, beds and cigarettes, as well as paying for sex and having sex outside marriage.[3] Medical visions of 'normal' sexuality tethered sex to reproduction and regarded sexual energy as something that needed to be disciplined and redirected into political and social work.[4] In early Soviet *kulturfilms,* endemic syphilis among indigenous populations was used as evidence of their 'backwardness' and need for state intervention to eradicate 'unhealthy' cultural practices.[5]

The death of Stalin in 1953 brought important shifts in the messages of sexual enlightenment as the Soviet regime shifted towards more subtle, but more pervasive, methods for disciplining and regulating the private lives of their citizens. Under the leadership of Nikita Khrushchev, social control pivoted towards the more mundane and ordinary aspects of everyday life.[6] Moral regeneration was also embedded within official policy, as enforcing 'communist morality' became a priority of the Party, state and various volunteer organizations.[7] Sex also became subject to communist morality in this period. The preservation of families became an objective of the Party discipline system, and individuals who engaged in queer sex, paid sex and sex that resulted in VD transmission were increasingly targeted by the authorities.[8] Beginning in the late 1950s, popular health magazines published educational articles to improve married women's knowledge of female methods of contraception and instructed men to 'protect' their wives from unwanted pregnancies by using condoms, refraining from using the withdrawal method, and even practising marital abstinence.[9] Under the conditions of Khrushchev's Thaw, the Soviet Medical Publishing House brought out a number of sex education manuals in the early 1960s that condemned sexual acts that allegedly endangered the collective by reducing labour reserves, encouraging irresponsibility, fracturing family relationships and impeding procreation, such as masturbation, homosexual sex and sex outside marriage.[10]

The shifting media landscape of the Brezhnev era made sexual enlightenment propaganda more pervasive as it became accessible to broader swathes of the population in various media forms. The number of newspaper articles on sexual health and morality penned by medical experts significantly increased throughout the 1960s and 1970s. From the mid-1970s, Party officials instructed venereologists to prepare radio and television broadcasts on VD treatment and prevention. By this point, the infrastructure for Soviet mass media had undergone explosive growth, which meant that radio and television were now staples of Soviet life. The number of radio sets in the USSR jumped from 3 million to 20 million over the course of the 1950s, and continued to grow to 70 million by the early 1960s and 95 million by 1970.[11] Television, once a novelty in the 1950s, became Soviet citizens' principal source of entertainment, propaganda and culture by the 1970s following enormous government investment in TV infrastructure and the mass production of television sets.[12] The number of televisions per Soviet family doubled between 1965 and 1970 from roughly one set per four families to one set per two families.[13] Media consumption in general was on the rise throughout the 1960s and 1970s, as Soviet citizens took more trips to the cinema, read more newspapers and magazines, watched more hours of television, and tuned in to more radio broadcasts than ever before.[14] Radio, television and print media were extremely popular, had established roles in the home and reached audiences across class, gender, ethnic, and generational lines, which made them key technologies for communicating ideas about health to the broader Soviet population. During the media boom of 1960s and 1970s, broadcasting sexual enlightenment brought state-approved ideas about sex, morality and sexual health into the homes of Soviet citizens with increasing frequency.

The development of Soviet sex education in Latvia

The Latvian SSR occupied a unique place on the USSR's cultural landscape. Latvia was a relatively young Soviet republic, as it was invaded and occupied by the Red Army (along with Estonia and Lithuania) in 1940 and forcibly incorporated into the USSR during the Second World War. Before Soviet invasion and annexation, public debates on sex education raged in interwar Latvia, driven by rising concern about low birth rates, high incidence of divorce and the destabilized sex ratio following the wholesale destruction of the First World War.[15] The 1920s were marked by simultaneous efforts to increase and restrict access to sexual knowledge to the Latvian population. On the one hand, medical professionals delivered public lectures on sexual hygiene for adults and limited sex education was included in the secondary school curriculum, but on the other, the sale of literature discussing issues related to sex (such as abortion, birth control and VD) was restricted to over 18s and these texts could not be publicly advertised in book shops.[16] The establishment of the authoritarian regime of Kārlis Ulmanis following his May 1934 coup ushered in a new era of pronatalism, with a blanket ban on abortion for social reasons and the circulation of information about contraceptives, alongside the introduction of a national eugenics programme, including eugenic abortions and sterilizations.[17]

Following Soviet invasion and annexation, the Latvian republic (along with the other Baltic republics of Estonia and Lithuania) formed part of the USSR's western periphery. This region had stronger links with the capitalist West than elsewhere in the Soviet Union, and therefore, had the reputation as a centre of illicit, criminal and anti-Soviet activity.[18] This reputation perhaps motivated Soviet leadership in Latvia to implement particularly stringent measures to address perceived sexual misconduct. The maximum prison sentence for sodomy was higher in the Latvian SSR than in the other Baltic republics.[19] The Riga police authorities also proposed the criminalization of female same-sex relations in the 1960s (although this idea was rejected by Moscow) and the city was home to the first ever Soviet vice squad, established in 1987.[20] Therefore, the dissemination of sexual knowledge in Soviet Latvia could have been influenced by state approaches to sexuality in the interwar period and concerns regarding the republic's reputation following Soviet annexation.

In the early 1960s, Soviet officialdom in Moscow turned their attention to mass sex education. Sociological and demographic studies on marriage and the family began to appear following the revival of both disciplines in the 1950s, and their results revealed high rates of divorce and falling birth rates in the western portion of the

USSR. Rising divorce and demographic decline deeply concerned policymakers and prompted calls for drastic state intervention to solve the problems of Soviet family life.[21] These trends were particularly pronounced in Latvia, where divorce rates were higher than the all-Union average and the fertility rate was amongst the lowest of all the union republics.[22] In Latvia, calls to solve issues related to marriage and the family were published in mass media. In early August 1964, the Soviet Latvian Russian-language daily newspaper *Sovetskaia molodezh'* (*Soviet Youth*) published long excerpts of the first Soviet public opinion survey conducted on love, marriage and sex under the direction of sociologist Boris Grushin.[23] Survey respondents lamented the lack of sex education and the detrimental impact that this had upon family life. The publication of Grushin's survey in Latvia generated a significant public response. The editors at *Sovetskaia molodezh'* received countless letters from concerned citizens, teachers, parents and venereologists calling for the introduction of youth sex education in the Latvian republic, some of which were published in full.[24] The editors even invited the Latvian SSR's Ministry of Education and Ministry of Culture to respond, after which both ministries issued statements agreeing that widespread sex education was urgently required for young people and promising that work to implement this would begin imminently.[25]

At the same time, an upsurge in rates of VD across the USSR also generated enormous official concern. In February 1963, the USSR's Ministry of Health issued an order chastising regional and republican health authorities for the sharp increase in VD cases. The Ministry claimed that the lukewarm commitment of republican ministries of health was to blame for rising rates of infection, as health authorities in republics, regions and cities were not adequately carrying out contact tracing, failing to conduct mandatory VD serological screenings of all hospital patients, or working with the police to ensure the prosecution of so-called 'malicious' transmitters of venereal infection.[26] Another crucially important factor seen to cause the increase in infection rates was the lack of 'sanitary propaganda', which had allegedly resulted in the widespread perception that venereal infections were not serious illnesses that required treatment in specialized clinics, and instead, diseases that could be treated outside the state healthcare system. The Soviet government enlisted medical workers to educate wider society through one-on-one patient consultations, the production and distribution of educational materials, or by organizing public lectures or film screenings at treatment clinics, universities, and workplaces.[27] These activities were collectively referred to in official discourse as 'sanitary-education work' and outlined as an important component of the labour obligations of medical personnel. The USSR's Ministry for Health monitored the amount of sanitary enlightenment work carried out across the Soviet Union, as republican ministries of health were required to send information about the number of public lectures, themed evenings, exhibitions, articles in the press and film screenings back to Moscow.[28]

Despite the Ministry of Health's warning, rates of venereal infection continued to climb across the USSR throughout the late 1960s and early 1970s.[29] The situation was particularly concerning in the Latvian SSR, where VD had increased sharply: between 1967 and 1973, incidence of gonorrhoea doubled and syphilis increased thirty-six times over.[30] By 1973, incidence of syphilis was almost four times higher in the

Latvian republic than the all-Union average, and Latvia had the second highest rate of gonorrhoea in the entire USSR.[31] To explain these extremely high rates, Latvian political leadership gestured to Latvia's reputation as a tourist destination and magnet for transient labour migration, as well as the 'moral promiscuity of individual citizens and prostitution'.[32] To prevent further reputational damage, Soviet Latvian leadership pursued an aggressive anti-VD campaign throughout the late 1960s and 1970s, which resulted in the establishment of institutions for forced VD treatment and 're-education' of individuals who refused medical intervention, increased police harassment of sex workers and gay men, and a significant upsurge in the number of individuals prosecuted for deliberately infecting another person with a venereal infection.[33] In 1973, the Latvian Republican Skin and VD Dispensary (*Republikāniskais ādas un venerisko slimību dispansers,* Republican VD Dispensary hereafter) was reopened in Riga after being closed down seventeen years earlier in 1956 when venereal diseases had been on the decline.[34]

Another core part of the anti-VD campaign in the Latvian republic was a renewed push for disseminating information on sexual health and sexual morality to adults and teenagers. In 1973, both the Latvian republic's Ministry of Health and Ministry of Internal Affairs wrote to the Central Committee of the Latvian Communist Party asking for assistance in developing anti-VD propaganda for newspapers, magazines, radio, and television.[35] At their meeting in May 1973, the Central Committee broadly agreed that mass media should be used as a medium for disseminating sex education to the population.[36] Soon after, doctors at the Republican VD Dispensary began to put together sex education materials in both Latvian and Russian, the latter in order to cater to the Latvian republic's predominantly monolingual Russophone population.[37] As these materials were drafted by medical professionals in response to rising rates of venereal infection, they focused almost exclusively on sexual health, rather than exploring other aspects of sex and sexuality.

Throughout the 1970s and 1980s, doctors at the Republican VD Dispensary prepared public lectures to be delivered at houses of sanitary enlightenment (*doma sanitarnogo prosveshchenie*), penned brochures and pamphlets, and wrote articles for publication in mass-circulation newspapers such as the Russian-language *Sovetskaia Latviia,* and Latvian-language *Rīgas Balss* and *Cīņa.*[38] In 1974, the Latvian minister for health developed a plan for the monthly screening of sex education films on television.[39] Before this point, films dealing with themes of sexual health and morality had primarily been screened at educational institutions, such as the Latvian Republican House of Knowledge (*dom znanii*).[40] Latvia's State Television and Radio Broadcasting Committee was initially reluctant to show anti-VD films on television because they were deemed to be unsuitable for women and children, but their reservations were quickly dismissed, and films began to be broadcast on television from the mid-1970s onwards.[41] The Russian-language popular science film *Bitter Chronicle* (*Gor'kaia khronika*) warned of the dangers of alcoholism and VD and was screened multiple times on TV RIGA throughout the late 1970s.[42] In addition to this, medical professionals also drafted scripts for radio on topics such as VD prevention and casual sex. Between 1975 and 1982, 170 of these lectures were broadcast on radios across the Latvian SSR.[43] Broadcasting sex education lectures on radio and television meant that state-approved ideas about sexual health and morality were beamed into the homes of residents of Soviet Latvia with increasing frequency. By 1963, around 77 per cent of the republic's population had access to at least one television channel, and this percentage likely climbed throughout the next decade as TV ownership exploded across the USSR.[44] Hundreds of thousands of residents of the Latvian SSR also had access to radio receivers and wired radios.[45]

While it is evident that there was a concerted effort to increase the availability of information about sexual health throughout the 1970s, this did not necessarily amount to greater access to sex education across the entire Latvian republic. Accessing information was largely dependent on whether an individual had access to a television, radio, or specific newspaper or magazine. There were some attempts to provide in-person sex education for adults and young people, but this was unequally distributed across the Latvian SSR. From the early 1970s, secondary schools in Riga reportedly all offered some form of 'moral education' for their pupils, but the topics covered varied widely from school to school and the classes were often optional.[46] Riga's middle school no. 66 embedded sex education within the curriculum for pupils from the first to tenth class, but this does not appear to have been widespread across the republic.[47] Latvia's Ministry of Education organized sex education film screenings at certain cinemas, but all of these were located in Riga.[48] Between 1975 and 1982, there were on average 136 public lectures per year on youth sex education across the Latvian SSR, but these tended to be held in cities (particularly Riga, Liepāja and Daugavpils), and some regions went years without a single lecture.[49]

Themes in Latvian sex education

Waging war on casual sex

In the Latvian SSR, sex education materials outlined specific sexual behaviours that were perceived to violate communist morality, while also emphasizing that Soviet citizens had a personal and societal responsibility to prevent themselves and others from contracting venereal infections. By including warnings about specific sexual behaviours that were deemed to be risky, medical professionals stepped outside their immediate area of expertise (venereology) and meshed discourses of health with discourses of morality. In newspaper articles, radio broadcasts, brochures and posters, venereologists aggressively pushed the idea that the only true way to avoid catching VD was to exercise sexual restraint and adhere to specific standards of sexual morality.

Casual sex in particular was demonized as a reckless activity infused with potent danger that almost always ended in VD. A Russian-language article prepared for publication in the journal *Veselība* (*Health*) by staff at the Republican VD Dispensary included case studies of VD patients (either real or fictitious, there is no way of knowing) whose engagement in casual sex ruined their entire life. There was Leonid V., a promising athlete on his way to becoming a record holder who cut his career short by engaging in casual sex with one of his 'admirers', catching gonorrhoea and leaving it untreated for several months.[50] Another man, Aleksandr T., became infertile and deprived his family of the 'happiness of having a child' following a drunken fumble with an unknown woman on a Riga park bench.[51] Darisa T. 'succumbed to a fleeting desire' with an acquaintance while her husband was out of town, which resulted in gonorrhoea, syphilis, infertility and divorce.[52] The article ended with the following take-home message: 'three stories, three human tragedies, and all one cause – CASUAL SEX'. By using relatable characters, these stories emphasized the danger posed to even 'respectable' Soviet citizens by failing to exercise restraint and deviating from the tenets of communist morality.

In line with sex education in other state socialist contexts, Soviet sex education materials presented succumbing to casual sex as a selfish and individualistic act that directly endangered the collective.[53] In a Latvian-language radio broadcast from November 1974 entitled 'It could have been otherwise, if only …', casual sex was discussed alongside other activities that apparently epitomized the 'uncontrolled, primitive satisfaction of base instincts', such as alcoholism, obesity and so-called 'nicotine mania' (*nikotīnmānijas*).[54] Articles addressed to young people described individuals with venereal infections as a 'burden to society, to their families, and to themselves', emphasizing the individual, collective and societal consequences of contracting VD.[55]

Venereologists added an air of scientific objectivity to explicit discussions of sexual morality. In a Russian-language newspaper article published in *Sovetskaia molodezh'*, Dr Zhukov (chairman of the Latvian SSR's Scientific Society of Dermato-Venereologists) pondered the differences between the concept of 'love at first sight' and deep, meaningful romantic connections. The first was dismissed as something 'primitive' that exclusively concerned sexual attraction and that was usually experienced 'in a drunken state'.[56] According to Dr Zhukov, drinking alcohol and succumbing to such sexual instincts carried the risk of impotence (*polovoi slabosti*) for young men. Rather than following through on feelings of 'love at first sight', Dr Zhukov recommended the 'harmless' and 'feasible' practice of sexual abstinence before marriage. Sexual energies could easily be suppressed by focusing on work, studies, physical culture and sports, all of which would lead to 'spiritual cleanliness' (*dushevnaia chistoplotnost'*).

Discussions of sexual abstinence as a method for preventing VD further illustrate the inseparability of discourses of health and morality in Soviet Latvian sex education materials. In the very few instances when contraception was actually mentioned, it was quickly dismissed as not entirely effective. The Latvian-language brochure 'Watch out for gonorrhoea!' instructed individuals to wash their genitals after sex, use condoms and to go to a clinic after sex with 'questionable individuals', but ended with the declaration that abstinence was the only guaranteed way to prevent contracting gonorrhoea.[57] A Russian-language newspaper article penned by venereologist G. Gertsmark underlined the idea that the only acceptable sexual intercourse was within marriage, declaring that 'spouses who remain faithful to each other will never contract a venereal disease'.[58] Rather than using modern barrier contraceptives, Soviet citizens were required to adhere to specific behavioural standards to prevent the spread of VD.

Abstaining from casual sex was presented as a collective responsibility shared by men and women. One Russian-language anti-VD pamphlet prepared for drivers of various forms of long-distance transportation by the Republican House of Sanitary

Enlightenment in Riga urged readers to 'remember the high moral character of the Soviet man' and to 'take care of yourself in order to protect your family and others from disease'.[59] Similar appeals to men to protect their families from VD appeared in numerous newspaper articles throughout the 1970s. This focus on men's behaviour reflects the greater significance Soviet officialdom ascribed to men's actions within the domestic sphere beginning in the Khrushchev era.[60] The focus on male sexual behaviour could also reflect broader concern about the 'crisis of masculinity' emerging in Soviet expert discourse and journalistic commentary from the 1970s onwards. Demographers and sociologists proposed health campaigns directed specifically at men to counter 'bad habits' and risky behaviours, like alcoholism, overeating and physical immobility, in order to address men's dwindling life expectancy, higher mortality rates and the more general post-war demographic imbalance.[61]

The war on casual sex was likely waged so decisively within Soviet medical discourse for a variety of reasons. First, the Soviet state incurred significant costs for children born outside marriage. Soviet family law only obliged fathers to pay child support if they were married to the mother of the child, if there was evidence that they had 'permanently' participated in the raising of the child, or if they acknowledged paternity themselves.[62] The state was financially responsible for children born out of casual or extramarital relationships, and millions of unmarried mothers were eligible to claim benefits.[63] Second, the number of registered abortions soared in the decades following the legalization of the procedure in 1955, and medical professionals and state officials alike worried deeply about the impact of extremely high rates of abortion upon women's health, particularly their future reproductive capabilities.[64] Third, there were chronic shortages of contraceptives that prevented VD transmission. In the mid-1970s, data from the Ministry of Health revealed that the actual supply of condoms available in the USSR did not satisfy the needs of the vast majority of the population.[65] The most commonly used contraceptive methods (induced abortion, the withdrawal method, the use of a menstrual calendar and vaginal douching) may have terminated or prevented pregnancy in some cases, but they did not offer any protection against VD.[66] The quality of barrier methods like condoms in the Soviet Union was also poor and usage remained low throughout the entire Soviet period.[67] Therefore, abstaining from casual sex was deemed to be the only reliable method for preventing the financial and physical consequences of unwanted pregnancy, as well as preventing the transmission of VD. In this context, doctors' expertise and authoritative voices were used to further broader state goals, such as addressing declining fertility and high rates of abortion.

The individual/national body

In Soviet Latvian sex education materials, the individual body and the national body were collapsed into one entity. As noted earlier, this had long been a feature of Soviet sexual enlightenment since its inception in the 1920s, but this device took on renewed significance in the context of the Brezhnev era. Declining birth rates at the all-Union level, and the knock-on effect upon the size of the labour force and military, were especially concerning for the Soviet government in the context of the Cold War.[68] Declining fertility also had profound ideological consequences. Soviet officialdom circulated carefully constructed images of the happiness and material comfort of Soviet citizens both within and beyond the borders of the USSR, but a communist state producing the conditions for population decline had the potential to undermine their efforts.[69] Demographic research conducted in the 1960s and 1970s also revealed worrying disparities in population growth. While birth rates were on the decline in western republics (including Latvia), they were on the rise in Soviet Central Asia.[70] Uneven population development had political implications, as it had the potential to encourage the development of national assertiveness amongst minorities and enable republican leaders to use their rapid population growth to demand additional allocations for their republics.[71] Throughout the Brezhnev era, the Soviet government addressed the problem of union-wide population decline and uneven population development by offering lump sum payments for new mothers, increasing government aid for single mothers and low-income families, and rolling out additional financial incentives for childbearing in low-fertility regions.[72] Population statistics were also subject to strict censorship in an effort to preserve the Soviet government's legitimacy in the eyes of domestic and international audiences.[73]

Anxieties about the national and ideological implications of declining fertility are evident in Soviet Latvian sex education materials. For example, a poster prepared for display in women's toilets and showers at industrial enterprises in the city of Daugavpils in 1972 included the following plea in block capitals:

> Dear women! Your health is in your hands, use it wisely for the benefit of the homeland, which needs a healthy generation of builders of communism.[74]

This statement reflects long-standing themes in Soviet pronatalist propaganda, whereby women were categorized as incubators for the next generation and women's contributions to the task of 'building communism' were framed around their abilities to bear and raise children.[75]

Concerns regarding the ideological implications of rising incidence of VD are also visible in sex education materials, wherein the sexual health of Soviet citizens was framed as another battleground of the Cold War. In 1973, Dr A. Miltiņš, chief physician at the Republican VD Dispensary, prepared a Latvian-language radio broadcast on incidence of VD in foreign countries, in which he provided detailed information on the rising rates of syphilis and gonorrhoea in the United States, Canada, and various countries across western and eastern Europe.[76] In the broadcast, Miltiņš claimed that VD was on the rise abroad because of the underfunding of venereological services and poor hygiene education (as well as the prevalence of extramarital sex, drug abuse, prostitution and homosexuality), omitting to mention that the picture was starkly similar in the USSR. Similarly, a Latvian-language newspaper article discussed how high rates of VD were 'understandable' in capitalist countries because of their 'social and moral peculiarities', but asked how Soviet citizens, who have 'learned to control the most complex apparatus and machines [could] be so helpless in their self-restraint and self-management?'⁷⁷ While the social and economic conditions of capitalism were seen as the cause of VD abroad, in the USSR it was individuals' failure to regulate their behaviour, fully participate in society and direct their energies to building communism that were the principal problems. When discussing how to combat VD, newspaper articles explained that merely avoiding casual sex was not enough, and instead Soviet citizens needed to root out those that were perceived to be the primary transmitters of infection. 'Society as a whole must denounce drunks, the idle, and amoral elements', one Latvian-language article explained, before encouraging Soviet citizens to report these 'perverted individuals' to their housing and workplace committees.[78] Another article instructed readers to create an 'intolerable environment' for 'drunks, parasites, and morally corrupted people'.[79]

In these articles and broadcasts, combatting VD was presented as an urgent necessity that required the active participation of all Soviet citizens. The framing of sexual health as a battleground between capitalist countries and the USSR and insistence on the eradication of VD as a necessary goal for wider society can be read as part of broader attempts by the state to mobilize citizens and revitalize the communist project at a time when waning faith in its promises had become increasingly pervasive.[80] In the Brezhnev era, mass media was one of the key arenas within which these attempts at mobilization took place.[81] Anti-VD newspaper articles and radio broadcasts articulated the need for society-wide mobilization to reduce rates of infection, as Soviet citizens were instructed to both adhere to specific standards of sexuality morality and call out those who did not.

Incentivizing/disincentivizing treatment

Sex education materials consistently emphasized the importance of expert knowledge and categorized the physician as the chief authority on matters of hygiene and sexual morality. Doctors at Latvia's Republican VD Dispensary wrote newspaper articles with titles like 'The Doctor's Advice' and 'Truth and Hearsay' with the aims of dispelling common misconceptions about VD transmission and encouraging those with symptoms to come to clinics immediately for treatment.[82] Similarly, a Latvian-language radio broadcast aired at 7.45am on 20 August 1974 reminded citizens that 'medicine is only truly powerful in the hands of a physician' and condemned the 'self-made doctors' who offered advice on VD treatment or sold antibiotics illegally outside the state healthcare system.[83] This discourse positioned medical professionals working within the state healthcare system as the chief purveyors (and therefore gatekeepers of) knowledge about venereal diseases, which in turn classified the ideal patient as a passive and obedient receptacle of instruction. Yuliya Hilevych and Chizu Sato have observed similar paternalistic rhetoric in discussions of abortion in popular health magazines, wherein a binary was established between doctors as 'agents of knowledge' on the one hand, and their uninformed, docile female patients on the other.[84]

Sex education was rife with warnings about the dangers of seeking treatment outside the state healthcare system. One Russian-language brochure produced for university students in 1974, entitled 'Beware of Becoming Infected with Gonorrhoea!', included several warnings against buying antibiotics through unofficial channels and stressed the importance of receiving treatment only from a qualified physician employed within a state facility. Students who self-medicated could not be sure that they were completely cured or even die because of an allergic reaction to antibiotics.[85] They could also allegedly become infected with syphilis as well as gonorrhoea, but the brochure did not explain how this was actually possible. Two Russian-language anti-syphilis newspaper articles prepared by a senior doctor at the Republican VD Dispensary included similar warnings. These articles contrasted the apparently ineffective self-treatment (*samolechenie*) with the effective medicine (*meditsina*), reflecting the long-standing denigration of folk and alternative medicine for the treatment of VD stretching back to the 1920s.[86] In scaremongering about self-medicating, medical professionals pushed messages that would presumably aid the state in its efforts to trace contacts of venereal patients and sources of infection, as well as prosecute those who 'maliciously' infected others. Individuals who self-medicated or received private treatment avoided the gaze of the authorities and sidestepped potentially awkward conversations with physicians about their sex lives, number of sexual partners and importance of adhering to standards of communist morality. This avoidance was evidently of concern to the authorities in the Latvian SSR, as in 1973, police in Riga and Jūrmala were instructed to identify individuals who had been treated by private doctors, alongside suspected homosexual men, brothel keepers, pimps and sex workers.[87]

Despite warning against the dangers of self-medicating, sex education materials drafted by staff at the Republican VD Dispensary arguably disincentivized infected individuals from seeking treatment through the state healthcare system. One article drafted for publication in the newspaper *Rīgas Balss* in late 1973 reassured those infected with venereal infections that they would be granted full confidentiality when they came to the clinic for treatment, but just a few sentences later insisted that patients were obliged to provide a full list of contacts to their physician in order to identify the source of their infection.[88] Another article in the newspaper *Padomju Jaunatne* (*Soviet Youth*) from October 1974 claimed that 'few contacts remained unidentified', as medical personnel and the police worked hard to trace suspected contacts even when VD patients could not provide a first or last name.[89] The article alleged that successful contact tracing could be performed with just physical descriptions of a contact, or a rudimentary map of the location in which the patient engaged in sex with the suspect. Medical personnel in the Latvian republic (as elsewhere in the USSR) were under immense pressure to identify and eliminate sources of infection and contacts, and were chastised by representatives of the Ministry for Health for their failure to do so.[90] Staff at VD clinics were given targets for the number of contacts to be identified per patient, and republican ministries of health were required to relay information about the annual average number of contacts identified within their particular republic back to Moscow.[91] Contact tracing hindered patient confidentiality as it made an individual's infection known to their sexual partners, as well as friends, colleagues, and relatives if they were living or working in close proximity. Providing the names of contacts also subjected these individuals to compulsory examination, and, if they refused, their forced transportation to a VD clinic by the police, or even criminal prosecution for evading VD treatment. These policies likely made VD patients reluctant to provide an accurate list of contacts when seeking treatment to avoid state interference into the lives of their sexual partners, friends, colleagues or relatives. Indeed, health authorities in the Latvian SSR (as in other republics and regions) reported low rates of contact tracing throughout the 1970s.[92]

Sex education materials were littered with constant reminders about the criminalization of VD transmission, which also likely disincentivized seeking treatment. One Latvian-language brochure entitled 'Venereal Diseases and their Prevention' included a lengthy discussion of all the different ways in which patients could be prosecuted under the Soviet anti-VD law and reiterated the fact that health authorities were legally obliged to perform compulsory examinations on any individuals believed to be contacts of the venereal patient.[93] In 1976, doctors at the Republic VD dispensary were asked to put together four hours of lectures on the theme of VD and their prevention to be delivered to university students in the Latvian SSR.[94] A substantial portion of one of the lectures was devoted to discussing the anti-VD law and the forced examination of suspected sources of infection.[95] Repeated reminders of the criminalization of VD transmission, coupled with the fact that suspected VD patients and contacts were subject to compulsory treatment and invasive examinations, would have arguably made treatment without the knowledge of the medical authorities particularly attractive.

Sex education also reinforced the stigma and shame associated with VD by insisting that they were illnesses primarily contracted by antisocial and amoral individuals. An anti-syphilis radio lecture from 1976 insisted that 'more often than not, venereal diseases affect people leading an immoral lifestyle: parasites, vagrants, and alcoholics'.[96] Newspaper articles included dehumanizing descriptions of individuals who were infected with VD. An article prepared for publication in *Padomju Jaunatne* in 1974 by a senior doctor at the Republican VD dispensary contained the following description of a suspected source of infection:

> The descriptions of casual acquaintances are sometimes so unappealing that the lack of disgust [that the patient felt during sexual intercourse] can only be explained by the patient's state of intoxication. Once he had sobered up, patient M. felt uncomfortable looking at the woman he had met while under the influence in a city park. 'I don't know her name, it was her who started it, she had bleached hair, a coarse voice, a kind of yellowish skin colour, red eyes, very drunk, and I've never seen her again'.[97]

The message that VD was predominantly spread by amoral people was pushed in sex education films. The short film *Reportage without Heroes* (*Reportazh bez geroev*) was first screened in the USSR in 1973 and first appeared on television in the Latvian SSR in December 1974.[98] The film opens with a hidden camera being installed at a VD clinic; a device intended to lead viewers to believe that they are observing genuine VD patients in conversation with a doctor. The VD patients in the film had either engaged in casual or extramarital sex with disastrous consequences. Doctors explain the law on VD transmission to insolent young people who dismiss the severity of their infections before presenting them with images of adults and babies with syphilitic lesions. During consultations, doctors are facing the camera, wearing white coats, and are bathed in light. In contrast, patients are only visible from behind and are often depicted as silhouettes, which served to underline the power imbalance between doctor and patient and 'radicalise the contrast between the ill and the healthy, knowledgeable and ignorant, advanced and backward'.[99]

The final patient in the film is a married man accused of infecting women across the Soviet Union while away on business trips. The man begins to tell the doctor that his 'intimate life' is none of her business when she interrupts him to say: 'No, you listen. You are socially dangerous. You are the source of infection for many women [...] What fate awaits your unborn child?' As this scene suggests, *Reportage without Heroes* reinforced the stigma and shame associated with VD by presenting a trip to a VD clinic as an unpleasant encounter in which patients were either devastated by their diagnosis or given the dressing down that they allegedly deserved by medical personnel. In the film, patients were also informed of the apparent common 'misconception' that VD treatment was straightforward and moralizing language permeated the doctor-patient consultation. Rather than encouraging people to go to their local VD clinic when they noticed signs of infection, films like *Reportage without Heroes* likely acted as a disincentive to seeking treatment through official channels and contributed to rising rates of VD.

Conclusion

Mass media was an important technology of sexual enlightenment in the Brezhnev-era USSR. In the Latvian SSR, sex education materials positioned medical experts working within the state healthcare system as the chief authority on matters related to both sexual health and sexual morality. Expert knowledge was entangled with broader political programmes, as doctors lent their authoritative voices to further state goals, such as prosecuting those who transmitted VD 'maliciously' and addressing declining fertility. In this context, medical experts played a key role in the articulation of specific ideas about sexual health that aligned with the pronatalist priorities of the Soviet government and addressed demographic decline in the western republics of the USSR. The role assigned to doctors at the Latvian Republican VD Dispensary required them to step outside their area of expertise (venereology) and discuss a broad range of issues related to sexual morality and sexual behaviour. Despite the push for mass sex education with the goal of reducing rates of VD, the messages pushed in articles, brochures, lectures, radio broadcasts and films were often in conflict with the broader public health outcomes that state officials set out to achieve. In casting syphilis and gonorrhoea as illnesses contracted primarily by amoral and antisocial individuals and constantly reminding their audience about the criminalization of VD transmission, the sex education materials prepared by staff at Latvia's Republican VD Dispensary disincentivized seeking treatment within the state healthcare system and likely contributed to high rates of venereal infection.

Notes

1. 'Ia emu doverilas", *Rīgas Balss*, 6 October 1973, 4.
2. Frances Bernstein, *The Dictatorship of Sex: Lifestyle Advice for the Soviet Masses* (DeKalb: Northern Illinois University Press, 2007), 103.
3. Ibid., 100–28; Tricia Starks, *The Body Soviet: Propaganda, Hygiene, and the Revolutionary State* (Madison: University of Wisconsin Press, 2008), 187–9.
4. Bernstein, *The Dictatorship of Sex*, 129–58.
5. Oksana Sarkisova, *Screening Soviet Nationalities: Kulturfilms from the Far North to Central Asia* (London: I.B. Tauris, 2017), 114–37.
6. Brian LaPierre, *Hooligans in Khrushchev's Russia: Defining, Policing, and Producing Deviance during the Thaw* (Madison: University of Wisconsin Press, 2012); Shelia Fitzpatrick, 'Social Parasites: How Tramps, Idle Youth, and Busy Entrepreneurs Impeded the Soviet March to Communism', *Cahiers du monde russe* 47.1–2 (2006): 377–408.
7. Deborah A. Field, *Private Life and Communist Morality in Khrushchev's Russia* (New York: Peter Lang, 2007), 24.
8. Edward D. Cohn, 'Sex and the Married Communist: Family Troubles, Marital Infidelity, and Party Discipline in the Postwar USSR, 1945–64', *Russian Review* 68.3 (2009): 429–50; Dan Healey, *Russian Homophobia from Stalin to Sochi* (London: Bloomsbury, 2018), 40–5; Rustam Alexander, 'Soviet Legal and Criminological Debates on the Decriminalization of Homosexuality (1965–75)', *Slavic Review* 1 (2018): 30–52; Siobhán Hearne, 'Sanitising Sex in the USSR: State Approaches to Sexual Health in the Brezhnev Era', *Europe-Asia Studies*, 74.1 (2022): 1793–1815; Siobhán Hearne, 'Selling Sex under Socialism: Prostitution in the Post-War USSR', *European Review of History*, 29.2 (2022): 290–310.
9. Yuliya Hilevych and Chizu Sato, 'Popular Medical Discourses on Birth Control in the Soviet Union during the Cold War: Shifting Responsibilities and Relational Values', in Ann-Kathrin Gembries, Theresia Theuke and Isabel Heinemann, eds., *Children by Choice? Changing Values, Reproduction, and Family Planning in the 20th Century* (Berlin: De Gruyter, 2018), 113–15.
10. Alexander, 'Sex Education and the Depiction of Homosexuality'; Vita Zelče, 'Dažas 60. gadu (re)konstrukcijas', *Latvijas Arhīvi* 3 (2003): 112–14.
11. Stephen Lovell, *Russia in the Microphone Age: A History of Soviet Radio, 1919–1970* (Oxford: Oxford University Press, 2015), 157; Kristin Roth-Ey, *Moscow Prime Time: How the Soviet Union Built the Media Empire That Lost the Cultural Cold War* (Ithaca: Cornell University Press, 2011), 11.
12. Roth-Ey, *Moscow Prime Time*, 181–3.
13. Christine E. Evans, *Between Truth and Time: A History of Soviet Central Television* (New Haven: Yale University Press, 2016), 4.
14. Roth-Ey, *Moscow Prime Time*, 14.
15. For a comprehensive overview of sex education in interwar Latvia, see Ineta Lipša, *Seksualitāte un sociālā kontrole Latvijā, 1914–1939* (Riga: Zinātne, 2014), 457–520.
16. Ineta Lipša, '"Over-Latvianisation in Heaven" – Attitudes towards Contraception and Abortion in Latvia, 1918–1940', in *Baltic Eugenics: Bio-Politics, Race and Nation in Interwar Estonia, Latvia, and Lithuania*, ed. Björn M. Felder and Paul J. Weindling (Amsterdam: Rodopi, 2013), 176–9.
17. Lipša, '"Over-Latvianisation in Heaven"', 186. On eugenic practices before and during the Ulmanis era, see Björn M. Felder, '"Mazvērtīgo samazināšana" – eiģēnika Latvijā',

Kultūras Diena (23 April 2005): 16–17 and Vita Zelče, 'Vara, zinātne, veselība un cilvēki: Eigēnika Latvijā 20. gs 30. gados', *Latvijas Arhīvi*, 3 (2006): 94–137.

18 Edward Cohn, 'A Soviet Theory of Broken Windows: Prophylactic Policing and the KGB's Struggle with Political Unrest in the Baltic Republics', *Kritika* 19.4 (2018): 769–92, 774; William Risch, 'A Soviet West: Nationhood, Regionalism, and Empire in the Annexed Western Borderlands', *Nationalities Papers* 43.1 (2015): 73–5; Ando Leps, 'Comparative Analysis of Crime: Estonia, the Other Baltic Republics, and the Soviet Union', *International Criminal Justice Review* 1 (1991): 81.

19 Healey, *Russian Homophobia from Stalin to Sochi*, 171; Ineta Lipša, 'Categorised Soviet Citizens in the Context of the Policy of Fighting Venereal Disease in the Soviet Latvia from Khrushchev to Gorbachev (1955–1985)', *Acta medico-historica Rigensia*, 12 (2019): 100 n. 20.

20 Alexander, 'Soviet Legal and Criminological Debates', 35; Alexander Hazanov, 'Porous Empire: Foreign Visitors and the Post-Stalin Soviet State', PhD dissertation (University of Pennsylvania, 2016), 214.

21 Healey, 'The Sexual Revolution in the USSR', 237–9.

22 Roland Pressat, 'Historical Perspectives on the Population of the Soviet Union', *Population and Development Review*, 11.2 (1985): 324, 326.

23 The survey was conducted by *Komsomolskaia Pravda* and directed by Grushin. More than 12,000 people participated. The results were originally published in the monthly magazine *Molodaia gvardiia*: B. Grushin, '"Slushaetsia delo o razvode …" O tak nazyvaemykh takzhe "legkomyslennikh brakakh"', *Molodaia gvardiia*, 6 (1964): 164–91 and 7 (1974): 255–82. Excerpts were published in two articles entitled 'Vtorzhenie v oblast' "stydnogo"' in *Sovetskaia molodezh*, 1 August 1964, 3, and 2 August 1964, 3.

24 'Esche odno vtorzhenie v oblast' "stydnogo"', *Sovetskaia molodezh*, 9 December 1964.

25 Aktual'nyi vopros', *Sovetskaia molodezh*, 8 January 1965, 2; 'Po sledam nashikh vystuplenii, edinyi tsentr nyzhen', *Sovetskaia molodezh*, 16 January 1965, 2.

26 Prikaz Ministerstvo Zdravookhraneniia SSSR ot 27/02/1963 'O meropriiatiiakh polikvidatsii zabolevaemosti sifilisom i rezkomu snizheniiu gonorei v SSSR'.

27 Field, *Private Life*, 58–60.

28 For example, the reports by the Estonian SSR (Gosudarstvennyi Arkhiv Rossiiskoi Federatsii, State Archive of the Russian Federation, GARF, f. R8009, op. 50, d. 4937, l. 148) and Lithuanian SSR (GARF, f. R8009, op. 50, d. 4937, l. 56).

29 There was an 11 per cent increase in the number of cases of gonorrhoea and syphilis across the USSR in 1968–9 and a 14 per cent increase in 1970–2, Rossiiskii Gosudarstvennyi Arkhiv Ekonomiki, Russian State Archive of the Economy, RGAE, f. 1562, op. 45, d. 5939, l. 35; RGAE, f. 1562, op. 45, d. 9813, l. 1; RGAE, f. 1562, op. 47, d. 1524, l. 9; RGAE, f. 1562, op. 48, d. 1943, l. 20. Certain regions experienced a rapid rise in the number of venereal infections in the late 1960s and early 1970s. For example, rates of gonorrhoea increased by 42 per cent in Khabarovsk region in 1967–8 (GARF, f. A461, op. 12, d. 131, l. 369), syphilis cases almost doubled in the Lithuanian SSR between 1973 and 1974 (GARF, f. R8009, op. 50, d. 4937, l. 52), and syphilis increased by over 600 per cent in Leningrad city between 1964 and 1967 (GARF, f. A461, op. 12, d. 131, l. 164).

30 Latvijas Nacionālais arhīvs, Latvijas Valsts arhīvs (Latvian State Archive, LVA hereafter), f. PA-101, apr. 37, l. 47, lp. 79.

31 GARF, f. R8009, op. 50, d. 4931, l. 30; LVA, f. PA-101, apr. 37, l. 47, lp. 79.

32 Hearne, 'Sanitising Sex in the USSR', 1805.

33 Hearne, 'Sanitising Sex in the USSR'; Lipša, 'Categorised Soviet Citizens', 109–12.

34 Lipša, 'Categorised Soviet Citizens', 112.
35 LVA, f. PA-101, apr. 37, l. 47, lp. 77, 82.
36 Ibid., l. 47, lp. 97, 103, 107.
37 The census of 1970 indicated that Latvian speakers comprised 56.8 per cent of the Latvian SSR's population and Russians made up 29.8 per cent. Latvijas PSR Ministru Padomes Centrālā Statistikas Pārvalde, *1970. gada Vissavienības tautas skaitīšanas rezultāti Latvijas PSR* (Riga, 1974), 108–9. The 1958 education reform allowed Russian-speaking children to drop the titular non-Russian language of their republic. Even though the reform was repealed in 1964, it enhanced the status of the Russian language in schooling and accelerated the decline of titular-language instruction. According to the 1970 census, just 18 per cent of Russians in the Latvian SSR could speak Latvian. On the reform, see Michael Loader, 'Latvia Goes Rouge: Language Politics and Khrushchev's 1958 Soviet Education Reform', in Michael Loader, Siobhán Hearne and Matthew Kott, eds., *Defining Latvia: Recent Explorations in History, Culture, and Politics* (Budapest: Central European University Press, 2022): 151–88.
38 LVA, f. PA-2141, apr. 3, l. 22, lp. 17, 97.
39 Ibid., lp. 95.
40 For example, the Russian-language film *Wasted Youth* (*Rastrachennaia iunost'*) was screened at the Republican House of Knowledge in Riga several times in the 1960s, 'V kinolektorii doma znanii', *Rīgas Balss*, 2 November 1964; 'V kinolektorii doma znanii', *Rīgas Balss*, 20 December 1966; 'V kinolektorii doma znanii', *Rīgas Balss*, 18 January 1967.
41 Lipša, 'Categorized Soviet Citizens', 117.
42 *Gor'kaia khronika* [Film] Dir. Arkadii Tsineman, USSR: Tsentrnauchfil'm, 1966. For screenings on Latvian television, see the following TV listings: 'Televidenie sreda 27 oktiabria', *Rīgas Balss*, 26 October 1976; 'Televidenie sreda 19 oktiabria', *Rīgas Balss*, 18 October 1977; 'Televidenie, piatnitsa 3 fevralia', *Rīgas Balss*, 2 February 1978; 'Televidenie sreda 26 aprelia', *Rīgas Balss*, 25 April 1978; 'Televidenie ponedel'nik 30 oktiabria', *Rīgas Balss*, 28 October 1978.
43 LVA, f. PA-2141, apr. 3, l. 22, lp. 145, 155, 158–9, 166, 173, 177, 179.
44 Sergei Kruk, 'Television Changing Habits: TV Programming in 1960s Soviet Latvia', in Stewart Anderson and Melissa Chakars, eds., *Modernization, Nation-Building, and Television History* (New York: Routledge, 2014), 89–109.
45 Kruk, 'Television Changing Habits'. On increasing radio listenership in the Latvian republic in the Brezhnev era, see Pekka Gronow and Jānis Daugavietis, 'Pie laika … Now Is the Time: The Singing Revolution on Latvian Radio and Television', *Popular Music*, 39.2 (2020): 274–5.
46 'V shkol'noi programme – "osnovy semeinikh znanii"', *Rīgas Balss*, 22 December 1980, 4.
47 LVA, f. PA-2141, apr. 3, l. 22, lp. 156.
48 Such as the Pioneris, Daile, Blāzma, Oktobris and Jugla cinemas, LVA, f. PA-2141, apr. 3, l. 22, lp. 156.
49 LVA, f. PA-2141, apr. 3, l. 22, lp. 145, 155, 158–9, 166, 173, 177, 179.
50 Ibid., lp. 122.
51 Ibid., lp. 123.
52 Ibid., lp. 124.
53 Mark Fenemore, 'The Growing Pains of Sex Education in the German Democratic Republic (GDR), 1945–69', in Lutz Sauerteig and Roger Davidson, eds., *Shaping Sexual Knowledge: A Cultural History of Sex Education in Twentieth Century Europe* (London: Routledge, 2009), 71.

54 LVA, f. PA-2141, apr. 3, l. 22, lp. 84. The inclusion of smoking in this list reflects broader currents in Soviet anti-tobacco materials, wherein tobacco use was presented as a learned behaviour that could be changed through strengthening willpower, rather than chemical addiction. For a detailed discussion, see Tricia Starks's chapter in this volume.
55 Ibid., lp. 82.
56 'Oshibka molodosti', *Sovetskaia molodezh'*, 20 February 1974, 4.
57 LVA, f. PA-2141, apr. 3, l. 22, lp. 37.
58 'Beregite zhizn', zdorov'e, liubov'', *Sovetskaia molodezh'*, 14 September 1973, 3.
59 LVA, f. PA-2141, apr. 3, l. 22, lp. 45.
60 Cohn, 'Sex and the Married Communist'; Amy E. Randall, 'Soviet and Russian Masculinities: Rethinking Soviet Fatherhood after Stalin and Renewing Virility in the Russian Nation under Putin', *Journal of Modern History*, 92 (2020): 892–4; Claire E. McCallum, 'Man about the House: Male Domesticity and Fatherhood in Soviet Visual Satire under Khrushchev' in Ilič, ed., *The Palgrave Handbook of Women and Gender*, 331–47.
61 Elena Zdravomyslova and Anna Temkina, 'The Crisis of Masculinity in Late Soviet Discourse', *Russian Studies in History*, 51.2 (2013): 13–34.
62 Bernice Madison, 'Social Services for Families and Children in the Soviet Union since 1967', *Slavic Review* 31.4 (1972): 836–8.
63 In 1957, 3.2 million unmarried mothers received government aid, and this number likely increased throughout the following two decades, Randall, "Abortion Will Deprive You of Happiness"', 24. On the system of payments, see Jerry G. Pankhurst, 'Childless and One-Child Families in the Soviet Union', *Journal of Family Issues*, 3.4 (1982): 508–9.
64 Mie Nakachi, *Replacing the Dead: The Politics of Reproduction in the Postwar Soviet Union* (Oxford: Oxford University Press, 2021), 187.
65 Andrej A. Popov, Adriaan Ph. Visser and Evert Ketting, 'Contraceptive Knowledge, Attitudes, and Practice in Russia during the 1980s', *Studies in Family Planning*, 24.4 (1993): 231–2.
66 Popov, Visser, and Ketting, 'Contraceptive Knowledge', 229. Larissa I. Remennick, 'Patterns of Birth Control', in Igor Kon and James Riordan, eds., *Sex and Russian Society* (Bloomington: Indiana University Press, 1993), 45–46. It is important to note that surveys on contraceptive use predominantly refer to married couples.
67 Hilevych and Sato, 'Popular Medical Discourses', 99–122; Amy Rankin-Williams, 'Soviet Contraceptive Practices and Abortion Rates in St Petersburg, Russia', *Health Care for Women International*, 22 (2001): 700.
68 Nakachi, *Replacing the Dead*, 201–2.
69 Hilevych and Sato, 'Popular Medical Discourses', 102.
70 Barbara A. Anderson and Brian D. Silver, 'Growth and Diversity of the Population of the Soviet Union', *Annals of the American Academy of Political and Social Science*, 510 (1990): 155–77.
71 Cynthia Weber and Ann Goodman, 'The Demographic Policy Debate in the USSR', *Population and Development Review*, 7.2 (1981): 287.
72 Nakachi, *Replacing the Dead*, 209–10.
73 Jessica Lovett, 'Turning Science into Fiction? Censoring Population Research in the Soviet Union, 1964–1982', *Contemporary European History* (2022): 1–20.
74 LVA, f. PA-2141, apr. 3, l. 22, lp. 47.

75 Tricia Starks, 'Fertile Mother Russia: Pronatalist Propaganda in Revolutionary Russia', *Journal of Family History*, 28.3 (2003): 411–42; Randall, '"Abortion Will Deprive You of Happiness!"'
76 LVA, f. PA-2141, apr. 3, l. 22, lp. 7–12.
77 'Atbildību, prasīgumu, dzīves skaidrību', *Cīņa*, 13 July 1973, 4.
78 LVA, f. PA-2141, apr. 3, l. 22, lp. 5.
79 'Chto nuzhno znat' o venericheskikh bolezniakh', *Rīgas Balss*, 28 August 1974, 6.
80 Alexei Yurchak, *Everything Was Forever, Until It Was No More: The Last Soviet Generation* (Princeton: Princeton University Press, 2005), 126–57.
81 Roth-Ey, *Moscow Prime Time*, 1–17.
82 LVA, f. PA-2141, apr. 3, l. 22, lp. 72, 129.
83 Ibid., lp. 71.
84 Hilevych and Sato, 'Popular Medical Discourses', 110–11.
85 LVA, f. PA-2141, apr. 3, l. 22, lp. 49.
86 Ibid., lp. 129, 149–50. Bernstein, 'Envisioning Health', 211–13.
87 LVA, f. PA-101, apr. 37, l. 47, lp. 89.
88 LVA, f. PA-2141, apr. 3, l. 22, lp. 3.
89 Ibid., lp. 80.
90 Lipša, 'Categorised Soviet Citizens', 98–9.
91 Hearne, 'Sanitising Sex in the USSR'. See for example, the report from the Moldovan SSR, GARF, f. R8131, op. 28, d. 6049, l. 20, the Lithuanian and Estonian SSRs, GARF, f. R8009, op. 50, d. 4937, ll. 52–6, 146–7.
92 GARF, f. R8009, op. 50, d. 4937, l. 71; GARF, f. A259, op. 46, d. 4716, l. 90; GARF, f. A259, op. 46, d. 5795, ll. 67–8; GARF, f. R8009, op. 50, d. 4937, ll. 52, 146–7; Rahvusarhiiv (National Archives of Estonia, ERAF) 1.20.17, lk. 5.
93 LVA, f. PA-2141, apr. 3, l. 22, lp. 32.
94 Ibid., lp. 54.
95 Ibid., lp. 57.
96 Ibid., lp. 148.
97 Ibid., lp. 81.
98 *Reportazh bez geroev* [Film] Dir. L. Gorin, USSR: Lennauchfilm, 1973; LVA, f. PA-2141, apr. 3, l. 22, lp. 95.
99 Sarkisova, *Screening Soviet Nationalities*, 122.

4

Health and heroism: Shifting patterns in late socialist Central Europe

Jan Arend

This chapter explores the shifts in the official discourse on mental health and the body that took place in the German Democratic Republic and Czechoslovakia in the 1970s and 1980s, and situates these discursive shifts in relation to the ideology of 'socialist heroism'. Examining stress care as a form of late socialist mind-body management, the contribution focuses on the emergence of a concern with stress and mental strain in popular health literature. The debate about stress broached issues like pressure to perform, fast societal change and the challenges linked to technological developments in the world of work. The advisory literature on stress management propagated such technologies of mind and body as autogenic training and yoga. In popular health literature, such practices were described as contributing to individual self-development while at the same time being part of a collectivist effort to increase human capacities more generally.

The chapter situates stress care within broader changes in mind-body management occurring in Western Europe and North America in the last third of the twentieth century. The stress debate was a transnational phenomenon observable on both sides of the Iron Curtain for it was an expression of superordinate developments. These included rising awareness of lifestyle-related health risks (like stress, lack of recreation or smoking) and the increasing dissemination of psychological guidebooks and self-help literature, as well as a growing interest in psychology as the foundation for health and personal success.[1] Furthermore, the concern with stress emerging in the 1970s was indicative, I argue, of changes in the sphere of socialist ideology. I show how the discourse of stress broke tacitly with central tenets of the narrative of socialist heroism, an ideology promulgated by state socialist regimes across the Eastern Bloc to mobilize performance and enthusiasm among their populations. By advocating 'gentleness' towards oneself, the discourse of stress care was clearly at odds with the propaganda of 'steely' socialist heroism. The fact that the concern with stress could be articulated in official sources shows that heroic propaganda was losing ground. At the same time, however, the practices and vocabularies of stress care contributed to the emergence of new models of 'adequate' behaviour that fulfilled similar functions as hero propaganda.

Health concerns in advanced industrial societies

What effects does life in developed industrial societies have on health? Since around 1960, this question was being discussed on both sides of the Iron Curtain by health experts, politicians and, gradually, by increasingly health-conscious strata of society. Heart conditions, high blood pressure, diabetes, lack of exercise, environmental toxins and cancer are but some of the ailments that gained public visibility across national borders during the second half of the twentieth century and pointed to a growing concern with the physical and mental consequences of advanced modernity.[2] Under the influence of a superordinate shift in values and structures, the 1960s saw the beginning of changes in various aspects of societal as well as individual approaches to health-related topics. In the context of this article, two aspects within this development are particularly significant. First, a new understanding of health-related risks gained traction during this time. Second, a pervasive notion of individual responsibility and self-care substantiated by psychological expertise began to be observable.

Although shifts in the understanding of and approach to health have hitherto primarily been studied in relation to Western societies, more recent works show that comparable but distinct changes occurred in state socialist countries like Czechoslovakia and the GDR.[3] The similarity of developments across East and West is in part owed to basic structural parallels between developed industrial societies. Knowledge transfers and entanglements also played an important role, however. Since experts in the field of health knowledge and health policy had been connected via international networks for some time before 1960, many debates were transnational and bloc-transcending. The World Health Organization (WHO) in particular provided an institutional setting for encounters between experts from both sides of the Iron Curtain. Such knowledge exchange considerably influenced the professional opinions of specialists from socialist countries such as the East German industrial hygienist, Siegfried Eitner, and the Czech specialist for internal medicine, Josef Charvát.[4]

In the 1970s, societal concerns about the risks associated with modern ways of living intensified. The so-called 'lifestyle diseases' like cardiovascular problems and diabetes began to attract increasing attention during this period. The contemporary rise in the incidence of such afflictions was attributed to the dangers of a modern lifestyle, characterized by lack of exercise along with unhealthy nutritional and consumption habits, as well as to harmful environmental influences in technologically advanced societies. This orientation towards risk detection somewhat blurred the boundaries of health and illness. Increasingly, healthy persons were no longer being viewed as free from disease, but as bearers of health risks.[5]

The concern with the danger of lifestyle diseases likewise began to inform public prevention measures in state socialist countries like Czechoslovakia and the GDR in the 1960s. The fact that numerous Czechoslovak and East German doctors and health-care politicians discussed the issue of health risks in international expert fora, especially the WHO, and introduced corresponding ideas and concepts into their domestic healthcare policy played an important role in this regard. For example, studies on the incidence of cardiovascular diseases were conducted in the GDR from the mid-1960s. During the 1970s, these studies achieved wide coverage by international standards, and by the 1980s around two-thirds of the GDR's population were participating in regular preventative health-monitoring programmes.[6]

Self-help literature was a key channel for the popularization of risk-oriented health concepts in state socialist countries and achieved high sales volumes. A prime example is the guidebook *Lebe ich richtig?* (*Am I Living Right?*), published in 1977 by the psychologist Peter Oderich, which praised autogenic training as a relaxation technique suitable for everyone and discussed the 'risk factors for a healthy, high-output and happy life' in great detail. Among other risk factors, Oderich's book listed mental stress, lack of exercise, smoking, an imbalanced diet and 'overstimulation' caused by watching television.[7]

The 1960s had seen more and more people consulting psychological self-help literature in Western countries as well as making use of the services offered by therapists and coaches. Under the influence of increasingly popularized expertise, individuals were regularly advised to engage in evaluation, introspection and self-optimization in order to achieve or maintain fitness in the professional and private spheres.[8] In Czechoslovakia and the GDR, the growth in the societal importance of psychological self-care manifested itself in an increased institutionalization of counselling and therapy beginning in the late 1960s. Popular psychology guidebooks and self-help literature offering strategies for maintaining emotional health and achieving success in one's professional and private life were published in larger numbers. Such publications primarily concentrated on issues like marital problems, alcohol abuse and smoking cessation.[9]

Symptoms such as chronic headaches, digestive problems, insomnia and erectile dysfunction also began to garner the attention of experts and the media.[10] These milder conditions, which were contemporarily referred to as 'neurotic' or 'psychosomatic', were now being taken seriously and addressed more frequently in the field of health care. Psychosomatic medicine became institutionalized, and numerous healthcare institutions like the Horní Palata day-care sanatorium for neurotic patients, established in Prague in 1969, or the Neuroseklinik Hirschgarten in Berlin, began to treat patients with mild psychosomatic afflictions.[11] Spas and baths increasingly turned their attention to mental and emotional wellbeing as well.[12]

The discourse of stress in East and West

It is no coincidence that a term previously used almost exclusively by experts in the fields of medicine and psychology came into fashion contemporaneously with the described shifts in health-related notions and practices – it was during the 1970s that 'stress' was transformed transnationally into a frequently used buzzword.[13] The widespread opinion that mankind had entered an age of stress pointed to fears about the physical and mental health-related consequences of an industrial society perceived as fast-moving and performance-focused.[14]

A concern with the issue of stress similarly emerged in state socialist Eastern and Central Europe.[15] The term was initially imported into the languages of the People's Democracies from the West by way of expert discourse.[16] In the context of state socialism, however, the topic of stress was problematic for ideological reasons. After all, it was not clear why stress should occur in a society that was, allegedly, free of labour exploitation. Up until the 1960s, we can observe an official discourse that negated the possibility of stress in a socialist society. Newspaper reports typically localized stress exclusively in the West – as a phenomenon characteristic of capitalist exploitation. This is not to say that state socialist experts refused to acknowledge instances of fatigue and exhaustion in their workforces. The relatively novel concept of stress, however, still regarded as 'foreign' by many, was used almost exclusively to describe life in the 'West'. The argument that socialist society was immune to stress, having eradicated the class antagonism and exploitation that produced stress-inducing working conditions, is frequently encountered in this context. Indeed, if stress was admitted to exist, its causes were typically located within the personalities of individuals rather than in the existing social order.[17] As Aleksandra Brokman's contribution to this volume similarly notes, the proponents of postwar Soviet psychotherapy tended to see mental health difficulties as problems to be solved by individual self-improvement rather than by changes in society.

In the late 1960s, however, discourses that acknowledged the existence of stress in socialist everyday life (both implicitly and explicitly) began to emerge in official literature.[18] Why did it become possible to discuss stress as a reality of life in state socialist countries? While the issue is complex, it appears that one explanatory factor was the discursive link established between stress and dynamic, modern societies. In contemporary East German and Czechoslovak accounts, stress was often portrayed as a side effect of technological progress and the accelerated rate of change in advanced modernity. To acknowledge the existence of stress in state socialism, therefore, was to imply that societies in the Eastern Bloc were developing as rapidly as their Western counterparts. Over the course of the 1970s and 80s, the term 'stress' made its way from the specialized vocabulary of doctors and psychologists to the state-run mass media. It eventually infiltrated the everyday language of the population as well – being deployed in the workplace, in the management of illnesses and in daily life.

The concern with stress became institutionalized in manifold ways in the illiberal, planned-economy context of late socialism. The practices and thought processes of personnel in manufacturing plants, for example, were increasingly characterized by anxieties about stress. Late socialist unionists, company physicians and occupational health and safety officials often worried about the physical and mental strain caused by new production technologies. Problems specific to the planned economy were also seen as a source of stress. A report compiled by the senior staff of the Karl Liebknecht transformer plant in Berlin in the mid-1960s, for example, noted that sick leave days taken by the plant's employees had increased. One reason for this development were 'nervous' gastrointestinal ailments among the workers. Employees suffered, the report continued, from mental strain resulting from the 'deficient, unrhythmic production process'. Planning problems were mentioned as causing a burdensome alternation of bustle and downtime. The report admitted that the workers were not resistant to stress and that widespread organizational problems in the planned economy resulted in psychosomatic strain and associated costs.[19] Concerns about stress pervaded the higher levels of government as well, for example, in the context of debates on the incidence of sick leave and the associated economic costs. During one discussion at the Czechoslovak Ministry of Health in 1972, for instance, 'increasing hecticness' and technological developments in the sphere of production were blamed for the contemporary rise in stress-induced neuroses.[20]

For a growing share of the population, personal lifestyles were also increasingly being marked by stress awareness and care. The latter provided one of the motives for people to seek rest and recreation in nature, for example, at dachas or garden plots. Guided by doctors, psychologists and self-help literature, socialist citizens suffering from psychosomatic afflictions like sleeplessness began to attribute such problems to stress much like their contemporaries in the West. One of many examples of contemporary engagement with the topic of stress is the 'clinic song' (*Kliniklied*) sung by patients at the Psychosomatic Department at the Heinrich Heine Clinic in Potsdam in the 1980s: 'Happily I sing my songs like the dear birds, for all my limbs are shaking after physiotherapy [...] Even my head is now clear, for the stress is gone!'[21] The Potsdam psychosomatic cures readily prescribed by doctors were taken up by various groups, including socialist functionaries, mothers working multiple shifts (especially in the Bitterfeld chemical industry), long-distance truck drivers and nurses. The song, an integral part of the spa treatment, refers to practices of attestation with which patients and medical professionals assured themselves of the anti-stress effect of such cures.[22]

Stress discourse and communist ideology: The case of socialist heroism

How did the discourse of stress – and the accompanying changes in official discourse on health and the body – relate to socialist ideology? To answer this question, I will focus on one classical narrative of Communist ideology, the narrative of socialist heroism. State socialist regimes and their intellectuals, initially in the Soviet Union in the interwar period, and then also in the newly founded People's Democracies in East-Central Europe after the Second World War, developed a classical narrative of socialist heroism that was transmitted to the populace through official channels and contributed to the mobilization of performance as defined by the respective regime. Within this narrative, which incorporated traits from Romanticism, certain qualities were ascribed to socialist heroes with a view to their function as role models for the population: He or she was 'hard', willing to sacrifice, selfless, took risks and was full of dedication to the rightful – socialist – cause. By abandoning their egos, socialist heroes assumed responsibility for the collective. Significantly, the socialist hero was associated with a distinct set of bodily and mental characteristics. For example, visual representations typically showed heroes with lean, fit and muscular bodies, while hero literature stressed their willpower.[23]

Already in the first socialist state, the Soviet Union, the idea of heroism had assumed a key position in culture and politics since the 1920s. Intellectuals like Maksim Gorky and Anatolii Lunacharskii who supported the Bolsheviks formulated central elements of the narrative of socialist heroism during this time. According to the visions of these fathers of the socialist hero concept, anyone could become a hero once the conditions of socialism were realized. In the transitionary period, however, distinguished individuals were required to blaze the trail into the utopian future.[24]

Hero propaganda began to become institutionalized in the Soviet Union in the 1930s. The title 'Hero of the Soviet Union' was awarded for the first time in 1934 to seven pilots who had rescued crewmembers of the expedition ship 'Cheliuskin', which had sunk in the Arctic Ocean.[25] Two years earlier, the Soviet writer Nikolai Ostrovskii had published the first part of his novel *How the Steel Was Tempered*, which featured the socialist hero Pavel Korchagin who sacrifices his health in the Civil War and in the process of 'building socialism'.[26] Over the course of the following years, a system of hero propaganda was developed that allowed state and party propagandists, educators and the mass media to introduce individual socialist heroes and their legendary deeds as well as a generalized idea of socialist heroism to the Soviet population in a targeted fashion. A number of different media, such as school textbooks, the press and cinema, were used to this end. Similar structures of hero propaganda were established in the newly founded satellite states in Eastern Europe after the Second World War.[27]

Socialist heroes made names for themselves in war, in sports and as cosmonauts. A particularly important site for the socialist hero narrative was the sphere of labour and production. Labour heroes broke records and seemed to suffer no fatigue while doing so. One example of this was the Soviet miner Aleksei Stakhanov, who was said to have extracted 102 tons of coal in a single shift in a hard coal mine in the Donets Basin in 1935.[28] The propagandistic dissemination of heroic stories had a number of different functions in state socialism – they legitimized communist rule and satisfied a general psychosocial desire for role models. In addition, heroic individuals exemplified a certain toughness in the face of austerity and sacrifice. The stories of labour heroes in particular served to activate and mobilize performance. This also applied to the title 'Hero of Labor' (later 'Hero of Socialist Labor') awarded to many meritorious workers.[29]

Researchers have convincingly demonstrated the considerable successes of heroism propaganda, particularly prior to the 1970s. Socialist heroes apparently enjoyed a high level of acceptance among the population, as evidenced by the fact that individuals like the GDR labour hero Adolf Hennecke received significant amounts of letters from audiences. The analysis of such letters shows that socialist heroes were viewed as advisory authorities and role models by a considerable part of the populace.[30] Heroes also frequently became the subjects of amateur poetry and collages. Their achievements motivated people to emulate them and engendered enthusiasm for the socialist cause. The mobilization of performance through the propagation of labour heroism was thus effective to a certain extent, and one could argue that the socialist hero narrative formed one of the pillars supporting state socialism as a relatively stable cultural and political project before 1970.[31]

Yet around 1970, if not earlier, a change started to manifest itself in the history of socialist heroism. It was during this period that the socialist hero narrative lost much of its societal lustre – the attractiveness of the behavioural model of the steely socialist hero began to wane. Scholars of socialist heroism argue that the excessive use of hero propaganda over the years caused its impact to wear off. According to this explanation, state socialism suffered from the fact that it had only limited performance incentives to offer its populations, and it therefore repeatedly attempted to propagate the behavioural model of the hero who was hungry for achievement and prepared to make sacrifices. In the words of historian Rosalinde Sartorti, this led to a 'continued process of demystification' that ultimately caused heroism to become a 'tedious and tiresome topic' for large parts of the population.[32] A further factor pointed to as a contributor to the demise of socialist heroism in various studies is the appearance of heroic figures symbolizing alternatives to the politics of the regime.[33] Numerous scholars see the decline of socialist heroism as a factor that contributed to the demise of state socialism as a whole.[34]

Contradicting discourses: Stress and heroism

While the narrative of socialist heroism and the discourse of stress were both part of official culture in the late socialist period in Czechoslovakia and the GDR, a comparison of the semantics of these discourses reveals fundamental tensions. One important point of comparison is differing approaches to the question of gender. While socialist hero propaganda explicitly included heroic female figures such as the young Soviet partisan Zoia Kosmodem'ianskaia, the discourse of stress was, in most instances, silent about the possibility of differences along gender lines. It appears that the discourse of stress (often generically male in its diction) masked unequal distributions of stress between men and women. Silent on the possibility of women experiencing greater levels of stress or being subject to different types of pressures, stress discourse rendered gender inequalities invisible.

The semantic differences between socialist heroism and the discourse of stress care are apparent in other respects. In his self-help book *Stress: Understanding–Recognizing–Overcoming*, Potsdam physician Dieter Seefeldt acknowledged that not everyone was able to 'jump out of bed' and engage in 'vigorous morning exercise' immediately upon the ringing of their alarm clock. He therefore advised:

> One can also begin with wriggling gymnastics in bed, with pleasurable stretching, extending, with a deep breath. Next the entire body is properly moved and massaged from head to toe. Slowly get up. Stretch and wriggle once more outside the bed[35]

Here we see – in a book published by one of the GDR's state publishing houses – gentleness and slowness recommended in regard to the reader's interaction with his or her own body and mind, along with a distancing from more 'vigorous' forms of activity. The discourse of stress in Seefeldt's book is clearly at odds with the ideas underpinning socialist heroism. Seefeldt's advice bears little resemblance to the 'steeliness' inherent in the traditional socialist hero, for whom activities like 'pleasurable' stretching and 'wriggling' would have been completely unthinkable. As this example suggests, the concern with stress spawned discourses and practices that were incompatible with the notion of socialist heroism and the earlier practices of 'working on the self' widespread during Stalinism – precisely because they were characterized by gentle self-care.[36]

The 1970s, and especially, the 1980s saw a propagation of exercise and relaxation techniques in state socialist countries that were similar to the abovementioned 'wriggling' gymnastics. These techniques included yoga, which was no longer repressed in the late socialist period despite its roots in spiritual traditions. Autogenic training, a relaxation technique based on autosuggestion, likewise enjoyed a growing popularity. Its practitioners were to induce tension relief themselves by reciting specific sentences like 'my body is becoming warm and heavy' in their head while lying down or sitting comfortably.[37] The reasons that led a certain share of the population to engage in such activities were diverse and included spiritual motives. The desire to practise these techniques of mind and body also derived in part from a rejection of state socialism. But more and more frequently, people sought tension relief as a result of a general concern with maintaining their own health and capacities. While this form of health awareness was not a mass phenomenon among late socialist populations, it did appeal to a growing segment of late socialist society as the latter became more differentiated in terms of lifestyle. Like in the West, activities including yoga and autogenic training fit into an established context of psychological expert knowledge popularized via self-help literature and popular media.[38]

Late socialist manuals and popular literature on yoga and autogenic training, much like other examples of stress management discourse, are characterized by a semantic logic that does not conform to the socialist hero ideal. Persons engaging in yoga and autogenic training were encouraged to focus their attention on their own experiences and sensations. They were to maintain a gentle, caring relationship with their own bodies. These stress-relief techniques were specifically intended to promote health and relaxed comfort.[39] The socialist hero, by contrast, served a cause greater than himself and his own body. He put his health and wellbeing at risk for this heroic (socialist) mission.

If putting one's health at risk was an appropriate behaviour for a socialist hero, what did the discourse of stress have to say on the issue of risk? As pointed out above, one context shaping the debate on stress in late socialism was a more general shift in health policy towards a risk-centred understanding of health. A large part of the population came into contact with the prevention campaigns launched by state socialist regimes in reaction to the threat of lifestyle diseases. In many cases, these prevention campaigns simply recommended avoiding risks. Following this logic, a healthy lifestyle was a low-risk lifestyle – which applied in particular to risk factors that could be avoided altogether, like smoking. A negative understanding of risk thus established itself. Whereas the socialist hero had been distinguished by a willingness to take risks, the socialist citizen educated by the prevention campaigns was supposed to avoid them.

The prevention campaigns did not encourage the complete avoidance of all types of risks, however. The discourse of stress was a prime example. A certain measure of stress was viewed as an unavoidable element of a healthy, productive life. Stress was also at times framed as a positive, energy-mobilizing force. Popular health literature therefore did not propagate the complete avoidance of stress, instead advising a sensible and measured approach to the risk it represented. A 1974 article on reducing the risk of heart attacks through changes to one's lifestyle featured in the popular Czechoslovak magazine *Vlasta* gave the following recommendation: 'Mental stress is necessary for physical toughening and the ability to perform. But in a measured fashion – as a garnish [...], not as a main course'.[40] Such texts postulated a sensible and measured handling of risks, which did not match the reckless bravery of the classic socialist hero.

Another concept that appeared in the early 1970s in popular health literature was that of 'one-sided strain' and mental-physical 'balance'. This terminology implied that it was important to find a middle ground between stress and recovery. The search for specific techniques of 'active regeneration' was key in this context.[41] More than before, mental stress experienced during the work process – caused by time pressure, the burden of responsibility and noisy work conditions – came to be viewed as significant alongside physical strain and exertion. A topical guidebook published in the GDR in 1973 characterized professionals talking shop during their lunch break as stress-inducing since workers were remaining mentally connected to the problems of their work. The guidebook recommended playing volleyball during lunch breaks as an escape. Similarly, the aforementioned stress-care guidebook by Dieter Seefeldt advocated midday naps at the workplace.[42] The concept of balance found concrete application in the shape of 'profession-specific compensation sports' as practised since 1969 at the Carl Zeiss Jena enterprise, where company physicians had determined that the staff of a female department was suffering from 'nervousness due to one-sided strain on certain brain areas'. The measures introduced to combat nervousness included gymnastics breaks with specific exercises that were designed to counterbalance habitual work movements.[43]

The assumption that labourers had a limited performance potential along with a pragmatic orientation towards sustainability were central to this concept of balance. Every worker was to perform at a level of intensity that he or she could maintain consistently over time following the active regeneration of body and mind. This, again, was quite at odds with the logic of the socialist hero narrative, which emphasized the ceaseless, record-breaking willingness of the hero to deliver. Simply put, the discourse of stress aimed to optimize performance while the socialist hero narrative tried to maximize it.[44]

Conclusion

What can we learn from analysing the discourse of stress in the late socialist GDR and the ČSSR in connection to ideological narratives such as socialist heroism? Late socialist authors of popular health literature did not refer to socialist heroism when writing about stress. Equally, propagandistic sources on the theme of socialist heroism mentioned neither stress nor the larger issues of health and body management. Yet the co-existence of these two discourses within the larger context of official language in late socialism is revealing. The discourse of stress and the discourse of socialist heroism both provided models of adequate behaviour and both could be put to use for the socialist cause of mobilizing labour performance. The two models of adequate behaviour were fundamentally contradictory, however. While socialist heroism advanced a model of reckless bravery and selflessness, the discourse of stress recommended gentle self-care in the aim of sustaining one's energies. The concern with stress observable in popular health literature thereby points to the waning influence of heroic propaganda in the 1970s and 1980s. The material analysed in this chapter suggests that shifts in official discourses on health and the body contributed to the decline of the ideology of heroism. New paradigms of behaviour established themselves under late socialism, coming to rival older heroic models.

Notes

1   M. Jackson, *The Age of Stress: Science and the Search for Stability* (Oxford: Oxford University Press, 2013); P. Kury, *Der überforderte Mensch. Eine Wissensgeschichte vom Stress zum Burnout* (Frankfurt: Campus Verlag, 2012); J. Arend, 'Ist Stress westlich? Zum zeitgeschichtlichen Ort der Belastungssorge', *Geschichte und Gesellschaft* 45.2 (2019): 245–74.

2   Cf. M. Harrison, *Disease and the Modern World 1500 to the Present Day* (Cambridge: Polity Press, 2004), 166–91. On the societal, economic and political processes of change that formed an important background for the described developments in notions of health, see also N. Ferguson, C. S. Maier, D. J. Sargeant and E. Manela, eds., *The Shock of the Global: The 1970s in Perspective* (Cambridge, MA: Belknap Press, 2011); A. Doering-Manteuffel and L. Raphael, *Nach dem Boom: Perspektiven auf die Zeitgeschichte seit 1970* (Göttingen: Vandenhoeck & Ruprecht, 2012).

3   For example, see also F. Bruns, 'Krankheit, Konflikte und Versorgungsmängel: Patienten und ihre Eingaben im letzten Jahrzehnt der DDR', *Medizinhistorisches Journal* 47 (2012), 335–67; L. Kalinová, *Konec nadějím a nová očekávání: K dějinám české společnosti 1969–1993* (Prague: Academia, 2012), 203–7; Viola Balz, 'Psychiatriereform in der DDR? Sozialpsychiatrie zwischen Innovationen, Mängelverwaltung und gesundheitspolitischen Präventionsprogrammen', in Annette Eberle et al. eds., *Menschenrechte und Soziale Arbeit im Schatten des Nationalsozialismus: Der lange Weg der Reformen* (Wiesbaden, 2019), 89–106; Eva Pýchová and Karel Dohnal, 'Koncepce veřejného zdravotnictví v České republice v historických souvislostech: Odkud vychází a kam směřuje tento obor?', in Hana Mášová, Eva Křížová and Petr Svobodný, eds., *České zdravotnictví: Vize a skutečnost* (Prague: Karolinum, 2005), 133–46.

4   C. S. Maier, 'Two Sorts of Crisis?: The "Long" 1970s in the West and the East', in H. G. Hockerts, ed., *Koordinaten deutscher Geschichte in der Epoche des Ost-West-Konflikts* (Munich: Oldenbourg, 2004), 49–62. On the networking between medical and psychological experts from the East and West, cf. B. Gausemeier, 'Von konditionierten Ratten und gestressten Werktätigen. Rudolf Baumann und der Stress – und Umweltdiskurs in der DDR', *N.T.M.*, 27 (2019): 311–41; J. Madarász, 'Prävention chronischer Herz-Kreislauf-Krankheiten: BRD, DDR und Großbritannien im Vergleich, 1945–1990', *Prävention und Gesundheitsförderung* 5.4 (2010): 315; Adéla Gjuričová, 'Bohatství pod neviditelným pláštěm? Psychoterapie v Československu po roce 1968', *Soudobé dějiny* 3 (2017): 319. See also the reference to the prevention concepts of the WHO in a lecture manuscript (mid-1960s) by Siegfried Eitner: Humboldt University Archive, collection 039001 (Charité, Department for Industrial Hygiene, 1959–70), folder 77 (Theoretische Arbeiten zum Krankenstand insbesondere in den Industriebetrieben der DDR), lecture manuscript 'Arbeitshygienische

Zielsetzung der Reihenuntersuchung'. On Charvát's participation in East-West professional exchange, see M. Franc, 'Doing One's Laundry in a Hotel Room: The Everydayness of Josef Charvát and Ivan Málek at Congresses and Scientific Conventions in Western Countries in the 1960s', in V. Dvořáčková and M. Franc, eds., *Science Overcoming Borders* (Prague: Masarykův ústav a Archiv AV ČR, v.v.i., 2018), 207–29. For the example of a conference, see V. Fencl, J. Cort, and J. Jirka, eds., *Prague Symposium – Pathogenesis of Essential Hypertension: The Joint WHO Czechoslovak Cardiological Society 1960 Symposium* (Prague: State Med. Publ. House, 1961).

5   R. A. Aronowitz, 'The Converged Experience of Risk and Disease', *The Milbank Quarterly* 87.2 (2009): 417–42.

6   Jens-Uwe Niehoff, 'Anmerkungen zu präventionskonzeptionellen Diskussionen in der DDR', *Jahrbuch für kritische Medizin* 31 (1999): 103–127; W. Süß, 'Gesundheitspolitik', in H. G. Hockerts, ed., *Drei Wege deutscher Sozialstaatlichkeit: NS-Diktatur, Bundesrepublik und DDR im Vergleich* (Munich: Hockerts, 1998), 55–100, 68; Madarász, 'Prävention chronischer Herz-Kreislauf-Krankheiten: BRD, DDR und Großbritannien im Vergleich, 1945–1990', 313–18; C. Timmermann, 'Appropriating Risk Factors: The Reception of an American Approach to Chronic Disease in the two German States, c. 1950–1990', *Social History of Medicine* 25.1 (2012): 157–74; L. Kalinová, 'Zdravotnictví (Healthcare)', in J. Kocian, ed., *Slovníková příručka k československým dějinám 1948–1989* (Prague: Ústav pro soudobé dějiny Akademie věd České republiky, 2006), 42–3.

7   P. Oderich, *Lebe ich richtig? Risikofaktoren in unserem Leben – Die Methode des autogenen Trainings* (Berlin: Dt. Verl. der Wiss, 1977), 23–70. See also the list of guidebooks and self-help literature on dealing with risk factors published in the early 1970s in Oderich's book: ibid., 124 and S. Trča, *Komplexní zdravotní výchova v rámci kardiovaskulárního a onkologického programu v okrese* (Prague: Dt. Verl. der Wiss, 1981).

8   J. Pfister and N. Schnog, eds., *Inventing the Psychological: Toward a Cultural History of Emotional Life in America* (New Haven: Yale University Press, 1997); N. Rose, *Inventing Our Selves: Psychology, Power, and Personhood* (Cambridge: Cambridge University Press, 1998); S. Maasen, J. Elberfeld, P. Eitler and M. Tändler, eds., *Das beratene Selbst. Zur Genealogie der Therapeutisierung in den 'langen' Siebzigern* (Bielefeld: Transcript Verlag, 2011).

9   On the history of mental health in socialist Eastern and Central Europe, see Aleksandra Brokman's chapter in this volume. See also G. Eghigian, 'Was There a Communist Psychiatry?: Politics and East German Psychiatric Care, 1945–1989', *Harvard Review of Psychiatry* 10.6 (2002): 364–68; S. Marks, 'Suggestion, Persuasion and Work: Psychotherapies in Communist Europe', *European Journal of Psychotherapy & Counselling* 20.1 (2018): 1–15; Gjuričová, 'Bohatství pod neviditelným pláštěm?' For contemporary examples of psychological advisory literature, see Siegfried Schnabl, *Nervös? Ursachen, Erscheinungsformen, Vorbeugung und Überwindung psychosozialer Gesundheitsstörungen* (Berlin, 1977); Stanislav Kratochvíl, *Jak žít s neurózou: Rady nemocným* (Prague: Avicenum zdravotnické nakladatelství, 1981). On therapeutic tobacco cessation, see Tricia Stark's contribution to this volume.

10 Numerous press articles from the 1970s and 80s address the problem of neurotic disorders, often making reference to a rising number of cases. See, for example, Anon., 'Autogenes Training für Gesunde: Psychische Spannungen auch ohne Medikamente zu beheben', *Neues Deutschland*, 8 November 1975; Z. Kukurová, 'Jako v království Šípkové Růženky: Elektrospánek v lázních Jeseníku navrácí zdraví a

dobrou mysl', *Pravda (Bratislava)*, 20 July 1978; Anon., 'Eigenschaften des modernen Patienten: Krankheitsbilder verwischen und sind schwieriger zu diagnostizieren', *Berliner Zeitung*, 27 December 1986.

11 On the institutionalization of psychosomatic medicine since the 1960s, see Dieter Seefeldt and Maria Ullrich, 'Das Anti-Streß-Programm: Eine Serie psychagogischer Vorträge innerhalb eines komplexen Therapieprogramms für funktionell-neurotische und psychosomatische Erkrankungen', *Zeitschrift für Physiotherapie* 32 (1980): 429–34; Jiří Kňazovčík, David Vačilja and Lukáš Záveský, *Dějiny Psychiatrické léčebny v Horních Beřkovicích v letech 1891–2011* (Horní Beřkovice, 2011); Anon., *Sedmdesát let psychiatrické léčebny v Kroměříži: 1909–1979* (Kroměříž: OÚNZ, 1979); M. Geyer, ed., *Psychotherapie in Ostdeutschland: Geschichte und Geschichten 1945–1995* (Göttingen: Vandenhoeck & Ruprecht, 2011), 112–14, 369–88, 565–8; A. Geisthövel, 'Karl Leonhard oder die Individualtherapie der Neurosen', in A. Geisthövel and B. Hitzer, eds., *Auf der Suche nach einer anderen Medizin: Psychosomatik im 20. Jahrhundert* (Berlin: Suhrkamp Verlag, 2019), 222–32; L. Malich, 'Kurt Höck oder der verordnete Aufstand des neurotischen Körpers', in A. Geisthövel and B. Hitzer, eds., *Auf der Suche*, 300–312.

12 See the overview of Czech spas with psychological and psychosomatic treatment options in the Czech National Archive, Prague, collection 966 (Ministry of Health of the Czech Socialist Republic, Meetings of the Ministerial Board, 1969–86), folder 42, document entitled 'Organizační uspořádání čs. státních lázní a jejich indikační zaměření', 10 February 1982. See Also Oldřich Grünner, *Lázeňské léčebné postupy v terapii neuroz* (Bratislava: Práca, 1967); A. Erbe and H. Hess, 'Die Häufigkeit neurotischer Störungen in einem Kneippsanatorium und daraus resultierende Konsequenzen', *Zeitschrift für ärztliche Fortbildung* 69 (1975): 1173.

13 On the history of 'stress' as a term of expert language even outside of the field of healthcare, see Jackson, *The Age of Stress*, 21–223; R. Viner, 'Putting Stress in Life: Hans Selye and the Making of Stress Theory', *Social Studies of Science*, 29.3 (1999): 391–410.

14 Kury, *Der überforderte Mensch*, 267–90; L. Haller, S. Höhler and H. Stoff, 'Stress – Konjunkturen eines Konzepts', *Zeithistorische Forschungen* 11.3 (2014): 359–81.

15 I treat this topic in more detail in: Arend., 'Ist Stress westlich?'; Jan Arend, 'Stress in the USSR: On the Dissemination of Health Knowledge in the Soviet Public Sphere, 1960s–1991', *Comparativ* 29.2 (2019): 91–104.

16 Such paths of transfer are traced for the case of the GDR in Gausemeier, 'Von konditionierten Ratten', 312, 320, 322–4.

17 The United States in particular was portrayed as a veritable land of stress in this regard. See, for example, Anon., 'Ještě jednou o infarktu', *Vlasta*, 6 November 1978.

18 For examples of media reports tacitly or explicitly acknowledging stress as a phenomenon of life in socialism, see Anon., 'Stress a agrese', *Mladý svět*, 15 February 1977; M. Pokorná, 'Dítě potřebuje klid', *Vlasta*, 28 September 1977; H. Henselin, 'Tragische Unfälle – eine Warnung. Gespräch mit dem Generalmajor Heribert Mally, Leiter der Hauptabteilung Verkehrspolizei im MdI, über den Ferienreiseverkehr', *Neues Deutschland*, 13 July 1985; Karl Hecht, 'Manches Wissenswerte über das "Salz des Lebens": Einige Überlegungen für praktische Verhaltensweisen zur Beherrschung des Stresses im täglichen Leben', *Berliner Zeitung*, 3 September 1988.

19 Berlin State Archive, collection C Rep 411 (VEB Transformatorenwerk 'Karl Liebknecht'), folder 1504, document entitled 'Bericht für L, W und BGL', 24 October 1964, sheets 1, 7–8 and 10.

20 Czech National Archive Prague, collection 855 (Government Office of the Czech Socialist Republic and Czech Republic, 1969–92), box 95lom7, folder 33, document entitled 'Návrh souboru opatření ke snižování absence pro nemoc', 28 December 1972. See also the discussion of 'risk workplaces' due to mental strain in the Czech National Archive, Prague, collection 966 (Ministry of Health of the Czech Socialist Republic, Meetings of the Ministerial Board, 1969–86), box 32, folder 6, document entitled 'Návrh koncepce oboru hygieny práce a nemocí z povolání', 12 December 1977.

21 'Fröhlich sing ich meine Lieder wie das liebe Vogelvieh, denn es zucken alle Glieder nach der Physiotherapie [...] Selbst im Kopfe ist es lichte, denn es hat sich ausgestresst!' Document 'Unser Kliniklied' (1980s), private archive Dr Johannes Kreissl, Potsdam. For further examples, see J. Arend., 'Ist Stress westlich?'. On the use of dachas in the late socialist period, see S. Lovell, *Summerfolk: A History of the Dacha, 1710-2000* (Ithaca, N.Y.: Cornell University Press, 2003), 197–208.

22 'Fröhlich sing ich meine Lieder wie das liebe Vogelvieh, denn es zucken alle Glieder nach der Physiotherapie [...] Selbst im Kopfe ist es lichte, denn es hat sich ausgestresst!' Document 'Unser Kliniklied' (1980s), private archive Dr Johannes Kreissl, Potsdam; Personal interview with Dr Johannes Kreissl, 6 June 2019. For further examples, see Arend., 'Ist Stress westlich?'.

23 On the socialist hero narrative, see K. Clark, *The Soviet Novel: History as Ritual* (Bloomington: Indiana University Press, 2000), especially 124–9; V. Macura, *Šťastný Věk: A jiné studie o socialistické kultuře* (Prague: Academia, 2008), 35–45, 96–104. On mental and bodily characteristics, see T. Clark, 'The "New Man's" Body: A Motif in Early Soviet Culture', in M. C. Bown and B. Taylor, eds., *Art of the Soviets: Painting, Sculpture, and Architecture in a One-Party State, 1917–1992* (Manchester: Manchester University Press, 1993), 33–50, 40–8.

24 The socialist ideology spoke of the 'New Soviet Man' in this context. See Günther, *Der sozialistische Übermensch: Maksim Gor'kij und der sowjetische Heldenmythos* (Stuttgart: J.B. Metzler, 1993).

25 See J. McCannon, 'Positive Heroes at the Pole: Celebrity Status, Socialist-Realist Ideals and the Soviet Myth of the Arctic, 1932–39', *Russian Review* 56.3 (1997): 346–65; J. Bergman, 'Valerii Chkalov: Soviet Pilot as New Soviet Man', *Journal of Contemporary History* 33.1 (1998): 135–52.

26 N. Ostrovskii, *Kak zakalialas' stal'* (Moscow: Molodaia gvardiia, 1934).

27 See, for example, E. Dobrenko and N. Jonsson-Skradol, eds., *Socialist Realism in Central and Eastern European Literatures: Institutions, Dynamics, Discourses* (London: Anthem Press, 2018).

28 See L. A. Kirschenbaum and N. M. Wingfield, 'Gender and the Construction of Wartime Heroism in Czechoslovakia and the Soviet Union', *European History Quarterly* 39.3 (2009): 465–89; L. H. Siegelbaum, *Stakhanovism and the Politics of Productivity in the USSR, 1935–1941* (Cambridge: Cambridge University Press, 1990); A. L. Jenks, *The Cosmonaut Who Couldn't Stop Smiling: The Life and Legend of Yuri Gagarin* (Ithaca, N. Y.: Cornell University Press, 2019). The cults surrounding the political leaders – beginning with Lenin – likewise exhibited signs of hero worship. See B. Apor, J. C. Behrends, P. Jones and E. A. Rees, eds., *The Leader Cult in Communist Dictatorships: Stalin and the Eastern Bloc* (Basingstoke: Palgrave Macmillan, 2004).

29 Hero propaganda did not always work entirely as intended by the system, however. The popular meanings of specific hero legends and the form of emulation that they inspired were shaped by a process of communication between the regime and the

people that the party cadres in charge of propaganda and education could not fully control. See S. Satjukow and R. Gries, 'Zur Konstruktion des "sozialistischen Helden". Geschichte und Bedeutung', in R. Gries and S. Satjukow, eds., *Sozialistische Helden: Eine Kulturgeschichte von Propagandafiguren in Osteuropa und der DRR* (Berlin: Links, 2002), 15–34. The acceptance of socialist hero figures also depended on the national context. Heroism had a specific place in the different national traditions and historical cultures. See, for example, D. Pratt, 'Troubles with History: The Anecdote, History, and the Petty Hero in Central Europe', in I. Kacandes and Y. Komska, eds., *Eastern Europe Unmapped: Beyond Borders and Peripheries* (New York: Berghahn Books, 2020), 133–50; H. Haumann, '"Held" und "Volk" in Osteuropa: Eine Annäherung', *Osteuropa* 57.12 (2007): 5–16.

30 S. Satjukow, '"Früher war das eben der Adolf …". Der Arbeitsheld Adolf Hennecke', in Gries and Satjukov, eds., *Sozialistische Helden*, 115–32.

31 McCannon, 'Positive Heroes', 359–63; S. Zwicker, *'Nationale Märtyrer': Albert Leo Schlageter und Julius Fučík: Heldenkult, Propaganda und Erinnerungskultur* (Paderborn: Schöningh, 2006), 189–235.

32 R. Sartorti, 'On the Making of Heroes, Heroism, and Saints', in R. Stites, ed., *Culture and Entertainment in Wartime Russia* (Bloomington: Indiana University Press, 1995), 176–93, 187. Similarly, Catriona Kelly writes the following with reference to the heroes of the socialist youth organizations in the Soviet Union: 'Increasingly, then, material about pioneer heroes had become the stuff of homework reading and nothing more'. See C. Kelly, *Comrade Pavlik: The Rise and Fall of a Soviet Boy Hero* (London: Granta, 2006), 215.

33 On alternative hero figures, see J. Kubik, *The Power of Symbols against the Symbols of Power: The Rise of Solidarity and the Fall of State Socialism in Poland* (University Park: Pennsylvania State University Press, 1994), especially 129–52; S. Stach, *Vermächtnispolitik: Jan Palach und Oskar Brüsewitz als politische Märtyrer* (Göttingen: Wallstein Verlag, 2016), 27–35.

34 Behrends, 'Helden und Heroismus', 14; R. Gries, 'Die Heldenbühne der DDR: Zur Einführung', in Gries and Satjukov, eds., *Sozialistische Helden*, 84–100, here 100.

35 D. Seefeldt, *Streß: Verstehen – Erkennen – Bewältigen* (Leipzig: Urania Verlag, 1989), 316. The book was first published in 1979. Cf. D. Seefeldt, *Stress – was tun? Anleitung zu Körper – und Nerventraining* (Berlin: Verlag Tribüne, 1979). See also L. Mojžíšová, *Aby nás záda nebolela. Díl 1. Cviky pro uvolnění a posílení krční páteře* (Prague: Ústav zdravotní výchovy, 1987), 3; L. Hruška, *Uvolňovací a posilovací cviky při bolestech páteře a svalstva* (Prague: Ústav zdravotní výchovy, 1987).

36 The notion of 'pleasure' in Seefeldt's language is notable and should be seen in the context of state socialist discourses on pleasure and the good life. For further detail, see D. Crowley and S. Reid, eds., *Pleasures in Socialism: Leisure and Luxury in the Eastern Bloc* (Evanston, IL.: Northwestern University Press, 2010).

37 On yoga in state socialism, see I. Costache, 'The Biography of a Scandal: Experimenting with Yoga during Romanian Late Socialism', in J. Furst, M. A. Fichter and J. McLellan, eds., *Dropping Out of Socialism: The Creation of Alternative Spheres in the Soviet Bloc* (Lanham: Lexington Books, 2017), 23–40; M. Tietke, *Yoga in der DDR: Geächtet, geduldet, gefördert* (Kiel: Ludwig, 2014), 63–141. On autogenic training, see W.-R. Krause, 'Hypnose und Autogenes Training in den 1980er Jahren', in M. Geyer, ed., *Psychotherapie in Ostdeutschland*, 555–7.

38 Personal interview with the East German physician and psychotherapist Karl-Heinz Bomberg, 18 January 2018. See also the recollections of Czech writer Daniela

Fischerová, who began practising Yoga around 1968: M. Vaněk, ed., *Obyčejní lidé–?! Pohled do života tzv. mlčící většiny* (Prague: Academia, 2009), Vol. 2, 186–90.

39 Milada Bartoňová et al., *Joga od staré Indie k dnešku* (Prague: Avicenum dravotnické nakladatelství, 1971); Horst Stahlberg, *Yoganastik für jedermann: 80 Übungen zur aktiven Gesunderhaltung* (Magdeburg: Volksstimme, 1978); Werner König, Gerhard Di Pol and Gerhard Schaeffer, *Fibel für autogenes Training Anleitung für Übende* (Jena: Fischer, 1979); Karel Vojáček, *Autogenní trénink* (Prague: Oddělení zdravotní výchovy Krajského ústavu národního zdraví, 1988).

40 Z. Fejfas, 'Zásady k omezení infarktu', *Vlasta*, 22 May 1974. See also P. Zemek, 'O věcech intimních', *Mladý svět*, 30 January 1973.

41 See, for example, Hans Arnold et al., *Die Komplexe sozialistische Rationalisierung in der Industrie der DDR* (Berlin: Verl. Die Wirtschaft, 1967), 74; E. Kersten, *Dritter Kongreß der Gesellschaft für Arbeitshygiene und Arbeitsschutz 1969, 21–4. Oktober 1969 in Potsdam: Arbeitshygiene und Arbeitsschutz im Prozeß der wissenschaftlich-technischen Revolution in der DDR* (Berlin: Verl. Volk u. Gesundheit, 1971), 36–7, 54, 67; Z. Bureš, *Psychologie práce a její užití* (Prague: Práce, 1973), 174–89; W. Hacker and P. Richter, *Psychische Fehlbeanspruchung, psychische Ermüdung, Monotonie, Sättigung und Stress* (Berlin: Springer, 1980).

42 J. Thamm, *Ausgleich und Entspannung* (Berlin: Verlag Volk u. Gesundheit, VEB, 1973), 22, 45. Seefeldt mentions that midday naps were prescribed by a company physician at a weaving mill near Zittau. See Seefeldt, *Stress – was tun?*, 108.

43 See Company Archive Carl Zeiss Jena, archive unit VA 01389 (Modell der Leitung des Teilsystems Körperkultur und Sport im Kombinat VEB Carl Zeiss Jena, 27 February 1969), sheet 20. On compensating sports at other companies in the GDR, see M. W. Johnson, *Training Socialist Citizens: Sports and the State in East Germany* (Leiden: Brill, 2008), 83–4, 141.

44 See, for example, the emphasis on the importance of sleep for heavily burdened executives in G. Thiele, *Das Zeitbudget in der Leitungstätigkeit* (Leipzig: DEU Leipzig, 1988), 18. See also K. Hecht, *Gesundheit und Menschenführung* (Leipzig: Urania-Verlag, 1969), 8; Haller, Höhler, and Stoff, 'Stress', 368.

Part Two

Practices

5

Work and therapy: Two visions of the Bulgarian New Man

Julian Chehirian

Introduction

This chapter examines work therapy as a technology of mind and body that was intimately connected to the politics and practices of building communism in Bulgaria. Work therapy was the foremost method of psychotherapy in psychiatric institutions for mentally and physically disabled people in the People's Republic of Bulgaria (1946–90). Tracing the relationship between therapeutic and non-therapeutic work, we will follow the parallel lives of Nikola and Dimitar Kazakov – two brothers, both artists. While connected by birth, artistic vocation and eccentricity, Nikola's and Dimitar's life trajectories were shaped by different institutional organs of the Bulgarian socialist State: for Nikola the psychiatric system, and for Dimitar the Union of Artists. Dimitar's work was lauded nationally and found its way to the Louvre; whereas Nikola, whom many artistic colleagues held to have been equally talented, was separated from art making – toiling instead on a pig farm as a psychiatric patient. Nikola has been forgotten. By examining Nikola's life through the prism of the Bulgarian State, however, we will see that Nikola's life is not *simply obscured*. Rather, its negativity can tell us something about the complex relationships between work, ideology and psychiatry in the recent history of Southeast European socialism. The Kazakov brothers are a revealing dyad across which to examine obverse incarnations of socialist subjecthood across the boundaries of mental illness and disability. These conditions, which have been less examined than physical disabilities in recent literature, raise provocative questions about the diversities concealed by the ideal of the Bulgarian 'New Man' – an embodiment of socialist maxims, and a modern subject achieved through the alternate path to modernity constituted by Soviet-style socialism.

Work was an overdetermined category in the Bulgarian socialist-era context, at once an action, an identity, a class and socio-political category; a driver of historical process; a form of sociality and a constituter of collectives – jointing individual action and collective purpose.[1] In the Bulgarian socialist republic, as in the broader Marxist-Leninist tradition, it was vested with transformative power, a quality made explicit through injunctions to contribute, through one's work, to the construction of communism.[2] The Bulgarian 'New Man' was to have a voluntarist character. And yet, participation in the building of communism was not voluntary. If work could transform individuals into a revolutionary working class – self-aware instigators of political emancipation from bourgeois rule – the opposite was feared. Inaction, resistance, dissent or action against the grain of revolution could imperil this process. In the earliest years of the regime, forced labour was envisioned as a method of ideological re-education. However, violence, starvation, disease, intimidation and backbreaking work quotas rather than re-education evolved into the reality of punitive labour in the People's Republic of Bulgaria. Lilia Topouzova has recently revealed that Bulgaria operated one of the most expansive and violent forced labour camp systems in Eastern Europe, which not only survived de-Stalinization but was re-invigorated in the mid-1980s in a campaign against Bulgarian Turks and the Muslim minority.[3] Work had these multiple meanings and valences in the politics of the socialist State.

Work therapy, I argue, is a form of labour qualification and exclusion that has remained obscured in our understanding of this period. Work therapy aimed to effect psychotherapeutic benefits for the individual, but also to increase the work ability of patients (*rabotosposobnost*).[4] This was believed to facilitate, furthermore, a process of social rehabilitation by inclusion in a workforce. Work therapy, however, proved to be a context of ideological qualification and social exclusion for individuals with mental illnesses and mental disabilities. As Claire Shaw has demonstrated in her work on deafness and disability in the Soviet Union, some disabled individuals saw labour capacity as a means of emancipation and agency. In the Bulgarian context, disability unions were active in representing workers with physical disabilities. This was not operative, however, for psychiatric institutions with work-therapy programmes. Mentally ill and mentally disabled patient-workers were excluded from key features of the society of socialist labour such as pay, participation in labour unions, inclusion in ritual celebrations of labour and additional trade-organized benefits in the form of programmes for personal finance and leisure. Psychiatric institutions functioned as spaces of exclusionary delimitation from the emancipatory ideals and infrastructure of socialist labour. Mandating work therapy for workers who the State saw as 'defective' and unfit for regular output, the State engineered not just individual workers, but also a distinct category of workers. Individuals in work therapy were outside labourers, captive to an institutional interior.

Nikola Kazakov's transition from worker to psychiatric inpatient to patient-worker is a cross-section of institutional conditions for individuals with mental disabilities. Nikola's first hospitalization extracted him from ordinary socialist labour and society and placed him in a facility that treated patients pharmacologically, and that lacked resources for psychotherapeutic care. He was severed from his ordinary socialist labour, but also from his artistic vocation and from his means for potentially therapeutic self-expression through artistic work during a prolonged period of psychiatric crisis. In this first period, we see psychiatric hospitalization as a state of exclusion from participation in the socialist State. After his escape from the first institution, Nikola was captured and assigned, out of expedience, to a social home for deaf individuals with developmental disorders closer to his hometown. This second institution was the first such institution in Bulgaria to initiate a programme for work as therapy. His assignment to unpaid work there will offer a complicated look at the intersection of disabilities within social care institutions.

The case study presented here may proffer insights into Soviet and socialist modernities by studying the interface of labour, ideology and psychiatry at a vulnerable fault-point – the lives of the ill and marginalized. For historians of science, the case study may raise important questions of individual agency on the side of patients and hospital directors, tempering tendencies for homogenizing analyses of transnational knowledge transfer.[5] By making use of not just institutional, but also oral history and visual sources, it aims to address a problematic silence of patient testimony in the archive. The first section provides an overview of the socialist-era psychiatry in Bulgaria and examines the implementation of work therapy in Bulgaria, while placing Bulgarian social homes for mentally ill and disabled individuals into a broader regional and historiographical context. The second and third sections examine the divergent dyad of Nikola and Dimitar, while placing Nikola's institutional experiences into historical context.

Note on method

This chapter attempts to address a silence that historians of psychiatry must reckon with – that of patient testimony.[6] To work within this silence concerning Nikola Kazakov's experience, I have conducted oral histories with three individuals who were involved with the deinstitutionalization and subsequent care of Nikola Kazakov. Their testimony has allowed me to corroborate details of Nikola's hospitalizations. The first individual is Georgi Todorov, an artist who was Nikola's caretaker and professional representative between 1995 and 1997. The second is Tzvetan Kolev, an artist and associate of Dimitar Kazakov who secured the installation of Nikola's and Dimitar's artwork in a permanent museum during his tenure as Director of the City Museum of Tryavna. The third is Lyuba Tsaneva, a curator at the City Museum of Tryavna and close friend of Dimitar, who was involved in Nikola's life post discharge. Nikola did not write much. However, he produced abundant visual testimony through a body of work that was inflected by the onset of his illness. His sculptures – effigies hand carved from knobby, knotted tree branches – articulate a seemingly somatized psychic distress (Figure 5.1). Axiniya Dzhurova, an art historian, notes how these figures keel, brace, recoil and silently gaze forward in their articulated postures.[7] Nikola's canvases, on the other hand, seem to reconstitute a lost pre-industrial social order – indexing a series of dislocations – from land, family, occupation and identity that comprised his position in socialist society. A subjective record of Nikola's illness is non-existent in written form, but Nikola left behind powerful traces of his experience that remain a part of a material-historical record. We must engage with these objects if we seek, as this chapter does, to understand Nikola's experience. Additional interviews with Filip Zidarov and Rumen Serafimov, both curators, and Orlin Dvorianov, an artist, aid in my contextualization of the structuring mechanisms of the Union of Bulgarian Artists.

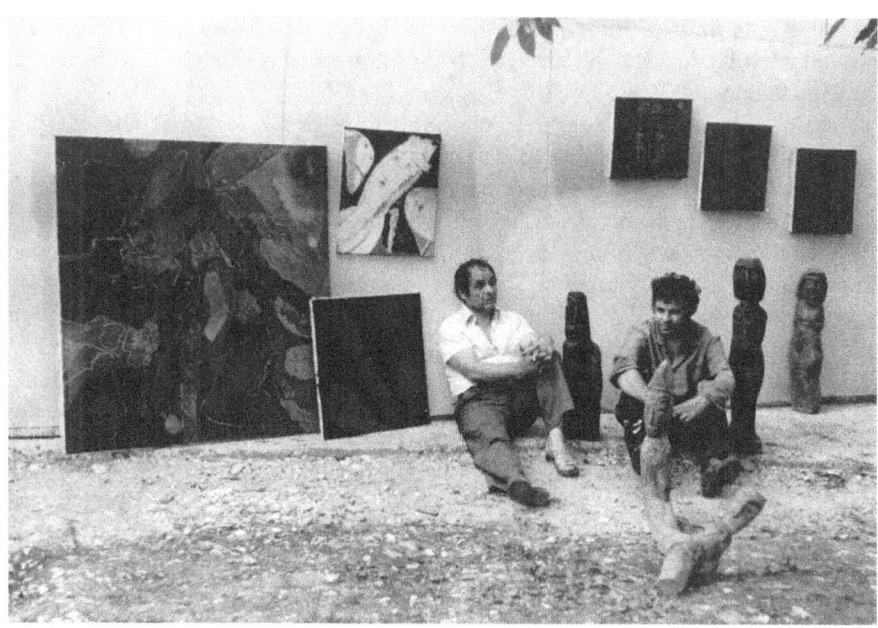

Figure 5.1 Dimitar Kazakov and Nikola Kazakov before the fire, 1979/80. Personal Archive.

Psychiatry, work and disability

As the history of psychiatry in Bulgaria is not well known, I will sketch its contours briefly. The Bulgarian psychiatric profession emerged at the turn of the twentieth century, stimulated by exchanges with German, Austrian and Russian universities.[8] The first dedicated psychiatric wards in Bulgaria were founded between 1880 and 1888.[9] The interwar period saw a national network of hospitals take form, and the postwar period a large-scale expansion of an outpatient clinic and dispensary network.[10] After 1947, the ascendant Communist Party abolished private medical practice, thus centralizing the administration of clinics, professional societies and university programmes. For Bulgarian inpatients from the late 1950s to the 1980s, psychiatric care consisted predominantly of pharmacological intervention.[11] In the early 1950s a series of scientific conferences in the USSR produced a sanctioned interpretation of Ivan Pavlov's scientific work on physiology.[12] The canonized Pavlovian view reified physiological factors underlying pathological conditions while devaluing non-empirical, subjective dimensions of human experience.[13] The Soviet debates were reflected in the recently established Bulgarian socialist republic, which appointed its own 'Pavlovian committee' to assess and implement the decisions of the Pavlovian sessions.[14] Between the mid-1950s and the late 1960s, the Pavlovian model dominated the field. Methodological diversification advanced in the 1970s and 1980s.[15] However, a nearly exclusive somatic emphasis in diagnosis and treatment continued as a norm in Bulgarian psychiatry. The apparent exclusivity of the Soviet approach in Bulgaria, however, did not prevent Bulgarian officials from developing vernacular adaptations of the Soviet approach to work therapy.

While the metamorphic and emancipatory promises of work were central to Marxist-Leninist ideation and Soviet rhetoric, the idea of work as transformative was not a Soviet innovation. The binding of work and transformation has earlier tendrils in the wake of the Enlightenment.[16] For Hegel and Marx, work *articulated* the subject into the world. For Michel Foucault, it disciplines.[17] With the perceived capacity for regulating its practitioners, work became a fixture of 'moral treatment' in the asylums of the late eighteenth and nineteenth centuries. Asylums organized environments for the rationalization of subjects through orderly architecture, simulated family units and the structured dispensation of time spent within their bounds. Hundreds of insane asylums built during the nineteenth century were conceived and designed based on the understanding that a rational environment could heal.[18] Asylum superintendents sought to organize patients into a productive rhythm of existence: farming, working with livestock, learning to operate machinery to produce goods in specialized workshops, or creating modest handicrafts. At the core of these practices lay the assumption that the individual was morally autonomous and governed by reason. The denigration of the latter was understood as treatable through exposure to exemplars of reason. Work, as it was understood, should restore productive capacity to individuals and to their society at large.

In post-Revolutionary Russia, work was not just a moral obligation but also an identity and a political obligation towards the State.[19] L.L. Rokhlin, a Soviet psychiatrist, argued that 'now, when, in our country, work has become the primary human need, the foundation and stimulus for creative life, one appreciates even better the psychotherapeutic importance of meaningful, purposeful and joyful work'.[20] The Soviet psychiatrist V.A. Giliarovskii 'valued the element of self-coercion in work, which, in his words, makes the patient overcome inner resistance', as Sirotkina and Kokorina write.[21] The Soviet person's contribution to building communism was above all their labour capacity. The New Soviet Person – as an ideal and archetype of revolutionary subjecthood – was capable not only of normal production, but of exceeding the limits of human capacity, such as with the norm-busting Stakhanovites.[22]

There were tensions between ideas of productivity, disability and social 'usefulness' in the Soviet context. Claire Shaw positions the deaf and deafened in a broader landscape of Soviet identities in relation to normative and able-bodied participation in the workforce.[23] Deafness 'did not preclude physical fitness or labour, key aspects of the theoretical makeup of the New Soviet Person'. It 'did not prevent an individual from wielding a hammer or working a metal lathe, nor, as the decades passed, did it impede deaf participation in the symbolic rituals of Soviet life'.[24] In what Lilya Kaganovsky articulates as a subversion of 'the cultural fantasy of virile, Stalinist masculinity', deafness, Shaw continues, occupied a 'distinctly liminal category' between Stakhanovites and disabled veterans.[25]

Unease about the centrality of improving work capacity to therapeutic work programmes predated the Soviet period in Russia, as in the case of Tsarist-era psychiatrist S.S. Stupin. As Sirotkina and Kokorina write, S.S. Stupin, 'the first psychiatrist in Russia to raise publically the issue of work for patients', argued that 'using patients' work to cover the hospital expenses [...] is incompatible with the idea of moral treatment'. The output of work therapy was, in fact, a significant means of subsistence for many institutions. Whereas predecessor therapeutic work innovators like the Tuke family of York conceived of patient work as non-productive and chiefly moral in significance, in the Russian case, 'work in practice became product-oriented as it often constituted the hospital's income'. Many Russian psychiatrists 'refused to give monetary reward to patients even when they used their labour'.[26]

While work therapy had emancipatory aspirations, its concretization in institutional practices occurred in a global context where, as Stephen Kotkin reminds us, socialist and capitalist states were competing in a geopolitical arena.[27] Gamarini-Kabala has argued that the idea of therapeutic work for mentally disabled children 'departed from its original emancipatory ideals and, in the end, reduced all human worth to the ability to perform productively'. The Soviet ideology of care for the mentally disabled reveals, for her, that labour was paradoxically 'a means of rehabilitation, a sign of integration, and a reason for exclusion'.[28] Aleksandra Brokman's contribution in this volume shows us that in Soviet psychotherapy, the value and significance placed on willpower in overcoming challenges was modulated in cases of chronic illness or disability, where acceptance was recommended as a way forward, contrasting the idea that all limitations could be transcended by volition.

The Soviet Union's 'productivist' and 'functionalist' policy on labour for the mentally disabled, as Sarah D. Phillips characterizes it, can help us understand its latency in the Bulgarian system. The prior approach was structured on the principle of hierarchical differentiation and ranking. Within a framework that linked disability status to work capacity, intellectually and mentally disabled individuals were 'excluded from the ranks of "invalids" and the concomitant benefits and entitlements'.[29] In Bulgaria, disabled individuals could participate in unions (e.g. Union of the Deaf, Union of the Blind) which participated in specially adapted work programmes such as in production-work cooperatives (*trudovo proizvoditelni kooperatsii*) and programmes for working from home (*nadomna rabota*) for those with limited mobility and labour capacity. Programmes for individuals with mental disabilities, however, were less flexible. In the absence of family care, individuals with mental disabilities were frequently institutionalized in long-term residential facilities, where work therapy, the primary form of psychotherapy (aside from pharmacological treatment), was implicitly linked to productive capacity.

Bulgarian health officials characterized the Soviet model of work therapy as highly effective and ideologically sound: furthering the goal of educating and disciplining mentally and physically disabled individuals into socially productive work. Work therapy was implemented in Bulgarian psychiatric hospitals and social homes with theoretical justifications adopted from Soviet exemplars.[30] In a 1956 Bulgarian psychiatric textbook written by V. A. Giliarovskii, the entire section on psychotherapy constitutes a description of 'work therapy'. Soviet psychiatrists, he writes, 'developed a special system – work therapy, which has a significant role in the fortification of mental (nerve-psychological) health. It plays a significant role in the treatment of neurotic states.' As Galiarovskii emphasizes, 'the goal of work therapy is to organize the working-life of the patient, to return them to socially beneficial work in the community'.[31] Anticipating the import that this rationale would have for Bulgaria, the author further stresses that 'scientific thought in this special field in Bulgaria and in the Soviet Union proceeds along the same pathways and is informed by the same theoretical foundation'.[32] In Bulgaria, however, a protracted debate ensued about the organizational and, indeed, managerial implementation of work therapy. Bulgarian officials in the health ministry and republic-ministerial committee debated whether and how to compensate patients for work performed. In a deviation from the Soviet model, which compensated patients for work, Bulgarian officials would rule against pay. This would give Bulgarian work therapy a different nature than Soviet work therapy.

The fire

In 1980, on a sparsely populated plateau on the outskirts of the capital of the socialist People's Republic of Bulgaria, a man in a woollen sweater climbed out from the second story window of an unfinished home and stood, somehow removed but also inescapably present, on a roof encircled by fire. Dark plumes of smoke rose at his feet, which threatened to stay affixed. This house, which Nikola Kazakov had nearly finished constructing for himself, and the rooms inside of it, joined other recent combustions in his inner world. For as the fire raged and as Nikola called for help, he saw images of others amidst the flames – the face of a recently estranged lover, of his recently deceased mother, and of his brother Dimitar. None were as close or as intimately available to Nikola Kazakov then as the heat.

Sparse plateaus such as this one were ushered symbolically into the centre with the ascension of the Bulgarian Communist Party to political power in 1947. The metamorphosis of this fledgling socialist republic from monarchy to a member of the international communist movement was supposed to register in such neglected locales of the country. A socialist modernization project accelerated to breakneck tempo was to leave no backwater untouched. Is the Bulgarian 'New Person' a meaningful category for historians of Bulgarian socialism? After all, in Bulgaria, state-socialism took root at the peak of Soviet Stalinism, and not in the heady era of early Soviet revolutionary and utopian imagination. And yet, I would argue, the powerful ambiguity of revolutionary disruption was live, as well as the transformations it brought about for ordinary people. Those who were to be renewed were recent inheritors of a nation that emerged from the Ottoman Empire just six decades prior (1878). No one was left untouched by these projects. The New Bulgarian People were not only agents of a future, but also subjects surveilled by a repressive State Security apparatus that aimed to ensure consent, or to engineer it if it was deemed to be lacking.

Nikola was born in 1935 in the small village of Tsarski Izvor in Central-Northern Bulgaria, his childhood marked by poverty and loss.[33] In his youth, Nikola was called 'slow' by some, an 'idiot' by others.[34] His passage through the institutions of youth further marginalized him. In primary and secondary school Nikola's classmates were younger with each passing year while he grew older. He 'went to school, worked the land, and shepherded cows'.³⁵ During two years of military service by mandatory conscription, his superiors treated him differently than others. He was kept out of the way of other soldiers, delegated to scrubbing mess halls or toilets while the other men flicked cigarettes between firing exercises 'against the capitalists' near the Greek border.³⁶

After fulfilling their military service, the Kazakov brothers initially went in separate directions. Nikola's older brother Dimitar Kazakov (1933–92) went off to study at the prestigious National Academy of Art. Nikola, on the other hand, returned home and apprenticed as a barrel maker.³⁷ Nikola soon decided that he, too, should like to become an artist. The young man began to take lessons in painting with an artist who taught painting to factory workers, and later, took instruction from the art professors Boyan Petrov and Nikola Arashev.³⁸ His early creations – a dim oil painting of a factory facade, a still life of a fruit platter – were described by his later friends and caretakers as 'dull' and 'unappealing', and unsuggestive of any particular skill or talent. By contrast his brother Dimitar would undergo training in the fine arts and become, in a matter of years, an artist of national significance, a figure in the 1970s rebellions against socialist-realist aesthetics by visual artists, and one of a small number of Bulgarian artists whose works are in the collection of the Louvre in Paris and the Pushkin Museum of Fine Arts in Moscow. Yearning to be closer to Dimitar, Nikola soon abandoned barrel making for day labouring on the outskirts of Sofia (moving to the capital itself required official permission or student status), gathering enough skill and materials to begin building his own house.³⁹

As a student at the Academy of Art, Dimitar Kazakov dodged opportunities to produce socialist paintings (of factories, of Lenin, of Georgi Dimitrov) for the proselytization of the working class. In developing a rather unique style and iconography – abstract in form but traditional in content – he was also able to dodge criticism for emulating the 'bourgeois decadence' of abstract painting that art critics associated with so much contemporary artwork produced in the West.⁴⁰ In Dimitar's paintings one sees mythological scenes at once evoking socialist modernist and western modernist aesthetics. His are modernist folk paintings. Space seems not to exist in any typical sense in his canvases – one can be looking onto a body from above and from below, from a side window and from the doorway. Perspective is multiple, and scenes are compound. Outsized faces of villagers project forward towards the viewer and converge with one another, seemingly occupying the same spaces at the same time.

The work of a professional visual artist like Dimitar was intimately tied to the cultural politics of building Communism. In crafting representations, whether in bronze, on canvas or mural, artists could educate, proselytize and provide the public with images of socialist values, ideals and role models. In the Bulgarian socialist republic, as in the broader Soviet-led bloc, the visual artist was in an esteemed and privileged, if highly regulated, situation of employment.⁴¹ This profession straddled the structure of the European fine art academy (with sections for painting, sculpture, graphics, textiles and so on at the National Academy of Art) and the socialist union structure that provided guide rails – a channel for professional maturation and support for artists (ranging from the youth-guild, known as the Union of the Young

Artist, to the Union of Bulgarian Artists).[42] Membership in the latter Union entitled member-artists to exhibit their work in the public system of galleries and museums, accept commissions from the State and to take advantage of other privileges including occasional residencies at art studios owned by the State, located throughout the country, as well as a coveted residence in Paris. An artist without a degree in the fine arts and without Union membership (like Nikola) could not show their work in public, sell it to the State or accept State commissions.[43] In short, one could be an artist only in one's self understanding – bereft of enabling frameworks for the social and financial structures of artistic labour.

Dimitar Kazakov was both breaking rules and following trends within the cultural landscape of 1970s and 80s Bulgaria, when earthy, folkloric identities and inheritances were articulated anew (or quite literally invented, such as *Le Mystère des Voix Bulgares*) and ethno-nationalist themes came to supplant Marxist-Leninist dogma to ballast the Party and the stagnating republic. Artistic labour – artistic production – and even politically ambivalent cultural labour like Dimitar's could be appropriated by the State towards its ends. And yet Dimitar asserted a high degree of autonomy with his work and was protective of his artistic freedom. His art was his work, and his artistic work was his profession – his role in society – unlike his brother Nikola, whose aesthetically similar work fell into the cracks of the State's labour and cultural management. If not for his brother's fame, Nikola would remain invisible.

One morning in 1980, Nikola was melting a solid block of tar to patch the roof.[44] The tar softened very gradually over the course of the early afternoon, with viscous black liquid pooling on the edges. As he turned his attention elsewhere, the solvent he had poured onto the tar caught fire and exploded.[45] In a painting from that same year entitled 'Recovery', Nikola's body, wrapped in bandages, occupies a central register. Above him, a doctor stands, superimposed onto a landscape that shows, in the upper left quadrant, a young woman, and below Nikola's body, in the lower left quadrant, the scene of the accident. Nikola dances amid the flames. Onlookers approach through the murk. In the upper right quadrant, a person – seemingly Nikola – lies on a stretcher. Nikola's burns healed over time. But he never fully recovered in psychological terms. His family found him aloof, unpredictable and impulsive.[46]

Whereas he previously painted with a cautious, hesitant hand, after the fire he seemed to work more quickly, intuitively and with greater abandon.[47] Slow, studied brushstrokes gave way to brisk, confident movements in his artwork. Where he once cautiously embarked upon each new work, now Nikola spread sheets of coarse paint on the canvas quickly and seemingly without concern for mis-steps, spreading dark, earthy tones as a seasoned farmer manipulates layers of tilled soil over a field. Nikola's paintings are often folkloric, featuring agrarian scenes, traditionally dressed villagers, thatched homes, fields in the throes of harvest and circle dances across the horizon. They conjure up idealized visions and recollections of Bulgaria's recently pre-industrial past. This constituted a deep reservoir of collective memory that socialism was to repave vigorously with industry. Georgi Todorov and Tzvetan Kolev both describe Kazakov's practice of sculpting wood out of gnarled, knobby branches.[48] With a wayward stroke of his knife, Nikola could call out of the wood anthropomorphic figures that were living and lifeless, communicative and inaccessible, like spirits liberated from a tree

(Figure 5.1). Nikola's sculptural works appear as bodies whose psychic experiences are conveyed through the body. His sculptures are visceral archives and documents – the rich body of traces and expressions that emerged from a cathartic period of creativity that would, however, soon come to an abrupt end.

By 1982–3 Nikola's mental condition deteriorated and his family could no longer care for him. A psychiatrist recommended that he be taken a village in the western foothills of the Rila Mountains in Kyustendil Province.[49] Nikola was admitted to the 'Home for Men with Mental Disabilities and Idiocy' in Pastra. The home – a long-term residential care facility – had been opened in April of 1980. It would house patients with both chronic mental and physical disabilities, as is often the case to this day with rural 'social homes' in Bulgaria. On 19 November 1980, the first eight residents were admitted. By 1 January 1981, Pastra had twenty-three staff members: one manager, two nurses, one accountant, one cleaner, one handyman, one driver, one cook, three kitchen workers and twelve nurses or orderlies.[50]

Patients at Pastra were subject to poor conditions. They were bathed by staff with hoses through the meshing of outdoor cages. Pastra remained in operation until 2012, when a case went before the European Court of Human Rights (Russi Stanev v. Bulgaria), and the facility was determined to have inhuman and degrading conditions. While year-end summaries between 1981 and 1986 note an annual visit by a psychiatrist, in a jarring, handwritten report in 1987, the director reports that 'since the time of the unveiling of this home, no psychiatrist has ever crossed over its threshold'.[51]

Nikola's treatment at Pastra was exclusively somatic. He was likely administered Chlorpromazine, a pharmaceutical first introduced in the Soviet Union in the 1950s. Benjamin Zajicek writes that this drug, known also by the brand name Thorazine, 'helped ameliorate the symptoms of psychosis: patients became calmer, hallucinations diminished, violent disturbance ceased'.[52] Medications produced tangible effects on patients. But they were not a complete solution to the home's management issues. Dozens of administrative orders called for the heightening of vigilance on the part of orderlies during shift transitions, and the strict forbidding of shift transfers without advance written permission from a supervisor. Of particular concern to supervisors was the repeated failure of their staff to prevent frequent escapes of patients from the hospital – between one and five escapes per year.[53]

A 1983 letter from the Municipal Council notifies the home that 'recently, more and more people lodged in the home are being seen in the village and on the road leading to the Rila Monastery, creating indignation in the local population and fear on the part of women and girls, because some of them undress and leave their clothing on the road'. 'We ask that you ensure that these people are not seen in the village and not allowed outside of the area of the home', the letter concludes.[54] In a sharper tone, in 1986, a Central State Security memorandum notified hospital administrators of sharpened security measures during the time of the 13th Party Congress of the Bulgarian Communist Party. In 'no case and under no circumstances' should any of the inpatients be permitted to leave the facility between 15 March and 15 April 1986, reads the letter from K. Stefanov of the Ministry of the Interior. The planned invisibility of the mentally ill towards visiting officials was a recurring phenomenon.[55]

One New Year's Day in the 1980s, Dimitar travelled to Pastra to visit. When he arrived, the staff on duty informed him that Nikola had escaped. This was not the first time. Someone had spotted a small campfire the previous night on a nearby mountain side. Nikola had developed an obsession with fires since the incident, and a taste for travel by train. Once boarded, he would typically be discovered days later in a distant part of Bulgaria.[56] This time Nikola would make it as far as Veliko Tarnovo – his home region. Out of expedience, the police took him to a nearby institution for the deaf and mentally disabled.

Therapeutic work

In 1987, Nikola Kazakov was permitted to leave the hospital in order to attend the opening of a permanent installation of his and Dimitar's artworks. The location of the museum is, to this day, the Museum of the Old Schoolhouse in the city of Tryavna. In the main hall of this wood and white plaster building is the largest collection of Dimitar's work, alongside five paintings and close to sixty wood sculptures by Nikola Kazakov. Tzvetan Kolev, then director of the museum, recalls that Nikola did not seem, initially, to recognize his work as his own. In 1990, a man named Georgi Todorov, captivated by the works by Nikola on display at the museum, learned of Nikola's whereabouts and drove to Tserova Koria – to a social home for the deaf and mentally disabled where Nikola spent the second chapter of his institutionalization. Ascending to the site of the facility, Georgi took in the sight of the building and its surrounding lands. A group of people were wearing identical clothing and moving in unison as if to a song unheard. They were cutting down tall grasses around the social home.

The State-wide provision of work therapy in socialist Bulgaria can be traced to Ordinance No. 666, calling for the formation of therapeutic work units (*trudovo-lechebni stopanstva*) and artisanal workshops in all Bulgarian psychoneurological institutions (e.g. psychiatric hospitals) and institutions for social care (social homes). This decision was finalized on 10 October 1953, and entered into effect on 1 January 1954. This ordinance originated in a report from Dr Peter Kolarov, the Minister of National Health and Social Services to the chairman of the Ministerial Council of the Republic. There Kolarov wrote that 'work therapy is one of the most effective and active methods for the treatment of mental illness'.[57] Additional justification, whether medical or neurophysiological, was, as usual, not offered.

The 'Home for the Mentally Retarded Deaf' in Tserova Koria was founded on 15 October 1963 as the first institution in Bulgaria for deaf individuals with developmental disorders and mental disabilities. It was also the first such facility in Bulgaria to develop a work-therapy programme. The institution was formed in a series of houses with an initial capacity of sixty beds and twenty-five staff members, including a director, an accountant, a doctor, a nurse, several orderlies, a cook and a cleaner. Work therapy was a core element of the institution from its founding: the Central Committee of the Union of the Deaf in Sofia purchased sixty decares of land from the village for its work-therapy programme.

While a small number of work-therapy programmes may have existed in a limited and self-organized form prior to Ordinance No. 666, Kolarov called for a broad expansion, thus 'applying the wealth of experience of Soviet medicine in our psychoneurological facilities and our facilities for social care' (as can be seen in Figure 5.2, which shows a therapeutic work unit at the Kalukovo psychiatric hospital in the 1960s). However, it becomes evident from the drafting and editing process that the Soviet model was not reproduced in the Bulgarian context. The ordinance would not be signed into action without a protracted debate on the level of the Ministerial Council. The main point of contention was whether or not patients involved in work therapy should be paid for their work. If they were to be paid, how much, and from which accounts? Kolarov argued that artisanal workshops as well as agricultural and animal husbandry cannot be organized and run in a fashion that meets the criteria for State-run enterprises (e.g. factories), because the work performed therein is by individuals who are 'defective to begin with', and further, because 'the goal is not to meet output norms, but is rather a therapeutic one'. It is unlikely that these programmes could be financially self-sufficient, Kolarov writes, without 'harming the therapeutic process, or without having negative consequences on the well-being of the pupils (patient-workers) in the social homes'.[58]

A special daily regimen was established for residents at Tserova Koria. The therapeutic work regimen was organized across two blocks (four hours, two hours) each day. The work-therapy programme expanded in the late 1960s to include not only farmwork (i.e. growing tomatoes, peppers, potatoes, cabbage, onion, corn), but also to include a weaving workshop for assembling brooms, baskets and braiding metal mesh for fences and a fabrication workshop (i.e. for producing items like jar

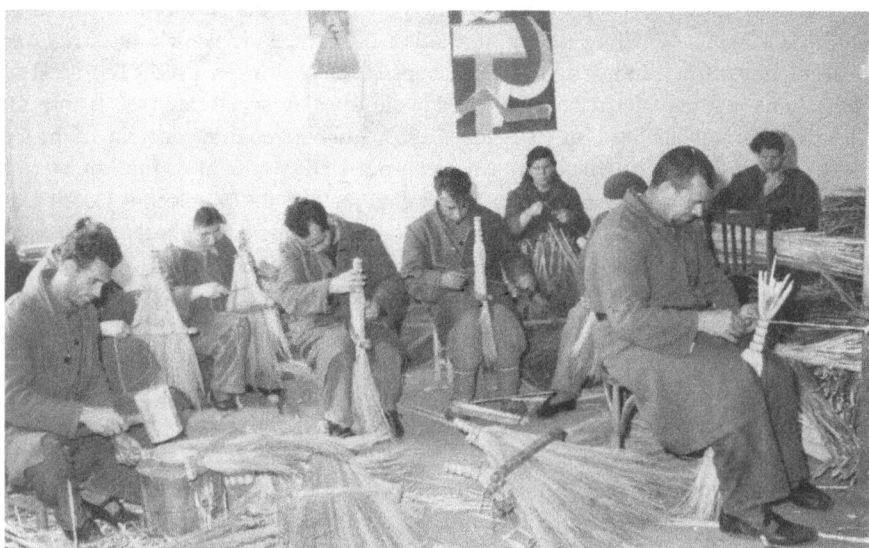

Figure 5.2 Work therapy with patients at the Karlukovo Hospital, 1960s. Personal Archive.

lids, machine washers and small aluminium parts). A 1966 order from the Ministerial Council specified output norms for these lines of production to the Union of the Deaf, which was responsible for their dissemination.[59] Nikola's work therapy at Tserova Koria included farm work and the production of basic goods. Archival photographs of work-therapy practices at psychiatric hospitals in Karlukovo and Lovech suggest that female and male patients performed certain productive tasks in tandem. The work that Nikola performed was generalized, bearing little connection to their prior education or labour specialization.

The debate at the Ministerial Council exposes the divergence between the Bulgarian and Soviet approach to work therapy. In the Soviet context, designated institutions for 'special funds' functioned as escrows or fiscal intermediaries for profits made from such facilities, which were set aside for the organization, maintenance and expansion of therapeutic production enterprises. Indeed, Sarah Marks shows that in the Soviet Union 'there were a number of schemes for the employment of psychiatric patients in agricultural colonies and in turbine factories built within the grounds of asylums, where payment in return for labour was a possibility, and patients could join trade unions'.[60] As Sarah Marks and Mat Savelli have argued, the assumption of a seamless transfer of medical practices from Soviet Russia to other Soviet republics and the socialist republics of Eastern Europe masks significant discontinuities and deviations in policy formulation and implementation.[61] In Bulgaria, such 'special funds' did not exist, and Kolarov's push for a compensation model was rejected.

The debate in the Ministerial Council highlights concerns both over imbuing work-therapy programmes with an expectation of output above all, and also over the question of how to incentivize workers to participate wholeheartedly in the work. On the one hand, there was a position that the work programme should not be funded at the expense of the institution, as the work performed cannot be expected to be productive and ensure financial subsistence. On the other hand, that profits made on goods produced by therapeutic workers should not go into the State budget, because that will rule out the possibility of paying, even at a reduced rate, for the 'work input' of mentally ill individuals in social homes. 'Without paying for the work of these individuals, there is no stimulus [incentive] for their participation in the work process, which has impacts upon the efficacy of the therapeutic results,' Kolarov writes.[62]

Kolarov's argument for the compensation of therapeutic workers was rejected, and no alterative model for compensation was developed. Lukanov, Deputy Chairman of the Ministerial Council, opposed Kolarov's proposition for paying for therapeutic work. 'Instead of paying for the labour of the sick', he asserted, periodic awards [bonuses] should be given for exemplary performance. Further justification is given in a subsequent report: 'It is wrong to pay for the work of the ill as is for normal workers because these individuals are being treated and because we are securing lodging, clothing, electricity and heating for them. The acquisition of habits for working [working discipline] should be achieved by pedagogic means. It is more educational to give periodic awards.'[63] As such, it was commonplace for patients to carry out unpaid labour, as illustrated in Figure 5.3, which shows an unpaid group of male patients producing clothes-pins in a therapeutic unit at the Regional Psychoneurological Hospital in Lovech in 1966.

Work therapy is education, and as such should not be compensated. This model of tutelage evokes the ambiguous position of therapeutic workers: not yet socialist workers, and perhaps (and indeed, in most cases) never to graduate to this status. Ultimately, it was decreed that proceeds from therapeutic enterprise's production should flow directly into the State budget, and that funds be set aside for these rewards. Furthermore, the size of the awards of the ill should not be proportionally more than 75 per cent of the bonuses given to a 'normal' worker performing the same work. Only 30 per cent of that bonus, however, should actually be given to the patient. The other 70 per cent should be retained by the institution for their care.[64]

A diachronic analysis of Tserova Koria brings out an important insight: building communism was as much a fiscal problem as an organizational one. While an emphasis on the cultural development (*kulturno-razvitie*) of workers is a common feature of memorandums from the late 1940s and onward, conditions of financing and leadership at this social home permitted such goals to be acted on only in the 1970s. Director Tsvetan Totev frequently noted, in year-end reports, the staff's difficulty in supervising residents in the evening. Arguments and physical fights broke out frequently, with staff injuries occurring. Totev stressed the need for additional forms of entertainment and programming to keep residents occupied.[65] Year after year, these recommendations were not implemented. As Slavi Slavchev took over the directorship during the mid-1970s, there is a discernible expansion in

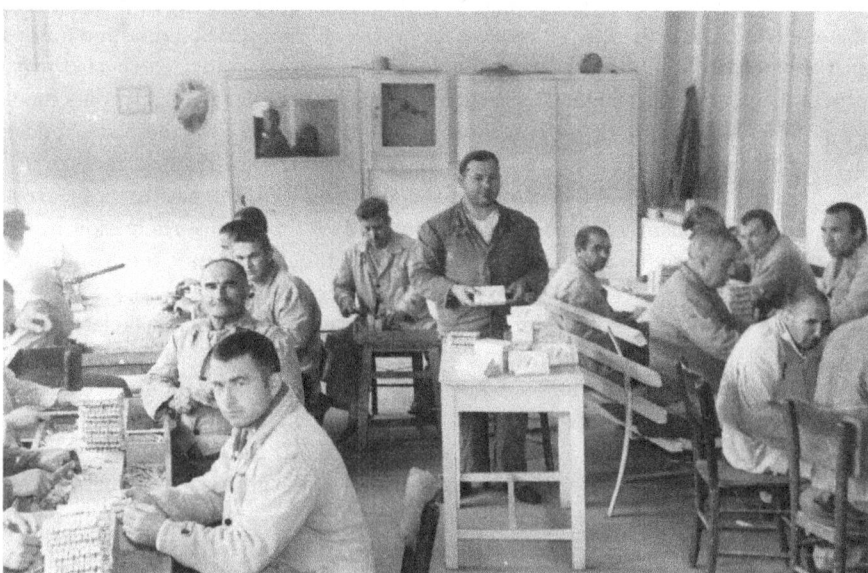

Figure 5.3 Work therapy by patients at Regional Psychoneurological Hospital in Lovech, 1966. Personal Archive.

the responsibilities of the institution beyond basic custodial care and work therapy. By the 1980s, institutional directives included ideological education (screening films, newsreels and political discussions), summer field trips to the Veselina River, the observance of residents' birthdays, decorating for holidays and efforts to keep residents in touch with families.[66] This points to a complex relationship between institutional financing, on one hand, and individual agency and leadership, on the other, which we risk overlooking.

Discharge

By 1993, Nikola likely had not made artwork in a decade. In consultation with his family, Georgi brought Nikola to an external consultation. The psychiatrist reduced his dosage to a third of his regimen and would recommend that Nikola be discharged from Tserova Koria. Figure 5.4 shows Nikola a year after his release. For a period of time

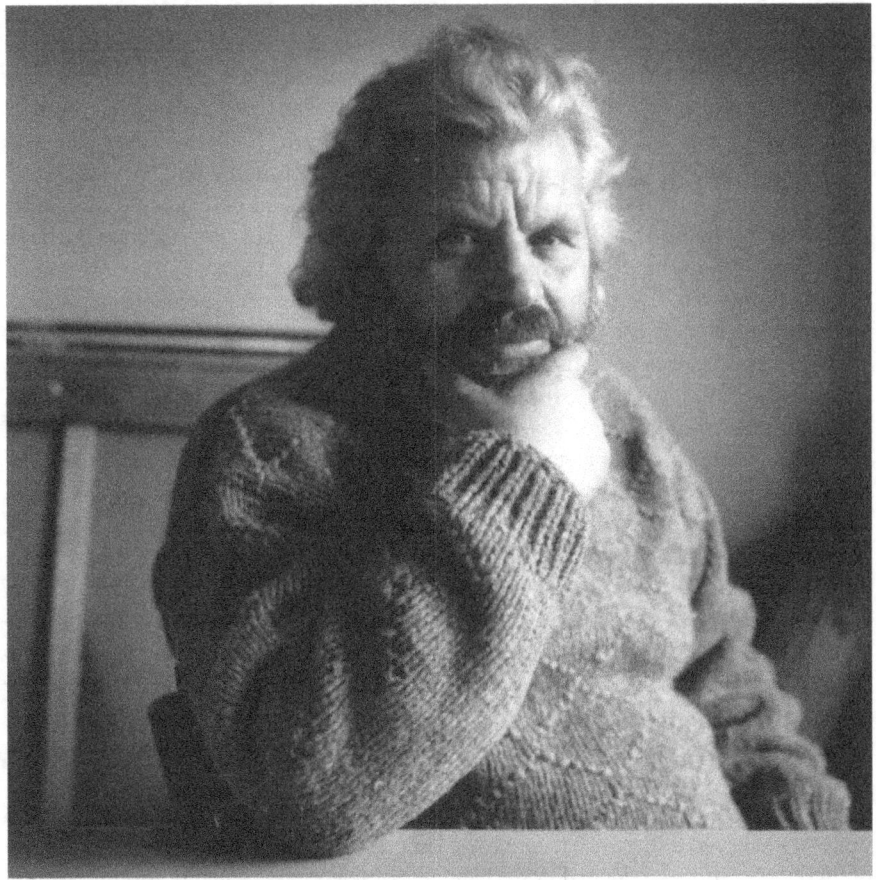

Figure 5.4 Nikola Kazakov a year after discharge, 1994. Personal Archive.

beginning on 14 May 1993, and ending in December 1995, Georgi lived with and took care of Nikola. During this time he encouraged Nikola to work, bringing him canvases, papers and supplies. But Nikola was unable to create much. He expressed little interest in creating art and had few recollections of his days of painting or sculpting. The psychiatrist who took care of Nikola at Tserova Koria confided in later years to Georgi Todorov that they may have made a mistake with Nikola. That they should have taken advantage of his inclination to express himself as a means of understanding what was going on for him – perhaps even helping him to work through his traumas. The use of visual art as a means of therapy appears not to have been a practice in Bulgarian psychiatry during this time. Nikola's treatment plan prescribed medications that had rendered him docile and inert, bereft of his artistic talents and unpaid for his labour.

Nikola's first hospitalization extracted him from ordinary socialist labour and society and placed him in a facility that treated patients pharmacologically, and that lacked resources for psychotherapeutic care. In this context Nikola Kazakov was severed from his ordinary socialist labour, but also from his artistic vocation and from his means for potentially therapeutic self-expression through artistic work during a prolonged period of psychiatric crisis. Nikola could no longer express his inner world visually. In this first period, we see psychiatric hospitalization as a State of exclusion from participation in the socialist State. After his escape from the first institution, Nikola was captured and assigned, out of expedience, to a facility for deaf individuals with mental disabilities closer to his hometown. The second institution was the first institution to initiate a programme for work as psychotherapy. Nikola's second hospitalization offers a different vantage point on work and psychiatry, illuminating the unequal provision of social services for disabled individuals in socialist Bulgaria: unions for the physically disabled, such as the Union of the Deaf, had substantial representation and organizational capacity relative to the conditions of institutional life for the mentally ill and disabled, for whom no similar representative organs existed.

Work therapy was a sublimation of the culture and politics of labour within a technology of mind and body. The therapeutic potential of work was rarely questioned, and its justification was typically linked to a vague hybrid of Marxist-Leninist and Pavlovian justifications for its purported efficacy. For individuals with physical disabilities, work adaptations or work at home programmes offered opportunities for empowerment and social inclusion through the workforce. In the case of work therapy as a psychiatric technology, however, the debates in Bulgaria reveal an internal understanding that uncompensated labour could be inimical to the broader goals of social inclusion. K. Lukanov's argument that work therapy is education that is not due compensation places psychiatric work therapy closer to labour re-education than to regular socialist work. An unpaid and unrepresented pool of labourers, the physically and mentally disabled, participated in the construction of a communist future, albeit as part of a workforce whose management was composed of psychiatrists and auxiliary medical staff in closed institutions.

Nikola's work therapy was organized in relation to the productivist mandates and norms established by the State through the Union for the Deaf. The therapeutic promise of these programmes, couched in the language of scientific rationality and therapeutic rehabilitation, could not exist independently of the State's demand for industrial output. Both ideology and economic planning circumscribed how work therapy could be imagined, developed and exercised in the Bulgarian context. Psychiatric work therapy was consummately socialist labour turned into a technology of mind and body, robustly implemented in disciplining work capacity according to the economic demands of the State. While Kolarov admitted that output could hardly be counted as the chief potential of work therapy, in the absence of a therapeutic programme tailored to individual needs and capacities, patient-workers were conducting standard labour in sequence with standardized production norms, without pay or representation. This paper has argued that a set of nominally therapeutic spaces of work existed as complex zones of inclusion and exclusion in relation to the broader emancipatory project of socialist state-building. 'Social homes' and psychiatric hospitals with work-therapy programmes for individuals with mental illnesses and disabilities existed as spaces of partial exclusion from the broader emancipatory vision of socialist labour.

Notes

1   I characterize work performed for state enterprises in socialist Bulgaria as 'socialist labour', acknowledging that while institutional structures were influenced by critiques of labour exploitation and alienation, they also did not achieve Marx's and Engels's vision of transcending labour in 'work'. As Christian Fuchs and Sebastian Sevignani have noted, in *The German Ideology* Marx and Engels asserted that communism would do away with 'labour', which is a 'necessarily alienated form of work, in which humans do not control and own the means and results of production', and which is a 'historic form of the organisation of work in class societies'. 'Work', by contrast, for Marx and Engels, as Fuchs and Sevignani argue, 'is a much more general concept common to all societies. It is a process in which humans in social relations make use of technologies in order to transform nature, culture and society in such a way that goods and services are created that satisfy human needs'. See Christian Fuchs and Sebastian Sevignani, 'What Is Digital Labour? What Is Digital Work? What's Their Difference? And Why Do These Questions Matter for Understanding Social Media?', *Open Access Journal for a Global Sustainable Information Society*, 11.2 (2013): 237–93. Was work for state-socialist enterprises 'work' or 'labour'? While I cannot resolve the longstanding debate over whether 'labour' was categorically different in the socialist bloc relative to that of liberal economies, I acknowledge it and choose to designate working for socialist enterprises as 'socialist labour', preserving the aspiration and paradox of a revolutionary vision – control by workers – that was not brought into being. As the means of production were owned and governed by the State under single-party rule, conditions for Marx's sense of alienation were preserved.
2   Stephen Kotkin argues that ideological categories were not simply static or repressive; they generated novel forms of identity and subjectivity. See his *Magnetic Mountain: Stalinism as a Civilization* (Oakland, CA: University of California Press, 1997).
3   Lilia Topouzova, 'On Silence and History', *The American Historical Review*, 126.3 (2021): 685–99. As Topouzova has argued, Bulgaria operated one of the most robust, violent and forced labour-camp systems in Eastern Europe, whose violence not only survived de-Stalinization but escalated in the late 1980s in a campaign against

Bulgarian Turks and the Muslim minority. See also: Mary Neuburger, *The Orient Within: Muslim Minorities and the Negotiation of Nationhood in Modern Bulgaria* (Ithaca, NY: Cornell University Press, 2011).

4   Work therapy differed from re-education through work. Work therapy was prescribed with therapeutic intentions for mentally ill and disabled individuals, whereas re-education through work was mandated for the reform of political prisoners. Re-education through work was a vision, in the very early years of the socialist State, for prisons and labour camps for those who were deemed, often extrajudicially, 'enemies of the state'. Their initial premise and arc of transformation, however, connects them. Both were conceived as a means of transforming subjects. The therapeutic potential of the prior was grounded in psychiatric terms, whereas that of the latter was grounded in ideological terms. The scientifically and ideologically 'therapeutic' intentions of each resolved into organizational problems seen as having administrative solutions. The outcome of the prior, diachronically, was a prioritization of productive capacity over therapeutic efficacy. The outcome of the latter was emphasis on productive capacity over the reforming of subjects. And yet, economic aims fell in deference to ideological aims, resulting in the rampant destruction of life.

5   An examination of the history of psychiatry in Bulgaria presents the possibility of tracing processes of transnational medical-scientific knowledge transfer in the context of modern East European state building, where European and Soviet modernities and interests competed for influence in an ethno-national state emerging from the Ottoman Empire, where in the decades after 1878, one can observe and track the emergence and, soon after, large-scale development of modern biomedicine.

6   In Nikola's case, there is hardly a profusion of biomedical or clinical documentation that silences him. It is more so the silence of underfunded and overstretched facilities, mismatched institutional assignments for his patient profile and a broadly silent social regard towards mentally ill and disabled individuals.

7   Authors Collective, *Orisiiata na Nikola Kazakov* (Sofia: Ko-op Galeriia, 2019).

8   Kiril Kirov, 'Bulgarian Psychiatry: Development, Ideas, Achievements', *History of Psychiatry*, 4 (1993): 565.

9   Georgi Koychev, 'History of Bulgarian Psychiatry', *Psychiatria Danubina*, 15.1–2 (2013): 61.

10 Kiril Milenkov and Christo Christozov, 'Mental Health Care in Bulgaria since World War II', *International Journal of Mental Health*, 20.4 (1991): 11–20.

11 Julian Chehirian, 'Excavating the Psyche: A Social History of Soviet Psychiatry in Bulgaria', *Culture, Medicine, and Psychiatry*, 42.2 (2017): 449–80.

12 G. J. Windholz, 'The 1950 Joint Scientific Session', *Journal of the History of the Behavioral Sciences*, 33 (1997): 61–81.

13 As recent scholarship has shown, however, the effects of this model were not uniform throughout the Soviet Bloc. See Sarah Marks and Mat Savelli, eds., *Psychiatry in Communist Europe* (London: Palgrave Macmillan, 2015).

14 The archives of the Ministry of Health include memos on the work of the Pavlovian Committee, the local propagation of Soviet medical discourse and ideology, as well as documentation of theses and academic courses on the Pavlovian Teaching. See 'Report on the work of the Pavlovian Committee' and 'Course on the Pavlovian Teaching – Theses', National Archives, Sofia, Fund 160, Archival Unit 14, Folders 48 and 99.

15 Hristo Hristozov, ed., *Psychotherapy – Methods and Tendencies* (Sofia: Medicine and Physical Culture, 2002).

16 Irina Sirotkina and Marina Kokorina, 'The Dialectics of Labour in a Psychiatric Ward: Work Therapy in the Kaschenko Hospital', in Marks and Savelli, eds., *Psychiatry in Communist Europe*, 28.
17 Ibid. Foucault emphasizes the deftness of work for disciplining: 'Work has a power to constrain which was superior to all other forms of physical coercion, as the regularity of hours, the demands it made on attention, and the obligation to achieve a result removed what would have otherwise been a harmful liberty of thought, fixing patients in a system of responsibility'. See Michel Foucault, *History of Madness* (London: Routledge, 2013), 485.
18 Carla Yanni, *The Architecture of Madness: Insane Asylums in the United States* (Minneapolis, MN: University of Minnesota Press, 2007).
19 For more on the relationship between work and identity, see Kotkin, *Magnetic Mountain*.
20 Ibid. Sirotkina and Kokorina, 'The Dialectics of Labour in a Psychiatric Ward', 28.
21 Ibid.
22 Lewis H. Siegelbaum, 'Okhrana Truda: Industrial Hygiene, Psychotechnics, and Industrialization in the USSR', in Susan Gross Solomon and J. Hutchinson, eds., *Health and Society in Revolutionary Russia* (Bloomington: Indiana University Press, 1990), 224–45.
23 Claire L. Shaw, *Deaf in the USSR: Marginality, Community, and Soviet Identity, 1917–1991* (Ithaca, NY: Cornell University Press, 2017).
24 Ibid., 4.
25 Ibid.
26 Ibid. Sirotkina and Kokorina, 'The Dialectics of Labour'.
27 Stephen Kotkin, 'Modern Times: The Soviet Union and the Interwar Conjuncture', *Kritika: Explorations in Russian and Eurasian History* 2.1 (2001): 111–64.
28 Maria C. Galmarini-Kabala, 'Between Defectological Narratives and Institutional Realities: The "Mentally Retarded" Child in the Soviet Union of the 1930s', *Bulletin of the History of Medicine* 93.2 (2019): 183.
29 Sarah D. Phillips,'"There Are No Invalids in the USSR!": A Missing Soviet Chapter in the New Disability History', *Disability Studies Quarterly*, 29.3 (2009). Philips cites Ol'ga Shek, 'Sotsial'noe iskliuchenie invalidov v SSSR', in Pavel Romanov and Elena Iarskaia-Smirnova, eds., *Nuzhda i Poriadok: Istoriia Sotsial'noi Raboty v Rossii, XX v.* (Saratov: Nauchnaia kniga, 2005), 375–96, and Elena Iarskaia-Smirnova and Pavel Romanov, '"A Salary Is Not Important Here": The Professionalization of Social Work in Contemporary Russia', *Social Policy & Administration* 36.2 (2002): 123–41.
30 Referred to as '*trudova terapiia*', '*trudovo-lechebnata terapiia*' and '*trudovo-lechebni stopanstva*'.
31 V. A. Giliarovski, *Psychiatry* (Sofia: Science and Art, 1956), 502.
32 Ibid.
33 Ibid. Authors Collective, *Orisiiata na Nikola Kazakov*.
34 It is possible that Nikola had a developmental disorder, though there is no concrete evidence of this having been medically diagnosed. Georgi Todorov, Personal Interview, December 2014.
35 Ibid.
36 Todorov, Personal Interview, December 2014.
37 Lyuba Tsaneva, Personal Interview, December 2014.
38 Ibid; Authors Collective, *Orisiiata na Nikola Kazakov*.
39 Tzvetan Kolev, Personal Interview, July 2014.

40 Filip Zidarov, Rumen Serafimov, Orlin Dvorianov, Tzvetan Kolev, Personal Interviews, July 2019.
41 Personal Interview, July 2019.
42 Filip Zidarov, Personal Interview, July 2019.
43 Ibid.
44 Todorov, Personal Interview, December 2014.
45 Kolev, Personal Interview, July 2014.
46 Todorov, Personal Interview.
47 Tsaneva, Personal Interview, December 2014.
48 Todorov, Personal Interview, December 2014; Kolev, Personal Interview, July 2014.
49 Ibid.
50 State Archive Kyustendil, Fund 1098, Folder 1, Archival Unit 5.
51 Ibid.
52 Benjamin Zajicek, 'The Psychopharmacological Revolution in the USSR: Schizophrenia Treatment and the Thaw in Soviet Psychiatry, 1954–64', *Medical History*, 63.3 (2019): 250.
53 State Archive Kyustendil, Fund 1098, Folder 1, Archival Unit 5.
54 State Archive Kyustendil, Fund 1098, Folder 1, Archival Unit 4.
55 For more on this, see ibid., and Chehirian, 'Excavating the Psyche'.
56 Todorov, Personal Interview, December 2014.
57 National Archive, Sofia, Fund 136, Archival Unit 13, pp. 12–13.
58 Ibid.
59 Veliko Turnovo State Archive, Fund 1231, Opis 1, Archival Unit 13, pp. 1–3.
60 Sarah Marks, 'Suggestion, Persuasion and Work: Psychotherapies in Communist Europe', *European Journal of Psychotherapy & Counselling*, 20.1 (2018): 1–15.
61 Ibid; Marks and Savelli, eds., *Psychiatry in Communist Europe*.
62 Veliko Turnovo State Archive, Fund 1231, Opis 1, Archival Unit 13. pp. 1–3.
63 Veliko Turnovo State Archive, Fund 1231, Opis 1, Archival Unit 13.
64 Ibid., pp. 1–3.
65 Veliko Turnovo State Archive, Fund 1231, Opis 2, Archival Units 1 and 4.
66 Ibid.

6

'Human capabilities are limitless': Will and self-improvement in postwar Soviet psychotherapy

Aleksandra Brokman

A textbook published in the Soviet Union in 1967 offered the following example to illustrate the methods and applications of psychotherapeutic treatment. Patient R., a teacher by profession, was referred for psychotherapy after experiencing an emotional breakdown as a result of a confrontation with an impudent pupil, to whom, in her volatile state and in response to his taunts, she awarded sixteen of the lowest grades. The therapist described patient R. as having 'hysterical character traits' such as egoism, emotional instability and a heightened sense of her own importance. He explained to his patient that her excessive behaviour was not caused by the pupil's insolence as such, but by her own personality traits, inability to control emotions and to think about her actions. The psychotherapist proceeded to analyse other situations from the patient's life in which those characteristics manifested and to teach her to always take a moment to calm down before responding to an insolent remark from a pupil, for example, by developing a habit of sliding her tongue along her teeth ten times before reacting. The aim of the treatment was to make R. realize her shortcomings and help her 'train her nervous system' so that she could better control her emotions.[1]

In 1983, during training camps in Dushanbe, Groznyi and Ufa, parachutists belonging to the Soviet national and the Russian republican teams were instructed in autosuggestion techniques. These therapeutic techniques were designed to improve the parachutists' performance through helping the athletes to control their bodily processes and sensations, to develop the characteristics believed to be indispensable for success in their sport and to overcome any psychological barriers. As a result, one of the participants managed to master the acrobatic manoeuvre he had been struggling with for some time, several athletes overcame the neurotic symptoms that used to impede their performance and all participants increased their confidence and self-control under stress and learned to regenerate their strength more effectively after long training. Many performed well at subsequent competitions.[2]

The cases provided above, while seemingly disparate, both illustrate how psychotherapy was practised and applied in the postwar Soviet Union, where it was envisioned and championed not only as a treatment but also as a means of improving performance and reducing the threat of mental illness in a wide variety of occupations and environments. The case of patient R. and the parachutists' training in autosuggestion techniques exemplify a trend that permeated Soviet postwar psychotherapy: an emphasis on the perfection and self-improvement of human beings. The emphasis on the perfection of the self and on the overcoming of both external obstacles and personal weaknesses had long been present in Soviet discourse.

The belief in the transformability of human beings was deeply ingrained in the ideology of the Soviet state, which from its early years sought to refashion its citizens into New Soviet Persons who would be characterized by discipline, commitment to revolutionary ideals, strong will and perfect control over their minds and bodies.[3] Individual self-improvement was actively encouraged as a path to becoming a conscious and purposeful Soviet citizen capable of always being in control of their actions and of refashioning the world around them.[4] While Soviet psychotherapeutic texts from the postwar period did not explicitly reference the model of the New Soviet Person directly, the thinking of their authors was visibly imbued with the intent to facilitate the self-transformation of people, both in clinical and non-clinical settings. Examining the self-improvement trend in medical discourse, this chapter explores applications of psychotherapeutic treatment in the postwar decades – a period that saw renewed efforts to popularize psychotherapy in Soviet medicine, the growth of the number of physicians trained in this discipline and, finally, psychotherapy's establishment as an officially recognized medical speciality in 1985.[5] This was a period when the theoretical basis and methods of Soviet psychotherapy, established in earlier decades, were being introduced into more and more medical institutions across the Soviet Union. Drawing largely on psychotherapeutic publications from the post-war USSR, this chapter explores the role that ideas about human transformation played in the theory and practice of psychotherapy.

The form of psychotherapy practised in the USSR differed from the psychotherapy practised in Western countries in both its theoretical background and in its dominant methods. Initially the development of this mode of treatment in Russia and the early USSR followed a similar path to the rest of Europe, with early psychotherapeutic methods relying on various suggestion techniques, hypnosis and 'moral treatment', and later with growing interest in psychoanalysis.[6] However, this began to change as the ideas of Freud fell out of favour with the Soviet authorities in the second half of the 1920s and were finally denounced as 'bourgeois' and 'anti-Soviet'.[7] In the place of psychoanalytic research, which largely came to a halt, Soviet psychiatrists continued to develop psychotherapeutic methods and schools that were losing popularity in Western Europe and North America. Consequently, post-war Soviet psychotherapy, as taught and practised, was comprised of markedly different methods to those in the West. In the absence of psychoanalysis, psychodynamic, behavioural or humanistic psychotherapy, approaches relying on suggestion (imparted under hypnosis or in the waking state) continued to be popular. They shared their dominant status with a multitude of modifications of autogenic training, originally developed in Germany by Johannes Schultz. Another very common psychotherapeutic approach was rational psychotherapy, based on persuasion therapy developed by an early twentieth-century Swiss doctor, Paul Dubois, which relied on the doctor using logical argumentation to gradually persuade patients to change their outlook and behaviour.[8]

Soviet psychotherapy also remained more unified than its Western counterparts. Irina Sirotkina has pointed out that physicians in late Imperial Russia and the early Soviet Union showed a much more eclectic approach to various psychotherapies than their colleagues from other European countries. Russian and Soviet doctors approached psychotherapeutic practices as complimentary rather than contradictory, developing various methods of psychotherapy alongside each other and seeking to combine them.[9] Eclecticism continued to characterize the work of Soviet physicians in the post-war period. Soviet doctors tended to deploy a combination of different therapeutic methods, being driven by the specific needs of the patient. Despite some differences in professional approaches and institutional application, Soviet post-war psychotherapy was largely unified in its theoretical background. Soviet psychotherapists emphasized the scientific nature of their treatments and the firm grounding of their discipline in human physiology, particularly in the theories developed by Ivan Pavlov.[10]

While a comprehensive outline of the Russian and Soviet physiological tradition is outside the scope of this chapter, one feature is particularly relevant to the present discussion. Soviet psychotherapists frequently expressed their commitment to the rejection of mind-body dualism. Although Soviet psychotherapeutic treatment was often aimed at what could be described as the 'psyche' – the sphere of emotions, personality traits and attitudes – the psychical realm was not seen by Soviet psychotherapists as an entity separate from the body. By contrast, the mental sphere was perceived as intricately linked to physiological processes, being shaped by them and capable of influencing bodily processes in turn. Psychotherapy was described as an 'active interference on the part of the physician into the state of the patient's cortico-subcortical dynamics' and was said to act 'through the psyche on the entire organism'.[11] Such a conceptualization of the discipline fitted into a broader trend of the Soviet psy-ences. In order to avoid succumbing to both mind-body dualism and so-called 'vulgar materialism', which saw the psyche completely reduced to physiological processes, the psy-disciplines generally explained consciousness as a 'property of a highly organised matter'.[12]

Both physiological symptoms and aspects of patients' inner lives were thereby considered objects of psychotherapeutic intervention and were frequently approached in similar ways. The picture of the mind-body relationship implicit in Soviet psychotherapy is further complicated by the emphasis that Soviet practitioners put on the will, which was presented as a crucial agent of self-transformation, capable of influencing and governing both the mental and the somatic spheres. This chapter argues that Soviet psychotherapists continued to espouse a particular version of dualism, placing the will on one side and the human organism (with its physiology, personality, emotions and thoughts) on the other. Psychotherapeutic techniques were aimed at helping patients exercise their will in order to achieve the desired transformation of the organism, which could manifest in the removal of an undesirable personality trait, a change of attitude towards one's illness or even in physiological transformation. Psychotherapists acted as guides and teachers in this process of self-improvement, identifying what change needed to take place and assisting patients with enacting it.

Teachers of life

Speaking at the All-Union Conference on Psychotherapy in 1956, Vladimir Nikolaevich Miasishchev, a Leningrad psychologist and one of the leading figures involved in popularizing psychotherapy in Soviet post-war medicine, described the role of the psychotherapist in the therapeutic process in the following way: 'Without exaggeration, it is right to declare that to an average patient the physician becomes a teacher of life. He must devote a great deal of attention to the re-education of the patient'.[13]

Miasishchev's view was by no means unusual. In the years that followed the conference, many of his colleagues emphasized re-education as an important part of the psychotherapeutic process and insisted that the physician performing such treatments was not only acting to remove symptoms but also to transform patients' outlook and behaviour. For example, in his 1962 book, Sergei Nikolaevich Astakhov, the author of several publications on psychotherapy, noted that all psychotherapeutic methods aimed to produce a 'change in the patient's attitude towards all the factors that contributed to the development of their illness' and to cultivate within them a 'correct attitude' towards their situation.[14] A very similar view was also expressed by another influential figure in the development of Soviet psychotherapy, Mark Lebedinskii – a Moscow-based physician and psychologist who headed the clinical psychology, psychotherapy and mental hygiene section at the All-Union Scientific Society of Neuropathologists and Psychiatrists (VNMONiP) between 1971 and 1978. Lebedinskii wrote that psychotherapeutic treatment 'ought to restructure, re-educate or eliminate all that might become a psychogenesis of a pathological construct in a person (an incorrect attitude towards themselves, illness, other people etc.)'.[15]

Patients' re-education and adjustment of their attitude towards themselves and their circumstances was an integral part of psychotherapy. In many instances such re-education constituted the core of how therapists sought to restore patients to health. This is well illustrated by the case study of a patient referred to as 'P', a medical student who began to stutter after a failed suicide attempt caused by his wife's decision to leave him for another man. The stuttering was so severe that patient P. could not even tell his story himself and had to rely on the assistance of his friends. The psychotherapist began the treatment by helping P. realize that his symptoms were the result of a psychical trauma caused by his divorce and suicide attempt. In addition to removing the patient's symptoms, the psychotherapist proceeded to inculcate P. with the belief that he was still young and had his whole life ahead of him: he would have an interesting, fulfilling job as a physician, would meet another woman and start a 'new, good family'.[16]

The removal of stuttering through hypnotic suggestion was but a small element in P.'s treatment. The core of the psychotherapeutic treatment received by patient P. and patient R., whose case study opened this article, was assistance in working on themselves. The aim of this process was to help patients perceive their situation in a new way and become better able to function in their workplace and everyday life. For R., this meant realizing that she was at fault for allowing herself to be ruled by her emotions and working to develop better self-control. For P., it was learning to look at his life in a more optimistic way and focusing on the future. Both patients, like many others treated by Soviet psychotherapists, were taught during the course of therapy how to change themselves and their outlook so as to lead better lives. The essence of psychotherapy was to teach patients a new and correct way of looking at themselves and their situation.

Instruction on how to live one's life and relate to one's circumstances is by no means unique to Soviet psychotherapy. Various forms of psychotherapeutic treatment developed around the world all postulated a certain vision of a 'good life' towards which patients or clients were to be guided.[17] What is distinctive about Soviet psychotherapy, however, is the firm and clear way in which its practitioners linked their discipline to pedagogy, frequently conceptualizing the final goal of treatment as successful re-education. While understanding psychotherapy as a medical procedure, Soviet psychotherapists did not draw a clear dividing line between medicine and education. Rather, Soviet practitioners believed themselves to be engaged in 'medical-pedagogical work', at times even openly drawing on the ideas of Russian and Soviet pedagogues.[18] The Ukrainian psychiatrist Aleksandr Slobodianik, for example, drew links between psychotherapy and the 'pedagogical principles' of the nineteenth-century Russian pedagogue Konstantin Ushinskii, as well as the prominent Soviet educator Anton Makarenko. Slobodianik made reference to a number of Ushinskii's ideas, including his view that upbringing was primarily meant to provide children with the necessary knowledge of reality to support the development of their personalities and 'mental strengths', and his emphasis on the importance of cultivating in children a sense of national, familial and personal duty and responsibility. While these principles of upbringing were applied to children, Slobodianik explained that they could also be applied to adults, 'especially those suffering from neurotic or mental conditions'.[19] He explained that since such conditions affected the psyche, it was necessary to 'rebuild the edifice of the subject's higher nervous activity' using the same rules and principles as in the upbringing of children, as well as the power of the collective, as recommended by Makarenko.[20]

The works of Makarenko proved particularly influential for psychotherapists who sought to re-educate patients through collective treatment.[21] Indeed, even when Soviet psychotherapists did not refer to pedagogical thought, they emphasized that their discipline was concerned with re-educating patients to facilitate their better adjustment to the circumstances of life and to society. Soviet psychotherapeutic treatment was closely entwined with re-educating patients and motivating them to engage in self-improvement. The emphasis on encouraging 'working on oneself' was not a new phenomenon in the Soviet discourse. Reshaping and perfecting oneself through the conscious effort of the will was encouraged by the Stalinist state and practised by people dedicated to Soviet ideology, who 'worked on themselves' to become better socialist subjects.[22] The growing perception of the self as 'an object to care about, to reflect upon, to perfect' was also a trend observed by Oleg Karkhordin in the postwar USSR.[23]

Contrary to the psychotherapeutic approaches popular in Western Europe and North America at the time, patients' desires regarding the goals of psychotherapy were not taken into consideration when determining the direction of treatment. In the second half of the twentieth century, paternalistic approaches to medicine in the West increasingly came under attack from patients' rights movements. A variety of psychotherapeutic approaches set the promotion of patients' autonomy and free choice as their main goal, and also adopted the practice of mutually determining the goals of psychotherapy with the client.[24] These trends were not paralleled in the USSR, however, where physicians remained deeply rooted in the paternalistic tradition.[25] In Soviet psychotherapeutic treatment, the direction of a patient's re-education and self-improvement was determined by the physician. Acting as the 'teachers of life', Soviet psychotherapists aimed their techniques at making patients more resilient, disciplined and determined to exercise their will to refashion themselves and overcome personal weaknesses. In essence, Soviet psychotherapists sought to cultivate the qualities that were ascribed to the New Soviet Person.

Mind, body and will

The materials prepared in the late 1970s to help university lecturers deliver courses on psychotherapy described the attitude that was to be cultivated in patients in the following way:

> The process of regaining health can be compared to a common struggle of doctor and patient against an illness. The course of illness and speed of recovery depend on the activity of the patient [...] It is necessary for every person to cultivate in themselves the characteristics of a fighter, so that they are ready to strive to overcome their illness, instead of being controlled by it. This in and of itself will be the patient's victory.[26]

Patients were expected to adopt an attitude of resilience and battle-readiness, and to focus their energies on cultivating the determination and willpower needed to overcome adverse situations such as falling ill. In order to get better, medical student P. needed to recognize that his stuttering was the result of a psychological trauma and work to reshape his outlook on life.[27] The importance placed on cultivating and exercising one's will can also be discerned in a case study of another patient described by Astakhov in the early 1960s: M., a shy nineteen-year-old student who developed a psychogenic condition which caused her to feel a need to urinate whenever she left the house. M.'s condition worsened until she stopped going out completely and neglected her studies. During treatment by rational psychotherapy, M.'s doctor explained to her that she suffered from a neurotic rather than an organic condition. Having described the root of her disorder, M.'s psychotherapist persuaded her that the success of her treatment depended on her own effort. Finally, the doctor helped M. to learn to control the pathological urge to go to the toilet by teaching her to exercise her willpower.[28]

For patient M., coming to understand her condition and cultivating the will to conquer her symptoms proved key to regaining health. This was true of many patients who received psychotherapeutic treatment. The exercise of willpower took a variety of forms, however. Psychotherapists acted as patients' teachers and guides. Accordingly, an important part of their role was to determine what exact kind of transformation was to take effect in the patient and to guide them towards that goal. While in the majority of cases the final goal was regaining health, chronically ill patients were instead encouraged to come to terms with their illness and to harness their will to proceed with their lives. This was clearly expressed by Lebedinskii who argued that while a neurotic patient should not be allowed to 'get used to' his condition and should be encouraged to focus his attention on fighting it, a patient with a permanent facial defect should be discouraged from fixating on it and guided towards finding meaning in his work and family life.[29]

The aforementioned examples all show Soviet psychotherapy's interest in influencing what is usually described as the mental sphere: attitudes, emotions, thoughts and personality traits. This is indeed representative of the majority of Soviet psychotherapeutic interventions. Despite practitioners' emphasis on the physiological basis of the treatments they performed, the practice of Soviet psychotherapy remained largely concerned with the psyche. However, this does not mean that we should dismiss psychotherapists' claims of rejecting mind-body dualism and approaching the human organism holistically. While psychotherapy usually focused on patients' outlook and inner lives, some psychotherapeutic methods and research practices were informed by a belief that the body and its physiological processes could also be influenced by verbal suggestion.

Since the 1920s, many psychotherapeutic experiments had focused on using verbal suggestion in order to exert influence on the human body – to slow or quicken the heart rate, to raise blood pressure, dilate or constrict pupils or alter blood sugar levels.[30] An important example of Soviet psychotherapy's attempt to influence not only the psyche but also the body can be found in one of its most common methods: autogenic training, during which patients sought to exert control over their organism through autosuggestion. Autogenic training was comprised of a series of exercises aimed at gradually inducing certain sensations and influencing specific bodily processes through the repetition of suggested formulas such as 'my right hand is very heavy', 'my left hand is very warm', 'my heart beats calmly and regularly' or 'my forehead is pleasantly cool'.[31] Each exercise was considered mastered when a patient was able to successfully effect the targeted change: a sensation of heaviness, a feeling of warmth (caused by the dilation of blood vessels and the increased flow of blood to a given part of the body) or a change in heartbeat. While the final goal of treatment was often the transformation of attitudes or personality traits, autogenic training began by teaching patients to exercise a certain level of control over their bodies.[32] Autogenic exercises were meant to help patients attain a state of relaxation and stabilize their emotions and 'higher nervous activity'. In addition, all exercises were accompanied by the formula 'I am completely calm', thereby also aiming at emotional transformation.[33] The assumption that the individual could exert an influence over their psychophysiology stood at the heart of autogenic training.

While there is some substance to Soviet psychotherapists' claims that they endeavoured to overcome mind-body dualism, these assertions still poorly reflected doctors' practical approaches to the human organism. An analysis of psychotherapeutic discourse and methodology reveals that Soviet specialists fell back on a different kind of dualism: one that placed a unified human organism (comprised of organic parts and physiological processes, as well as emotions, thoughts, behaviours and attitudes) on one side, and the will, on the other. This dualistic point of view is implicit in the writings of Soviet psychotherapists and can be discerned in the importance that they placed on the will. As such, 'will-organism' dualism provides a more suitable lens for discussing Soviet psychotherapy than either 'mind-body' dualism or 'monism'. The former fails to explain practitioners' commitment to influencing both human physiology and the psyche through psychotherapeutic methods, while the latter does not do justice to Soviet psychotherapists' emphasis on human will or their purported rejection of 'vulgar materialism'.

The concept of the will was crucial for Soviet psychotherapy's goal of transformation and self-improvement. Indeed, Slobodianik described it as the 'motor of human activity' which allowed people to shape and reshape the world around them, arguing that the cultivation of such volitional characteristics as 'initiative, self-reliance, purposefulness' should be a priority for a psychotherapist.[34] However, Slobodianik added that the burden of this task should not rest entirely on the shoulders of practitioners. Each patient should be responsible for cultivating their own will, in preparation for a more self-reliant life. Slobodianik asserted that this could be done through the patient striving to become more like a carefully chosen role model, keeping a diary with reflections on their progress, or performing mental exercises for stimulating willpower. While such exercises in will cultivation were part of the normal upbringing process for Slobodianik, patients exhibiting signs of an insufficiently developed will were to be helped by the psychotherapist.[35]

The importance of a strong will for Soviet psychotherapy is also visible in how it was conceptualized in relation to hypnosis – a treatment ostensibly at odds with cultivating patients' willpower. As Anna Toropova shows in her chapter in this volume, in the early Soviet period hypnosis was indeed often associated with the suppression of the will, leading some practitioners to dismiss it as incompatible with the revolutionary project.[36] However, by the postwar period hypnosis had become established as one of the main methods of psychotherapy, practised by the same doctors who emphasized the importance of willpower. While hypnosis continued to be described as a state of increased suggestibility, the possibility of it having a negative impact on willpower was dismissed. Postwar texts on hypnosis referred to this idea as a misconception and asserted that hypnotherapeutic treatment not only did not weaken patients' will but actually restored and strengthened it.[37] To be sure, such assertions failed to explain how exactly hypnosis contributed to strengthening patients' will. Yet the cultivation of the will was simply too important a goal for Soviet psychotherapy to continue to entertain previous doubts about hypnotherapeutic methods.

A strong will was seen as a prerequisite for mastering one's behaviour and attitudes, and thus for overcoming an illness. Patient M., for example, overcame her compulsive urge to go to the toilet through learning to exercise her willpower. M.'s treatment largely focused on strengthening her ability to use her will to resist the pathological urge and to gradually overcome it altogether.[38] Similarly, patients suffering from insomnia were to learn to help themselves fall asleep by exercising their will through autosuggestion formulas. Alcoholic patients, with the help of a psychotherapist, strengthened their will until they were able to use it to resist the urge to drink.[39] While developing a strong will was not considered to be sufficient for overcoming alcohol addiction on its own, it was nevertheless suggested as an important part of treatment, to be used alongside other therapies.[40] Tricia Starks notes in her chapter in this volume that the strengthening of patients' will was the foundation of many Soviet tobacco-cessation therapies. While in the 1960s the evolving understanding of tobacco dependency led to more attention being given to chemical therapies, the references to willpower continued to resurface, particularly in the context of failed quitters.[41]

Soviet psychotherapeutic discourse conceptualized the will as an agent of self-transformation, through which people could assert control over their body and mind. This was clearly visible in the basic exercises comprising autogenic training, which taught patients to purposefully shape their sensations and to influence their physiological functions and emotional outlook. Other autosuggestion formulas proposed by Soviet psychotherapists also reveal a belief in the dominance of human will over both psyche and physiology. For example, the following formula was proposed for patients suffering from angina pectoris, tachycardia and other heart conditions:

> I am calm ... All my muscles are relaxed, blood vessels in my body have dilated ... I feel a pleasant warmth in my left hand ... My heart beats regularly, calmly ... The flow of blood to my heart improves ... My heart is working completely calmly, regularly, without problems. I do not feel my heart at all.[42]

A different example of a therapeutic autosuggestion formula was proposed to help patients master and redirect their compulsive thoughts:

> I am always calm ... I feel an increase in my strength and energy ... I have power over my thoughts and feelings ... I control myself without any effort ... I can easily concentrate on any thought ... I am confident of my strengths and abilities. I can overcome any difficulties and find a way out of any situation ... I have entirely gotten rid of all unpleasant sensations, compulsive thoughts and misgivings ... I am always calm and confident of my strengths.[43]

Such formulas did not simply describe physiological processes and psychological states, but were expected to function as commands given by a patient to their own body and mind. Thus, psychotherapists believed that the repetition of 'my heart beats regularly' sent the body a message that caused the heartbeat to become more regular and calm. The phrase 'I have power over my thoughts and feelings' aimed to submit the individual's perceptions and emotions to the control of the will. Both bodily and mental processes were conceptualized as, at least to an extent, subject to the will, which could be mobilized to transform them in the way recommended by a psychotherapist.

The view of the human organism that emerged from Soviet psychotherapy positioned the will above both physiology and mind. While the will was said to be a part of the psyche, in practice it was treated as at least partially separate from the mental sphere and its role in the psychotherapeutic process was distinctly different from that attributed to the rest of the psyche. The will was ascribed an ability to exert influence over both body and mind. While thoughts, attitudes and feelings were seen as something that could be re-structured and transformed, and physiological processes as something that could be influenced, the will was the agent responsible for this transformation. The training of the will during psychotherapeutic treatment was to strengthen this resource and to direct it towards influencing the rest of the organism in the desirable way.

The process of strengthening and applying the will to the improvement of oneself and the cultivation of one's capacity to withstand external circumstances was supported and guided by a psychotherapist, who acted not only as a physician but also as a 'teacher of life'. However, Soviet psychotherapists were clear that while they could direct their patients towards developing initiative, self-reliance and self-control, they could not exercise their will for them. Ultimately, patients were expected to commit to overcoming the adverse situation that befell them and fight against their condition through the effort of their own will. In fact, the failure of psychotherapeutic treatment was sometimes directly attributed to the patient's failure to exercise their will independently.

Writing about the attitudes towards mental disorders in the United States, Tanya Marie Luhrmann has noted that, unlike patients with physical illnesses, the sufferers of mental illness were often seen as responsible for their condition: 'If something is in the body, an individual cannot be blamed; the body is always morally innocent. If something is in the mind, however, it can be controlled and mastered, and a person who fails to do so is morally at fault.'[44] A similar distinction in the attribution of blame can be observed in the attitudes of Soviet psychotherapists towards conditions that affected human psychophysiology, as well as towards defects of the will. The former generally did not cause blame to be ascribed to the suffering individual – the patients afflicted by such conditions were thought to be morally innocent. For example, the psychotherapist's assessment of patient R., who as a result of family conflicts developed 'hysterical traits' and psychogenic blindness, did not attribute personal responsibility to R. when treatment through hypnotic suggestion failed. The failure was simply presented as a sign that a different therapeutic approach needed to be found to free R. from the condition that affected his body and his personality.[45]

Patients were blamed, however, for their lack of will to commit to treatment. For example, Astakhov was clear that no treatment – not even pharmacological therapies – would help smoking and alcohol addicts unless they focused their will on getting better and showed it 'not through their words, but through their deeds'.[46] Similarly, the failure of treatment through autosuggestion was sometimes explained as a result of the lack of a sufficiently strong will on behalf of the patient.[47] Transformation and self-improvement required effort. The guidance of the psychotherapist was to help strengthen and cultivate the will, but was not thought sufficient to overcome deficiencies in the patient's will. The will was treated as responsible for the perfection of the organism. Those who cultivated and applied their willpower could transform themselves into fighters ready to defeat illness and overcome personal flaws. Those committed to self-improvement could become more in control of their bodies, thoughts and emotions. Those who failed to do so, however, could be dismissed as not being committed enough to mastering their minds and bodies. The will of such patients was seen as too weak to attain the necessary transformation, thereby rendering these individuals morally at fault.

Psychotherapy for champions

While the belief in the close intertwinement of the restoration of patients' health and self-improvement was central to Soviet psychotherapy, its emphasis on self-perfection was most pronounced in psychotherapeutic applications outside the clinic, especially in the training of athletes. Psychotherapeutic techniques were taught to athletes preparing for sporting competition in order to improve their performance through increasing their control over their bodies and minds. The work with parachutists described in the opening paragraphs of this chapter was part of a project led by M. Ia. Bondarchik at the Laboratory for Medical and Biological Scientific Research into Technical and Military-Applied Sports, which investigated the application of psychotherapeutic methods in sport. The stated goals of Bondarchik's project included: increasing mental fortitude, optimizing performance and training methods through psychotherapeutic techniques and speeding athletes' recovery from mental and physical tiredness.[48] Over the course of the project, athletes were also assisted in improving their concentration, eliminating harmful habits such as drinking or smoking and in shortening their reaction time.[49] Psychotherapeutic techniques were used to teach athletes how to develop greater resilience and self-control, to push beyond their limits and thus to achieve better results in competition.

Bondarchik's project was neither the only nor the first instance of psychotherapy being applied for the purpose of training Soviet athletes. On the contrary, Bondarchik's work was firmly grounded in a trend that had been developing within Soviet psychotherapy over the postwar decades. Researchers and practitioners in the field began to take an interest in using psychotherapeutic methods to improve sporting performance already in the 1950s. While physical culture and sport were presented as vital activities in strengthening the bodies and minds of the Soviet population from the early years of the USSR, after the onset of the Cold War, sporting competitions emerged as a key battleground in the clash between socialism and the capitalist West.[50] The securing of sporting victories became crucial; to outperform competitors and bring home more medals was to prove the superiority of the socialist system.[51]

The increased importance assigned to sporting successes drew some psychotherapists, who looked for ways of applying their methods and knowledge outside the clinic, to focus their research on working with athletes. It also shaped psychotherapists' priorities. To be sure, the prevention of neurotic and mental disorders, the usual argument given for using psychotherapeutic methods in work with the healthy population, was still studied and discussed. Yet the improvement of athletes' strength, resilience and results clearly began to take precedence. While early research conducted in the 1950s had used hypnosis to put athletes into an appropriate 'combative state' and to help them experience less tiredness, ultimately it was various forms of autosuggestion and suggestion in an awake state that became the most popular in the work with athletes.[52] The significant advantage held by suggestion over hypnosis was that after instructions and appropriate formulas were provided by a psychotherapist, they could be administered by coaches and by the athletes themselves, ideally several times a day.

Since the athletes' bodies were the instruments through which they achieved their victories, the suggestion and autosuggestion formulas recommended during their training focused much more heavily on bodily sensations and physiological processes. Psychotherapeutic techniques were to improve athletes' control over the body and their ability to perform well and recover quickly. Such techniques were not expected to replace physical training. Rather, suggestion and autosuggestion formulas were to supplement training programmes by focusing the athlete's will on improving the performance of their body.

Arkadii Timofeevich Filatov of the Ukrainian Institute for the Advanced Training of Physicians, one of the most prominent psychotherapists engaged in the training of athletes who participated in their preparation for the 1980 Moscow Olympics,[53] recommended the following formula to help sportsmen and women relax and recover after a competition or intensive training:

> Every nerve cell and every nerve in your body relaxes and rests. You feel a pleasant warmth and heaviness in your entire body ... The feeling of heaviness is brought about by the widening of the blood vessels in your body. The blood vessels in your muscles and in all other parts of your body have widened. The blood washes away from your muscles the substances produced during their intensive work ... The blood brings nutrients to every muscle cell of your heart. Your heart is getting stronger, its endurance increases ... Your muscles are resting and getting stronger. Their strength and endurance increase.[54]

Just like other verbal suggestion formulas, this was not simply a description of physiological processes but a command. The repetition and visualization of such formulas was supposed to induce or to quicken the described processes and to increase athletes' awareness and mastery over their bodies. The suggested formulas also reminded athletes that there were no limits to human self-perfection: 'The greater the effort, the greater man's abilities become. What used to be the world record, today is just the beginner level in many sports. Human capabilities are limitless here.'[55]

Psychotherapists occasionally engaged in direct attempts to improve specific abilities of the human body through autosuggestion. A.A. Martynenko, for example, used autogenic training to cultivate quick reflexes in competitors in motorcycle sport. His version of the training was supplemented by the visualization of a race from start to finish at the speed dictated by the metronome. It included the following formula:

> My self-confidence is unwavering. I make decisions quickly, without hesitation. My movements are confident and well-coordinated. I assess all situations in an

instant ... I am confident, composed, careful. I am in harmony and ready for action. My muscles obey my will.[56]

This formula was meant to build confidence in one's ability to control one's reactions and to perform well during a race, which in turn was expected to translate into an actual improvement in one's results. Thus, the athlete's reflexes would be improved by their effort to transform both their perception of their abilities and their actual abilities through their will, with the will being able to influence both mind and body.

The influence exerted on the mind was intended to psychologically prepare athletes for competitions, removing all barriers that could limit them, such as the anxiety provoked by performing in an unfamiliar stadium or feelings of anxiousness before the start of the race. However, psychotherapists also sought to achieve a more profound transformation in their athletes. Filatov expressed the belief that psychotherapists should aim to stimulate harmonious personality development and to encourage athletes to work to perfect themselves, arguing that it was his professional duty to 'use all the means available to him in order to stimulate this self-perfection'.[57] Autosuggestion and suggestion formulas were to help athletes transform themselves into better composed, more adaptable and more confident people. Filatov recommended that athletes repeat the phrase 'I can be unwaveringly self-confident' during their autosuggestion sessions, and additionally prescribed the following formula:

> Self-confidence is not a characteristic people are born with, and has to be developed. The level of self-confidence depends on whether it has been nurtured. Human capabilities are limitless here. People who are born shy, if they systematically work on themselves, can become confident, decisive and resilient.[58]

The formula also contained a description of how athletes' work and commitment to autosuggestion was bearing fruit and indeed making them more confident.[59] Just like formulas describing physiological processes, it was an instruction meant to direct changes in athletes' attitudes and emotions. In both cases, human capacity for change and growth were said to be limitless. The human will could reshape both mind and body, and it was the psychotherapist's task to encourage athletes to exercise this willpower and to direct their efforts towards self-improvement.

Conclusion

Konstantin Ivanovich Platonov, sometimes hailed as the father of Soviet psychotherapy who outlined its theoretical and physiological basis, insisted that words, the main instruments used by psychotherapists, were one of the main tools that could be used by physicians to restore patients to health, alongside medication, surgery or physiotherapeutic procedures.[60] His statement was often referenced by other researchers and practitioners writing about psychotherapy. Words were described as instruments that could be wielded like a scalpel and administered like medicines to induce physiological changes in the human organism, while psychotherapeutic sessions were compared to surgery to emphasize the precision and preparation they required.[61] Soviet psychotherapists' use of such imagery in talking about their discipline is revealing. First, it is yet another illustration of psychotherapy being conceptualized as a method that addressed not only the psyche but the whole organism. Second, such imagery put emphasis on the expertise required to conduct psychotherapeutic treatment.

Psychotherapy was primarily envisioned as a form of medical treatment and the majority of changes that its practitioners sought to enact aimed to restore patients to health. Suggestion and autosuggestion formulas were to remove symptoms and enable patients to get back to their daily activities. However, Soviet psychotherapy was not envisioned solely as a means to treat illness. Physicians who worked to popularize psychotherapy in the USSR searched for different applications for their methods, often outside the clinic. Soviet psychotherapists sought to prevent neurotic and mental health disorders, to make people better adjusted to their working environment and to improve their performance in sport and in other types of work. Both inside and outside the clinic, Soviet psychotherapy included an element of striving to transform people and encouraging their self-improvement. The physicians who administered psychotherapeutic treatments determined the direction of change and assisted what was seen as the growth and perfection of the patient. Words were the instruments for this procedure. The suggestion and autosuggestion formulas provided to patients and to athletes were the means of influencing their bodies and minds in a precise manner. Psychotherapy was not just a method of treatment but also a technique for transforming people into more resilient, controlled, confident and ultimately better individuals.

An important factor in that personal transformation was the will, which needed to be applied by patients in order for their self-improvement to be successful. The emphasis on willpower is visible in the writing of both psychotherapists working in the clinic and those who focused on preparing athletes for competitions. Soviet psychotherapists did not draw a clear dividing line between the mind and the body when it came to exerting psychotherapeutic influence. Both psychical and physiological processes could be subject to the will. While treatments directed at the psyche were much more common, psychotherapy was also used to help people improve their bodily capacities. Such an approach was in keeping with Soviet practitioners' assertion that they rejected mind-body dualism, yet also reflected the privileged place given to willpower in the process of transforming patients' bodies and minds. The will was treated as an agent of change, capable of influencing physiological processes, thoughts and emotions. It was described as a part of the psyche but it was treated differently than the other parts of the mind. Consequently, neither mind-body dualism nor its rejection offers a sufficient explanation for how Soviet postwar psychotherapy approached the human organism. Instead, psychotherapeutic discourse reveals a different dualism present in the thinking of Soviet physicians: a dualism that placed the will and the rest of the human organism into a binary opposition. The latter was the object of psychotherapeutic influence, while the former was the agent of change and self-perfection. It was through cultivating and applying their will that patients were to overcome their harmful habits and thinking patterns, defeat their illnesses, achieve better results in work and in sport and, ultimately, become more in control of their bodies, thoughts and emotions.

Notes

1 I. F. Miagkov, *Psikhoterapiia: Rukovodstvo dlia studentov meditsinskikh institutov i vrachei* (Moscow: VNMONiP, 1967), 33.
2 Gosudarstvennyi Arkhiv Rossiiskoi Federatsii (GARF), f. r-9552, op. 15, d. 14, ll. 34–5, 77.
3 B. Jungen, 'Frozen Action: Thoughts on Sport, Discipline and the Arts in Soviet Union of the 1930s', in N. Katzer, et al., eds, *Euphoria and Exhaustion: Modern Sport in Soviet Culture and Society* (Frankfurt: Campus Verlag, 2010), 61–79; Catriona Kelly, 'The New Soviet Man and Woman', in Simon Dixon, ed., *The Oxford Handbook of Modern Russian History* (Oxford: Oxford University Press, 2013).
4 R. Bauer, *The New Man in Soviet Psychology* (Cambridge, MA: Harvard University Press, 1952).
5 Aleksandra Brokman, 'Creating a Medical Speciality: Psychotherapy in the Post-War Soviet Healthcare System', *Journal of Health Inequalities*, 5.2 (2019): 203–9.
6 Irina Sirotkina, *Diagnosing Literary Genius: A Cultural History of Psychiatry in Russia, 1880–1930* (Baltimore: Johns Hopkins University Press, 2002).
7 For a detailed analysis of the reception and fate of psychoanalysis in the USSR, see A. A. Etkind, *Eros of the Impossible: The History of Psychoanalysis in Russia* (Boulder: Westview Press 1997); Martin A. Miller, *Freud and the Bolsheviks: Psychoanalysis in Imperial Russia and the Soviet Union* (New Haven: Yale University Press, 1998).
8 Aleksandra Brokman, 'The Healing Power of Words: Psychotherapy in the USSR, 1956–1985' (PhD thesis, Norwich: University of East Anglia, 2018).
9 Sirotkina, *Diagnosing Literary Genius*, 104–105.
10 Brokman, 'The Healing Power', 48, 62–70.
11 K. I. Platonov, *The Word as a Physiological and Therapeutic Factor: The Theory and Practice of Psychotherapy According to I.P. Pavlov* (Honolulu: University Press of the Pacific, [1959] 2003), 423; V. E. Rozhnov, 'Meditsinskaia deontologiia i psikhoterapiia' in V. E. Rozhnov, ed., *Rukovodstvo po psikhoterapii* (Moscow: Meditsina, 1974), 18–25, 22.
12 This view of the psyche was based on Engels's concept of various levels of reality, according to which each level had its own laws guiding the motion of matter. Since something new was added at every level, the laws of the higher level of reality could not be explained by the laws of the lower one. Consciousness was viewed as resulting from a higher level of organized matter and thus could not be simply explained by the laws governing lower levels, including physiology. See: J. A. Gray, 'Attention, Consciousness and Voluntary Control of Behaviour in Soviet Psychology: Philosophical Roots and Research Branches', in N. O'Connor, ed., *Present-Day Russian Psychology: A Symposium by Seven Authors* (Oxford: Pergamon, 1967), 1–38; T. R. Payne, 'The "Brain-Psyche" Problem in Soviet Psychology', *Studies in Soviet Thought*, 7.2 (1967): 83–100.
13 V. N. Miasishchev, 'Certain Theoretical Questions of Psychotherapy', in R. B. Winn, ed., *Psychotherapy in the Soviet Union* (New York: Evergreen Books, 1961), 2–19, 13.

14 S. N. Astakhov, *Lechebnoe deistvie slova* (Leningrad: Gosudarstvennoe izdatel'stvo meditsinskoi literatury, 1962), 69.
15 M. S. Lebedinskii, *Ocherki psikhoterapii* (Moscow: Meditsina, 1971), 6.
16 K. M. Varshavskii, *Gipnosuggestivnaia terapiia: lechenie vnusheniem v gipnoze* (Leningrad: Meditsina, 1973), 99.
17 L. J. Kirmayer, 'Psychotherapy and the Cultural Concept of the Person', *Transcultural Psychiatry*, 44.2 (2007): 232–57.
18 V. N. Miasishchev et al., *Osnovy obshchei i meditsinskoi psikhologii* (Leningrad: Meditsina, 1975), 187.
19 A. P. Slobodianik, *Psikhoterapiia, vnushenie, gipnoz* (Kyiv: Zdorov'ia, 1983), 88.
20 Ibid.
21 Tsentral'nyi arkhiv goroda Moskvy (TsAGM), f. r-533, op. 1, d. 158, l. 4.
22 J. Hellbeck, *Revolution on My Mind: Writing a Diary under Stalin* (Cambridge, MA: Harvard University Press, 2006).
23 O. Kharkhordin, *The Collective and the Individual in Russia: A Study of Practices* (Berkeley: University of California Press, 1999), 5.
24 E. Erwin, *Philosophy and Psychotherapy: Razing the Troubles of the Brain* (London: Sage Publications, 1997); C. P. Bankart, *Talking Cures: A History of Western and Eastern Psychotherapies* (Pacific Grove: Brooks/Cole, 1997); S. Joseph, *Theories of Counselling and Psychotherapy: An Introduction to the Different Approaches* (Basingstoke: Red Globe Press, 2010).
25 R. T. De George, 'Biomedical Ethics', in L. R. Graham, ed., *Science and the Soviet Social Order* (Cambridge, Mass: Harvard University Press, 1990), 195–224
26 V. V. Voskresenskii, *Psikhoterapiia i psikhoprofilaktika na sluzhbe zdorov'ia cheloveka* (Krasnodar: Obshchestvo Znanie RSFSR, 1977), 24–5.
27 Varshavskii, *Gipnosuggestivnaia terapiia*, 99.
28 Astakhov, *Lechebnoe deistvie*, 22–5.
29 Lebedinskii, *Ocherki*, 400–1.
30 Lebedinskii, *Ocherki*; Platonov, *The Word*.
31 Ia. R. Doktorskii, *Autogennaia trenirovka* (Stavropol: Stavropol'skoe knizhnoe izdatel'stvo, 1978); A. M. Sviadoshch, 'Autogennaia trenirovka' in Rozhnov, ed., *Rukovodstvo*, 90–101.
32 Doktorskii, *Autogennaia trenirovka*, 25–33.
33 Ibid.
34 Slobodianik, *Psikhoterapiia*, 88–9.
35 Ibid., 90.
36 Anna Toropova, 'Rest for the Brain' or 'Technology of the Unconscious?': Hypnosis in Early Soviet Medicine and Culture', in this volume.
37 G. Ia. Avrutskii, A. A. Neduva, *Lechenie psikhicheski bol'nykh: rudovodstvo dlia vrachei* (Moscow: Meditsina, 1981); N. Spiridonov, Ia. Doktorskii, *Gipnoz bez tain: vnushenie, gipnoz, autogennaia trenirovka* (Stavropol: Stavropol'skoe knizhnoe izdatel'stvo, 1974).
38 Astakhov, *Lechebnoe deistvie*, 22–5.
39 Varshavskii, *Gipnosuggestivnaia terapiia*, 38–39.
40 TsAGM, f. r-533, op. 1, d. 158, l. 4.
41 Tricia Starks, 'Soviet Pioneers in Smoking Cessation: From Group Therapy in the 1920s to Cytisine in the 1970s', in this volume.
42 Miagkov, *Psikhoterapiia*, 95. It must be noted that although psychotherapists prepared suggestion and autosuggestion formulas for patients suffering from heart

conditions and other physical illnesses, they did not expect their methods alone to cure organic disorders. Soviet specialists stressed that psychotherapy was to be administered alongside other treatments, in order to increase patients' determination to recover, and thus also their chances for recovery.

43 Doktorskii, *Autogennaia*, 42.
44 T. M. Luhrmann, *Of Two Minds: The Growing Disorder in American Psychiatry* (New York: Knopf, 2000), 8.
45 Lebedinskii, *Ocherki*, 265–6.
46 Astakhov, *Lechebnoe*, 94.
47 Miagkov, *Psikhoterapiia*, 96.
48 GARF, f. r-9552, op. 15, d. 14, l. 4.
49 Ibid., 45–6, 57.
50 S. Grant, 'Bolsheviks, Revolution and Physical Culture', *The International Journal of the History of Sport*, 31.7 (2014): 724–34.
51 M. O'Mahony, *Sport in the USSR: Physical Culture – Visual Culture* (London: Reaktion Books, 2006); E. E. Redihan, *The Olympics and the Cold War, 1948–1968: Sport as Battleground in the U.S.–Soviet Rivalry* (Jefferson, NC: McFarland & Company, 2017).
52 GARF, f. r-7576, op. 7, d. 223, ll. 3-6.
53 GARF, f. r-8009, op. 50, d. 8665, l. 109.
54 A. T. Filatov, *Emotsional'no-volevaia podgotovka velosipedistov* (Kyiv: Zdorov'ia, 1975), 43–4.
55 Ibid., 45.
56 A. A. Martynenko, 'Mototsikletnyi sport' in A. T. Filatov, *Emotsional'no-volevaia podgotovka sportsmenov* (Kyiv: Zdorov'ia, 1982).
57 Filatov, *Emotsional'no-volevaia podgotovka velosipedistov*, 82.
58 Ibid., 29.
59 Ibid.
60 Platonov, *The Word*, 8.
61 Astakhov, *Lechebnoe*, 3; Rozhnov, 'Meditsinskaia', 23.

7

Soviet pioneers in smoking cessation: From group therapy in the 1920s to Cytisine in the 1970s

Tricia Starks

Therapeutic tobacco-cessation techniques emerged in Russia before tobacco was considered addictive. The connection of nicotine and dependency is a relatively recent development. In 1957, the World Health Organization decided to term smoking a 'habit' rather than an 'addiction', not revisiting the question until 1964 when they conceded there might be other factors involved.[1] It was not until the 1970s that global researchers proposed that smoking was more than a habit and dependent upon chemical reinforcements that evinced significant withdrawal symptoms. Only within the last few decades have understandings of nicotine dependency broadened to a vision of an array of biopsychosocial prompts that tangle up chemical and physical issues with the social and cultural.[2] Soviet medical authorities began the first national anti-smoking programmes and created the first publicly funded tobacco-cessation clinics in the 1920s, well before these modern ideas of tobacco use and dependency. Instead, Soviet anti-tobacco authors depicted smoking cessation as entirely dependent upon the will of the smoker, which could be cultivated and trained. From the 1920s to 1970s, such concepts guided arguments on how to best achieve tobacco cessation. Relying upon the will denied biochemical addiction and dismissed psychosocial prompts as irrational and inconsequential. Instead of seeing smokers as bodies in space and culture with a broad array of physical, sensorial, and chemical experiences, the problem of continued smoking was reduced to an issue of will and outlook.

When smoking became nothing but the will, techniques for quitting followed predictable routes for strengthening it. Early cessation therapies relied on creating new conditioned reflexes, with the help of hypnosis, suggestion, and/or aversion therapies that incorporated tinctures and mouth rinses to make smoking unpleasant.[3] Although these innovative clinics sunk from view, the 1920s cessation techniques carried on after smoking risk was reconceptualized in the wake of large-scale epidemiological studies in the 1950s that connected smoking and lung cancer and after newer ideas of addiction developed. Soviet postwar understandings of tobacco danger and cessation techniques relied upon ideas developed in the 1920s. The emphasis upon nicotine, however, as a slow poison to the system opened the door to using other innovative chemical therapeutics like cytisine that instead of creating aversion to tobacco supplanted nicotine cravings. Many of these therapies have become prominent today.

This essay outlines Soviet attitudes towards nicotine and tobacco dangers from the 1920s into the 1970s and the cessation therapies promoted by Soviet medical authorities. The changing concept of how to treat tobacco use connects not just with ideas about the will and new chemical therapies, but also with anxieties about popular health and rising tensions from modern life. Smoking connected into these general concerns as well as a worry over the declining health of Soviet men and their decreasing life spans. Even as new concerns emerged, however, the continued emphasis upon willpower showed the longevity of ideas of how to fight tobacco use.

Although Soviet anti-smoking authors quickly incorporated Western attacks on tobacco into their established campaigns, the Soviet medical and state authorities did not react quickly. Motions against smoking such as official announcements, labelling and advertising bans as deployed in Britain and the United States took some time to take hold in the USSR. Soviet cessation techniques continued to rely upon methods and arguments used since the 1920s. The Soviet emphasis on the chemistry of tobacco, and especially the poison nicotine, led to unique answers to tobacco danger. The Soviets developed chemical therapies that mimicked nicotine and saw remarkable success.

Nicotine and nerve danger

Nikolai Semashko, the first Commissar of Public Health for the Bolsheviks, put forward a plan to stamp out tobacco use in the revolutionary state in 1920. His plan was multifaceted, attacking tobacco agriculture, production, trade and export, but he was unable to get it implemented.[4] He did, however, as head of a state agency devoted to public health and unified, universal, prophylactic care, embark upon a national anti-smoking propaganda campaign unprecedented in its scope. Massive amounts of posters, pamphlets, films, slides and lecture materials accompanied the general campaign to instil healthier habits in the population and fight infectious diseases and other public health problems.[5] Nestled within this flurry of propaganda were messages of anti-smoking and against other bad habits considered 'lifestyle illnesses'.[6] Lifestyle illnesses were those threats to health centered on habits, cultural practices and, in most cases, ignorance of what medical authorities considered correct, rational and hygienic living. These illnesses encompassed everything from drink and tobacco to use of faith healers and village wise women or sexual habits considered instrumental to the spread of syphilis.[7]

Smoking was extremely widespread in revolutionary Russia. On the eve of the First World War, observers considered Russians inveterate smokers, indulging in tobacco even more avidly than alcohol. Most males were believed to smoke and to go through at least a pack a day of the peculiar Russian cigarettes called papirosy or to smoke an equivalent amount of the rough, nicotine-heavy Russian tobacco called makhorka.[8] The use of quicker acting, inhaled tobacco along with the high nicotine leaf likely caused more intense dependency for the mass of the population in Russia earlier than in other markets that used tobacco in snuff, chaw or pipes.

Semashko based his attack on decades of anti-tobacco work in Russia and Europe that detailed the corrosive effects of the alkaloid on the nervous system and its role in the development of neurasthenia. After the revolution, Semashko took this concern for nicotine, and bolstered by a perceived epidemic of nerve disease, went on the offensive against smoking. Semashko and other anti-tobacco authors readily connected smoking to the wave of neurasthenia diagnoses in the 1920s. A 1920 piece for service members stressed that smokers often suffered from neurasthenia or 'inflammation of the nerves'.[9] A 1925 pamphlet noted that smokers had general degradation of the nervous system, weakness, poor reflexes, weak memory, cloudy thinking and impotence.[10] Another of the same year connected smoking to mass neurasthenia among office workers.[11] A 1925 pamphlet argued that tobacco use led to degradation of higher nerve function.[12] As the 1926 *Why Is Tobacco Dangerous?* noted, the gradual onset of tobacco poisoning on the nerves was hidden by the initial burst of energy from smoking. But then dizziness, headaches, problems of sight and hearing and harm to nerves began 'and it stands clear that for nerves tobacco is a very harmful and dangerous item, which people all by themselves happily poison themselves'.[13]

The intensity of anti-tobacco and anti-nicotine rhetoric declined in the 1930s due to several major transitions. First, while Lenin had been a staunch anti-smoker, Stalin smoked both pipes and papirosy. Anti-tobacco rhetoric, and discussion of how nicotine enslaved the user or weakened their potency, was not as easy to make. Further, Semashko's removal as head of the Commissariat of Health left a void in leadership of the anti-tobacco campaign.[14] While anti-tobacco literature aimed at women and children continued to come out, other essays, pamphlets and posters reduced to a trickle. Similarly, the innovative dispensary-based group therapies were no longer publicized. Finally, just as alcohol production increased to serve as a cash cow for the state in the drive for industrialization, so too did Anastas Mikoian, the Commissar of Food Industry, call for increased tobacco production to bring in money and satisfy demand from workers for more smokes.[15]

It would be after the Second World War before researchers anywhere moved to conceptualize smoking as creating chemical dependency. Though not beholden to the same market pressures as in the West, the Soviets did not accept tobacco compulsion as an addiction for other reasons. Soviet authors, while employing the term habit most often to refer to smoking, complicated the understanding of smoking by layering the term habit with implications from the works of Ivan Pavlov and his concept of the conditioned reflex. As Anna Toropova explains in her essay for this volume, Pavlovian concepts influenced many fields including those for creating new behaviours. Anti-tobacco authors used the concept of the Pavlovian conditioned reflex, that is, over time, tobacco use became a habit cultivated through repetition of physical movements and regular stimuli, to explain the long-term effects of regular poisoning with nicotine as a stimulus to poor habits that, cultivated, nurtured and repeated, became and embedded in personal behaviours and then society as a whole. Cessationists argued that just as smokers had been slowly turned into habituates they needed to be trained into new behavioural patterns that did not include smoking. The multi-edition early 1950s pamphlet *On the Dangers of Smoking* noted the deep roots of tobacco use in Soviet society and culture at all levels and the difficulty in fighting it, 'The fight with tobacco smoking requires large labors. Smoking has travelled deeply into our lives, becoming an everyday occurrence. Most men smoke, many women, and even a few youths.'[16]

Arguing for the deeply embedded nature of smoking, the author concluded:

> Smokers must understand that in smoking a large role is played by not so much the accustoming to the narcotic as much as accustoming to the very process of smoking, to papirosy, to pipes. Therefore, those who wish to quit must refuse the habit of smoking, which is an artificially acquired, conditioned reflex, and to restore the protective reflex – the body's protests to a violently injected poison – nicotine.[17]

Despite acknowledging a chemical component to tobacco use, the author discounted any talk of nicotine being like narcotics as there were no symptoms of tobacco withdrawal (*tabachnogo goloda*) and the action of nicotine was violent. Instead, a smoker should be easily able to quit if they understood why to do so.[18]

The 1960s and 1970s continued the emphasis on nicotine as damaging to nerves and the heart, readily sliding into prevalent ideas regarding health stressors. In 1960, A. N. Bakulev's entry for *The Big Medical Encyclopaedia* forwarded the picture of smoking as reflex that had developed in the 1920s concluding that 'Smoking of tobacco (*nikotinizm*) is one of the most widespread types of narcomania and includes a large mass of users; it therefore can be termed a quotidian narcomania'. He emphasized the repeated actions of smoking as important to the development of the habit, because 'The process of smoking tobacco consists of the sucking action and the sensation of taste'. Despite this, he argued that 'Smoking of tobacco does not appear a physiological necessity of the organism; it is more closely a pathological act'.[19]

Collective therapies

Despite the anxiety over smoking in the 1920s, anti-tobacco authorities noted a general lack of literature on the issue and even the 'contempt' for the question. Dr A.G. Stoiko, in an extensive 1928 overview of cessation therapies, contended that this distaste was born not of the severity of the problem, but lack of success. He argued that 'Tobacco therapy is studied generally with little desire, and the cause of that comes from, of course, its difficulty'. Stoiko pointed to problems not in science or medicine, but society as it surrounded the smoker with 'a whole mass of negative suggestions (spoken in the language of psychology) or conditioned stimuli (in the language of reflexology) that hinder the ability to extinguish, an often very lasting, conditioned reflex'. Stoiko pointed out that instead of reinforcing cessation, all around the smoker, society 'reinforces the conditioned reflex, (with) the wide reach of tobacco advertisements standing on every corner, and the papirosy sellers everywhere as well'. Despite this, Stoiko set out to show the way forward by outlining persuasion, hypnosis and suggestion; targeted therapy; and self-suggestion. Persuasion, he clarified, meant attendance of a patient to doctor's advice on how to easily live without tobacco. Among cessation theorists, the irrationality of smoking retained constant emphasis. This reflected the influence of the Swiss theorist Paul Charles Dubois who advocated for the rational treatment of nervous disorders with 'persuasion therapy' that entailed appeals to patients that engaged them logically.

Stoiko was more positive on suggestion therapy than hypnosis, which he said was effective in curing alcoholism but not tobacco use. He argued that where the alcoholic was susceptible to hypnosis, the smoker was not as nicotine did not make patients pliable. Further, the hypnosis patient was 'passive' waiting for the doctor to do all the work and 'gives nothing of himself', which Stoiko found useless for cessation.[20] As Anna Toropova's essay in this volume illustrates, hypnosis therapy was much debated as to its success and its mechanisms in the 1920s. Not surprisingly, others countered Stoiko and considered hypnosis highly effective in fighting tobacco use. Dr V.N. Zolotniskii argued in his *On the Danger of Smoking Tobacco* that 'one of the more hopeful means for quitting smoking is therapeutic hypnotic suggestion'.[21] Others similarly saw the value of the technique.[22]

Stoiko's techniques utilized foreign and domestic inspirations. German psychotherapist Wladimir G. Eliasberg (1887–1969) served as the source for the concept of 'targeted therapy' where smokers established a base line of pulse, blood pressure and other data at a first visit, and then by monitoring changes over time they could appreciate health improvements. Stoiko considered this method to be quite successful as 'The sick by himself, not through a book and not through a doctor's lecture comes to know the danger of smoking'.[23] This appeal to the rational reflected the ideas of Dubois while the method of autosuggestion came from the work of the French psychologist and pharmacist Emile Coue de la Chataigneraie (1857–1926). Coue, who found hypnosis an imperfect method of affecting behaviour change, instead proposed a modified version of suggestion therapy for conscious patients. Stoiko and others championed this form of therapy over hypnosis.

Stoiko reserved most of his discussion for 'collective psychotherapy', a unique approach to cessation from the Soviets. He began by arguing that tobacco acted upon the body in ways differently than morphine, opium, or even alcohol. He pointed out that since nicotine was a poison, it did not have withdrawal effects; instead manifesting in complaints of 'a psychological character', the only commonality of which was a feeling that 'something is not right'. He concluded, anecdotally, that when he himself had quit smoking, and deprived himself of the 'neurological hammer' his 'head worked poorly or got lost somewhere in the rhetoric'. From this he said it was obvious that the least active force in tobacco use was the physiological effect on the body. Stoiko depicted these hurdles to quitting as entirely psychological in nature. He noted the existence of 'imaginary danger' such as the belief among some smokers that quitting suddenly might shock the heart or nervous system. He suggested smokers got trapped in a mental loop, where they believed that it would be difficult to quit and therefore through mental reinforcement they were unable to quit. He cited as evidence the difference between successful and unsuccessful attempts – 'In only one way are they different than people who have quit – they do this easily because they believe in the ease of it'.[24]

Stoiko focused on the 'collective method of psychotherapy' which he argued was the 'most rational' choice because it addressed the 'social character' of smoking. By hearing from those who had quit, comparing themselves to successful non-smokers, working with others and hearing how the collective disliked smoking, tobacco users could build from others the will to quit. Without any symptoms of chemical withdrawal for tobacco, and without a recognition of biological dependency on nicotine, tobacco use was simply a cultivated action for authors that was reinforced by social and cultural cues. Strengthening the will, through techniques such as rational suggestion and behaviour modification, became the preferred means of Stoiko and others. Such dependency upon the will to override problems continued throughout the Soviet period, as seen in later cessation therapies and as outlined in the work by Brokman in this volume where she shows how Soviet post-war experts built on early ideas about the will as capable of 'influencing and governing both the mental and the somatic'.

The overwhelming numbers seeking treatment influenced Stoiko's choice of collective therapy as it most effectively used the doctor's energy so that many could be healed at once. To demonstrate the techniques, Stoiko brought up the implementation of the work with its first group of twenty to fifty people. He noted that the patients had been chosen from a common social group so that their days would be filled with reinforcement. This was desired, he noted, but not required. He recommended a quick succession of lectures, on basics of reflexology, tobacco danger, the social character of smoking and danger to others from tobacco. Lectures ended with a period of collective suggestions. To carry on the therapy outside the dispensary, patients were urged to create a meeting circle of like-minded individuals.[25]

Group therapy in the style outlined by Stoiko became the basis of an incredibly popular programme from the Moscow Regional Health Department in the late 1920s. Spurred by the perceived crises of smokers, the dispensary system of treatment expanded to address tobacco use. The dispensary was an outpatient facility that combined doctor care with home visits from nurses and sanitary propaganda. Dispensaries operated for alcoholism, tuberculosis and other diseases. The connections of smoking with alcoholism and tuberculosis made this an ideal fit.[26] The programme was incredibly popular and smokers overwhelmed the system so that if in 1924 there were 30–40 people signing up a month, they soon climbed into the thousands.[27] In 1928, 8,000 smokers flooded the system before enrolments were cut off.[28] According to one report, when fully instituted, the dispensary, group therapy and anti-smoking approach could reach 40–50 per cent effectiveness.[29] An incredible success rate given that even today, cessation attempts are only successful 5 per cent of the time.[30]

Therapeutic suggestion, guided by a physician and practised en masse and in private, constituted the major form of treatment by the group. These statements focused upon the problems of smoking or its repellent aspects, and users were to repeat these to themselves in groups and then throughout the day. It was not a new technique. A 1919 pamphlet outlined a full set of considerations that smokers should keep in mind, 'Daily and always we must think of all the unpleasantness and bad outcomes of smoking for our health and those around and also the money spent on smoking, the damage to work [so that] papirosy call to mind a feeling of revulsion'.[31]

Other therapies also proved popular in the period, indicating that many did wish to quit smoking. The 1920s chemical therapies in tobacco cessation were limited to medicines that made smoking taste unpleasant. This use of chemicals, however, still fits within the parameters of reflexology, but as a negative stimulus for discouraging repeated behaviour. This made it back into advice literature in the 1930s and appeared in pamphlets to the 1960s and later.[32] Some were not chemical but behavioural. For instance, the 1964 pamphlet *The Green Death* praised an inventive wife who threw two kopeks out the window, 'methodically and silently', every time her husband lit up until the negative impression finally induced him to quit.[33]

Social and chemical reflexive therapies continued to be discussed in popular health journals in the 1930s, but the dispensary method for smoking cessation and mass sessions disappeared. The retreat from public cessation came with a general decline in anti-tobacco propaganda. Anti-smoking rhetoric from the 1930s until the 1960s focused on women and children and quitting was rarely discussed. Changed global attitudes towards smoking and the rise of tobacco-related illness in the USSR pushed cessation back into the spotlight. This different scientific and social terrain did not, however, change the therapies and attitudes advocated by Soviet authorities.

Bakulev's 1960 entry for *The Big Medical Encyclopaedia* detailed most expansively cessation therapies and showed the development by the Soviets of the concept that social and cultural stimuli reinforced smoking behaviour. To address the problem, Bakulev advocated a variation of the 1920s dispensary methods. Utilizing a strong understanding of cultural and social cues, as well as a feel for the sensory attractions of the habit, Bakulev concluded:

> The psychology of smoking and its fixation is aided by the so-called weapons of production in the means of appealing packs, carved pipes, pleasant mouthpieces. No small meaning comes in the pretty packaging cladding a pack of papiros and such. In addition, the process of smoking for some smokers transforms into a special ritual: the manner of smoking and the holding of the papirosy, kneading and tapping with the fingers to drop the ash, the manner of exhalation of the smoke and such. All this becomes attractive and tempting for those beginning to smoke and opens before them a curtain on still unknown pleasures, even though the first attempt of smoking calls forth disgust for the taste.[34]

Bakulev's nuanced discussion of smoking's matrix of compulsions was reflected in a more encompassing understanding of the difficulties in quitting. For the Soviets, social life hindered and culture complicated quitting when all around there were incitements to smoke. When such a patient comes in, according to Bakulev, they ask for the doctor to impose his power upon them, saying in effect, 'Operate on me as you need, hypnotize me, suggest me what you will so that I do not smoke, but I cannot achieve anything by myself.'[35]

To help strengthen the smoker's will, Bakulev used chemical and psychological therapies based on cultivating a conditioned reflex. Silver nitrate solution, which made smoke taste unpleasant, would use adverse stimuli to mould behaviours. Hypnosis and suggestion would rely upon creating new reactions. He added in the idea of gradual reduction through rationing out the smokes with continued use of suggestion. Bakulev emphasized the role of the individual in cessation but also stressed the way that medical professionals must facilitate and encourage patients.[36] According to the

1960 pamphlet *Quit smoking!*, quitting was easy as, 'According to data … 71.2% of smokers easily quit smoking, not experiencing in this any unpleasant associations'. While some might experience 'fatigue, cravings for tobacco, a few apathy, distraction, sleep disturbance and a few strengthened cough', these were fleeting. Instead, smokers should quit immediately, though the author provided only reasons why to do this and no advice on how – a startling omission for a pamphlet entitled *Quit Smoking!*[37]

By the 1960s, Western findings on the carcinogenic dangers of smoking had become more accepted in Soviet medical literature and joined the already established rhetoric on the dangers of tobacco, nicotine poisoning, nervous disorders, and heart dangers. This echoed a general concern for the stressful effects of modern life on health, as outlined Jan Arend's essay in this volume, and an emerging fear for male health in particular.[38] A 1965 manual from the Ministry of Health and Sanitary Enlightenment Institute 'written with doctors from many specialties (therapists, neuropathologist, psychiatrists, chemists, etc.)' embraced Western understandings of tobacco danger:

> From the American medical report 'Smoking and Health' (published in January 1964) it is seen that smoking does not just engender cancer of the lungs but has a significant effect on mortality from other illnesses. According to the data, smokers die from different diseases at a rate of ten times more often than non-smokers and heavy smokers even twenty times more often![39]

Unlike previous specialized publications, which dismissed the problem of cessation as a simple question of developing the will, this 'instructional-methodological' publication argued that many smokers saw the danger but could not quit without a doctor's help, since 'The healing of tobacco smokers appears a difficult task requiring the correct path and a complex and strictly individualized therapy'.[40]

The manual detailed doctor-supervised treatment for those in 'light or middle stage tobacco intoxication' which would work for most utilizing mouth washes, vitamin therapy and aversion therapy (using ipecac, apomorfin or emetin to induce unpleasant experiences). For aversion therapy, under a doctor's supervision, medicine was administered until the onset of nausea, at which point the doctor directed the patient to smoke, then, 'With every vomit the patient takes a drag of tobacco smoke and this simultaneously inspires disgust in the smoker to tobacco smoke and smoking tobacco'.[41] This mirrored anti-alcohol treatments of the time that employed purgatives. The completed course resulted in lowered blood pressure according to the author. Given the traumatic procedures, this was not surprising.

In addition to aversion methods, the pamphlet gave detailed instructions for 'substitution' therapy using lobeline or tsititon. For lobeline it was a two- to three-week course of therapy with intramuscular injections of a 1 per cent solution two times daily – one after breakfast (9.00–10.00 am) and one around dinner time (5.00–6.00 pm) administered under a doctor's supervision. Adverse reactions included complications for arteriosclerosis and alterations in the brain, heart, liver, and nerves.[42] Tsititon had a ten- to twenty-one-day course with injections or could also be taken orally when dissolved in water. The recommendations pointed out that some might simply reduce tobacco intake or might return. In the first case, the user should go through the treatment again after a month and a half or so. In the latter, they should return immediately to the doctor. The author argued that properly administered clinical use showed 'the marked advantage in the use of tsititon'.[43]

The past figured heavily in the instructions on quitting – either in terms of the therapies recommended or in a general attempt to educate smokers as to the origins of their problem. A 1958 essay in the magazine *Health* used anti-smoking rhetoric from the 1500s, while another article in the same year on 'How I Quit Smoking' helpfully included information from the seventeenth century.[44] From the archaic, the author moved humorously through to his own experience with familiar approaches to cessation – compensatory sweets, slow reductions in use and the old standby of smoking enough in one time to get sick (which ended with a neighbour calling the fire brigade).[45] Reflecting the emphasis upon tobacco use as a conditioned reflex, yet still singing in the key of previous methods, the 1959 pamphlet *Smoking Is Dangerous* advocated immediate quitting and argued that no more than two to three days of discomfort, perhaps some weakness or a headache, would follow but that the quitter would need to maximize their will and get help from a supportive group of fellows as 'A person who is quitting smoking will still long be under the power of reflexes and earlier acquired habits'. If this proved insufficient, suggestion, hypnosis, silver nitrate or other chemical helpmates might be employed to strengthen the resolve of the smoker to quit.[46]

History grounded anti-tobacco works, and historic arguments, grafted to newer science, explained tobacco's attractions. One of the more ubiquitous was the explanation of the compulsion to tobacco use as a learned behaviour that became ingrained in the user; that is, a conditioned reflex. 'Habits are second nature', repeated many a pamphlet over the decades, using the contention of Marcus Tullius Cicero (106–43 BCE) from his essay 'The Ends of Good and Evil' where he built upon the concepts of Aristotle (384–22 BCE) regarding behaviour. In the hands of cessationists, Cicero's maxim became a support for the idea that tobacco use was like any other 'bad' habit such as biting one's nails, poor diet or sleeping in late.[47] Such downplaying of the origins of tobacco's pull melded easily with reflexology's emphasis upon conditioned responses and downplayed depictions of smoking as a chemical addiction.

Older therapies, older arguments and older theories continued to feature in diagnoses of the smoker – especially in the character of the failed quitter. Neurasthenia, which had fallen from fashion in the West, still appeared in Soviet contexts. The 1960 pamphlet *Alongside the Smoke of the Papirosy: Health Vanishes* underscored the connection between the two, scathingly commenting, 'The only ones who cannot quit smoking are those weak-charactered, will-less people, suffering from some illness like neurasthenia – itself an outgrowth of smoking'. New propaganda joined the mix, like the methods featured in Siobhán Hearne's essay. For example, by the 1970s, sanitary propaganda included a full menu of anti-drinking, anti-smoking films to try out on the captive audience including *Two Habits (Alcohol and Smoking)* (1970); *The Business of Tobacco* (1972); *The Danger of Smoking* (1975); *Smoking leads to …* (1978); *Don't Smoke* (1978) and *Passive Smoking* (1978).[48] But despite the new mediums, to fix the neurasthenic required older messages including, 'systematic study of sport, high-grade physical labor, hardening (*zakalka*) the organism, which helps the smoker to seriously strengthen their health and become a physically and psychically (*dukhovno*) strong person. That will in its turn helps to a marked extent the fight with smoking.'[49] Strengthening the will, especially for children, had been a long-time halt upon the development of neurasthenia and smoking compulsion according to first tsarist and then Soviet cessationists and continued to be so in the postwar era. As Brokman demonstrates, fighting to strengthen the will in the postwar world became a means of fighting all sorts of psychological and neurological problems.[50]

The therapies used within the Soviet context, despite their specific connections to reflexology or neurasthenia, did mirror the emphases found in other countries on communal support, group support and the psychology of smoking. The first British anti-smoking clinic was set up at the London School of Hygiene and Tropical Medicine in 1957 and other clinics followed using combinations of the Alcoholics Anonymous model as well as counselling, group meetings and hypnotherapy – all techniques the Soviet had used for decades. The therapeutic style, which depended upon convincing individual smokers of the rational problems with their habits, assumed that smokers had the time to attend meetings and appointments and also the recourse to trained, medical authorities for support.

New chemical therapies

The 1965 Soviet publication *On the Dangers of Smoking (Lecture Outlines)* from the Sanitary Enlightenment Institute hinted at an evolving understanding of tobacco dependency. Arguing that clinical research showed that 'habit' might describe the relationship of about a third of smokers to tobacco, for the remaining two-thirds there were 'visible consequences' from quitting including irritability, insomnia, fatigue and weakened immune responses. The severity of these physical responses indicated that there was something more to smoking than just a habit like biting nails – 'the need to smoke in these people is more associated not with a habit, but with a disease predilection (*pristrastiem*)'.[51]

No smoker wanted to repeat the revolting experience of the first smoke, argued the author, but 'predilection' developed sometime after the 'second, third, tenth, even a hundredth *papirosa*'. The markers of greater dependency on tobacco did not set in at the same point for all, but eventually they might develop a true '*tabakomaniia*'. This could come on quickly, just like with morphine, and distinguished smoking from slower developing dependencies, like that for alcohol. The pamphlet introduced not just a view of tobacco dependency as more than habit but included ideas of some new chemical therapies that were being developed that might be of use, including atropine (a product out of Armenia that was not mentioned in any other literature), lobeline (an alkaloid from lobelia with action similar to nicotine, also known as 'devil's tobacco') and tsititon (also known as cytitonum, a solution of cytisine alkaloid or under the brand name Tabex, hereafter cytisine). Unlike earlier tinctures and mouth coatings, tsititon did not fight tobacco use through aversion but acted like nicotine and decreased biochemical prompts to smoking. These chemical aids were not to be used in isolation, but alongside other techniques already proposed – groups, new environments, physical culture, self-suggestion, hypnosis and mouth washes.[52]

Cytisine emerged as a therapy in Eastern Europe in the wake of the Second World War. During the war, in response to tobacco scarcity, smokers turned to other leaf, such as maple trees, to fill papirosy.[53] The leaves of the golden rain tree (*cytisus laburnum*) had been used as a tobacco substitute and the aftereffects had been recognized as decreasing nicotine cravings. It is now understood that cytisine stimulates breath and circulation and acts as an agonist of nicotine receptors (a substance that initiates a physiological response when combined with a receptor).[54] The molecular structure of the chemicals of tobacco and the golden rain tree leaf were remarkably close (Cytisine – $C_{11}H_{14}N_2O$; Nicotine – $C_{10}H_{14}N_2$). The similarities had been noticed earlier. A 1912 animal experiment had found that the alkaloid cytosine created the same responses as nicotine.[55] According to N. A. Ponomareva's 1965 commentary on the drug and cessation therapy, 'The preparation tsititon was developed in 1941 by the VNIKhFI im. S. Ordzhonikidze (All Union Scientific Chemical Pharmaceutical Research Institute in the name of S. Ordzhonikidze) and approved by the Pharmacology committee of NKZ SSSR (People's Commissariat of Health of the USSR).'[56] Despite this early entrée of the drug into the East European scene, it would not be until 1978 that the global tobacco industry would identify cytisine as a substance that closely mimicked the effects of nicotine and later still before Western cessation therapies would regularly incorporate it.[57]

In fact, 1965 proved a watershed year for the treatment in Eastern Europe and the Soviet Union when Tabex, a derivative of the leaves, was first tested in Bulgaria and East Germany. While success was reported, there were also adverse effects including changes in taste and appetite along with dry mouth, headache, nausea, irritability and constipation. It was counter-indicated for those with arterial hypertension. As its effect on circulation increased blood pressure, the testing of cytisine took place alongside anabasine (another alkaloid with close relationships to tobacco) and the results did not separate out the two nor was the study double blind or in line with a number of research strategies in the West. These findings were therefore not readily incorporated into Western research protocols.[58] According to a review written in 2006, this led to a sad situation that 'an apparently effective smoking cessation drug that has been used for decades in Germany and Eastern European countries remained unnoticed in other countries'.[59] This misses the even earlier 1941 advent of the drug according to Ponomareva's revelation by the Soviet Union's research establishment. The lag had great consequence. According to a 2014 study, the use of cytisine in smoking cessation 'almost doubles the chances of quitting at 6 months'. In sum, cytisine shows better results than nicotine replacement therapy though it does carry more adverse effects and has been little used in the West despite these unparalleled positive results.[60]

Conclusion

The early Soviet antipathy to smoking resulted in early, and innovative, approaches to smoking cessation that built on the work of Russian and Soviet specialists with unique attitudes towards behaviour modification and the role of the collective in both fostering and discouraging behaviour. Approaches emphasized the danger of the poison nicotine, encouraged collective group therapy, and paid attention to the many ways that social and cultural connections could further tobacco use. At the same time, the prevalence of therapies dependent on either positive reinforcement or aversion therapy reflected the strength of reflexology among the Soviets. While Soviet support for cessation waned under Stalin, it remerged in the 1960s and returned to their communal and reflexology roots. The continued attention to the poison of nicotine, along with wartime experience, left the Soviets more open to alternative chemical therapies. Experimentation in this direction led to the creation of the cytisine-based drug Tabex, which has seen remarkable success.

Notes

1. Robert N. Proctor, *Golden Holocaust: Origins of the Cigarette Catastrophe and the Case for Abolition* (Berkeley: University of California Press, 2011), 237–8.
2. John A. Dani and David J. K. Valfour, 'Historical and Current Perspective on Tobacco Use and Nicotine Addiction', *Trends in Neuroscience* 34.7 (2011): 383–92; M. A. Russel, 'Cigarette Dependence: I. Nature and Classification', *British Medical Journal* 2 (1971): 330–1 and 'Cigarette Smoking: Natural History of a Dependence Disorder', *British Journal of Medical Psychology* 44 (1971): 1–16.
3. Emma Widdis, *Socialist Senses: Film, Feeling, and the Soviet Subject, 1917–1940* (Bloomington: Indiana University Press, 2017), 11–14; Daniel P. Todes, *Ivan Pavlov: A Russian Life in Science* (Oxford: Oxford University Press, 2014), 464–81; Jennifer J. Carroll, *Narkomania: Drugs, HIV, and Citizenship in Ukraine* (Ithaca: Cornell University Press, 2019), 11.
4. Tricia Starks, 'Red Star/Black Lungs: Anti-Tobacco Campaigns in Twentieth-Century Russia', *Journal of the Social History of Alcohol and Drugs* 21.1 (Fall 2006): 50–68.
5. Tricia Starks, *Cigarettes and Soviets: Tobacco in the USSR* (DeKalb: Northern Illinois University Press, 2022), 17–27.
6. Susan Gross Solomon, 'Social Hygiene in Soviet Medical Education, 1922–1930', *Journal of the History of Medicine and Allied Sciences* 45.4 (1990): 607–43; and 'David and Goliath in Soviet Public Health: The Rivalry of Social Hygienists and Psychiatrists for Authority over the Bytovoi Alcoholic', *Soviet Studies* 41.2 (1989): 254–75.
7. Tricia Starks, *The Body Soviet: Propaganda, Hygiene, and the Revolutionary State* (Madison, WI: University of Wisconsin Press, 2008).
8. Lev Borisovich Kafengauz, *Evoliutsiia promyshlennogo proizvodstva Rossii (posledniaia tret' XIX v.–30-e gody XX v.)* (Moscow: Epifaniia, 1994), 166, 198, 265; V. A. Kholostov and G. L. Dikker, 'Tabachnaia promyshlennost'' za 50 let sovetskoi vlasti', *Tabak* 4 (1967): 8; Jack E. Henningfield, Emma Calvento and Sakire Pogun, *Nicotine Psychopharmacology* (Bethesda, MD: Springer, 2009), 62–63; 468–9.
9. Ia. A. Violin, *Tabak i ego vred dlia zdorov'ia* (Kazan: Shtaba zapasnoi armii, 1920), 11. Nikolai Krementsov, *Revolutionary Experiments: The Quest for Immortality in Bolshevik Science and Fiction* (Oxford: Oxford University Press, 2014), 27–8.
10. Ia E. Shostak, *Kurevo* (Ul'ianovsk: izd. Ul'ianovskogo Gubzdravotdela, 1925), 11.
11. I. G. Uporov, (Dr) *Tabak, evo kurenie i vliianie na organizm* (Sverdlovsk: Izd. Sanepida Sverdlovskogo okzdravotdela, 1925), 12.
12. A. P. Nechaev, *Tabak i ego vliianie na umstvennuiu deiatel'nost' vzroslykh i detei* (Moscow: Zhizn' i znanie, 1925), 5.

13 I. M. Varushkin, *Pochemu vreden tabak* (Moscow: Gosizdat, 1926), 13.
14 Christopher M. Davis, 'Economics of Soviet Public Health, 1928–32: Development Strategy, Resource Constraints, and Health Plans', in Susan Gross Solomon and John F. Hutchinson, eds., *Health and Society in Revolutionary Russia* (Bloomington, IN: Indiana University Press, 1990), 146–172, 156; and his *Economic Problems of the RSFSR Health System, 1921–1930* (Birmingham: University Centre for Russian and East European Studies, 1978), 58–64.
15 A. Mikoian, 'Zadachi tabachnoi promyshlennosti', *Tabachnaia promyshlennost'* 8 (1931): 4–7. Malinin, *Tabachnaia istoriia*, 155–6; Igor Bogdanov, *Dym otechestva, ili kratkaia istoriia tabakokureniia* (Moscow: Novoe literaturnoe obozrenie, 2007), 194–5; A. V. Malinin, *Tabak: O chem umolchal Minzdrav* (Moscow: Russkii tabak, 2003), 109.
16 V. G. Arkhangel'skii (kand.dok.nauk), *O vrede kureniia*, 2-oe izd. (Moscow: Medgiz, 1951), 3. The 1950 run had 50,000 copies and the 1952 and 1953 editions both had 100,000.
17 Arkhangel'skii, *O vrede kureniia*, 19.
18 Ibid., 20–2. On nicotine withdrawal's insignificance, see I. V. Strel'chuk, *Klinika i lechenie narkomanii* (Moscow: Medgiz, 1949), 203–5.
19 A. N. Bakulev, 'Kurenie tabaka (nikotinizm)' in *Bol'shaia meditsinskaia entsiklopediia* (Moscow: Sovetskaia entsiklopediia, 1960), 1051; on postwar therapy see Aleksandra M. Brokman, 'Creating a Medical Specialty: Psychotherapy in the Post-War Soviet Healthcare System', *Journal of Health Inequalities* 5.2 (2019): 203–9.
20 Dr A. G. Stoiko, 'O lechenii tabakokureniia i kollektivnoi psikhoterapii ego, kak osobom metode', *Voprosy narkologii* sbornik vol. 2 (1928): 84.
21 V. N. Zolonitskii, *O vrede kureniia tabaka* (Moscow: G. F. Mirimanova, 1925), 20.
22 N. K. Bogolepov, *Voprosy nevro-psikhiatricheskoi dispansernoi praktiki* (Moscow: Moskovskii gorodskoi otdel zdravookhraneniia, 1936), 62–3.
23 Stoiko, 'O lechenii', 84–5.
24 Ibid., 86–7.
25 Ibid., 88.
26 Susan Gross Solomon, 'David and Goliath in Soviet Public Health: The Rivalry of Social Hygienists and Psychiatrists for Authority over the Bytovoi Alcoholic', *Soviet Studies* 41.2 (1989): 263; Kathy S. Transchel, *Under the Influence: Working-Class Drinking, Temperance, and Cultural Revolution in Russia, 1895–1932* (Pittsburgh: University of Pittsburgh Press, 2006), 83–9; Mary Schaeffer Conroy, 'Abuse of Drugs Other than Alcohol and Tobacco in the Soviet Union', *Soviet Studies* 42 (1990): 447–80.
27 Zababurina, 'Boremsia s narkotizmom', *Za novyi byt* 8–9 (1925): 17.
28 'Khronika: K bor'be s kureniem', *Gigiena i zdorov'e rabochei i krestianskoi sem'i* 14 (1928): 14.
29 A. S. Sholomovich, 'Bor'ba s kureniem i lechenii kurel'shchikov', *Voprosy narkologii sbornik* 2 (1928): 82–3.
30 Kathleen Sebelius, *How Tobacco Smoke Causes Disease: The Biology and Behavioral Basis for Smoking-Attributable Disease; a Report of the Surgeon General* (Rockville, MD: U.S. Department of Health and Human Services, 2010), 105–6.
31 A. Polianskii, comp. *Deistvie tabachnago dyma na zhivotnykh i cheloveka (Stoit'-li kurit? Kak rekomenduetsia kurit'?)* (Novonikslaevsk: Tip. Soiuz-Bank, 1919), 15.
32 'Novosti: Meditsiny i zdravookhraneniia', *Gigiena i zdorov'e rabochikh i krest'ianskikh semei* 5 (1938): 17;" P. Goncharov, 'Bros'te kurit'' *Gigiena i zdorov'e rabochikh i krest'ianskikh semei* 16 (1938): 16; Aleksandrov, *Zelenaia pogibel'*, 90.

33   Aleksandrov, *Zelenaia pogibel'*, 88.
34   Bakulev, 'Kurenie tabaka (nikotinizm)', 1052–3.
35   Ibid., 1056.
36   Ibid., 1056–7. See a 1949 description of this in Strel'chuk, *Klinika i lechenie narkomanii*, 205.
37   L. P. Zaits, *Brosaite kurit'!* (Sverdlov: Sverdlovskoe knizhnoe izdatel'stvo, 1960), 19. Tir. 7,000.
38   See for example, Boris Urlanis 'Beregite muzhchin!' *Literaturnaia gazeta* 24 July 1968, 12.
39   N. A. Ponomareva, *O lechenii lits, kuriashchikh tabak (instruktivno-metodicheskoe pis'mo)* (Moscow: Rosglavpoligrafproma, 1965), 2–3.
40   Ibid., 2–5.
41   Ibid., 8–9.
42   Ibid., 9.
43   Ibid., 9, 14.
44   V. S. Grashul', 'Kurenie i rak', *Zdorov'e* 12 (1958): 22–3; E. Shatrov, 'Kak ia brosal kurit'', *Zdorov'e* 5 (1958): 23.
45   Shatrov, 'Kak ia brosal kurit', 23.
46   V. M. Banshchikov, *Kurit' vredno!* (Moscow: Medigiz, 1959), 30–5; quotation p. 30.
47   A. V. Chaklin, *Vrednye privychki i rak* (Moscow: Znanie, 1969); Elsewhere see Boginskii, *Tabak i ego kurenie*, 9.
48   State Archive of the Russian Federation (GARF), f. 8009, op. 50, d. 9265, l. 68; for reviews of some of these, see V. Lagutina, 'Novye filmy', *Zdorov'e* 3 (1971): 32.
49   I. P. Bazhenov, *Vmeste s dymom papirosy: Ukhodit zdorov'e* (Moscow: Medgiz, 1960), 26–7. tir. 125,000.
50   A. V. Suvorov, *Vospitanie voli i kharaktera: V pomoshch uchiteliu* (M: Narkompros RSFSR, 1941), 2; Torfimov, *Tabak – vrag zdorov'ia*, 37.
51   V. A. Bogoslovskii, *O vrede kureniia (Konspekt lektsii)* (Moscow: Institute Sanitarnogo prosveshcheniia, 1965), 21.
52   Ibid., 22–9.
53   A. V. Malinin, *Tabachnaia istoriia Rossii* (Moscow: Russkii tabak, 2006), 202; Harrison E. Salisbury, *The 900 Days: The Siege of Leningrad* (New York: Harper and Row, 1969), 424.
54   Jean-François Etter, 'Cytisine for Smoking Cessation: A Literature Review and a Meta-Analysis', *Archive of Internal Medicine* 166 (2006): 1553.
55   H. H. Dale and P. P. Laidlaw, 'The Physiological Reaction of Cytisine, the Active Alkaloid of Laburnum (*Cytisus laburnum*)', *Journal of Pharmacology and Experimental Therapeutics* 3 (1912): 205–21; R. B. Barlow and L. J. McLeod, 'Some Studies on Cytosine and Its Methylated Derivative', *British Journal of Pharmacology*, 35 (1969): 161–74.
56   Ponomareva, *O lechenii lits*, 14.
57   Jean-François Etter, 'Cytisine for Smoking Cessation: A Literature Review and a Meta-analysis', *Archive of Internal Medicine* 166 (2006): 1553–9. Formula Ponomareva, *O lechenii lits*, 14. A contrast to perceived backwardness elsewhere for Soviet science; Anna Geltzer, 'Stagnant Science? The Planning and Coordination of Biomedical Research in the Brezhnev Era', in Dina Fainberg and Artemy Kalinovsky, eds., *Reconsidering Stagnation in the Brezhnev Era: Ideology and Exchange* (Lanham, MD: Lexington Books, 2016), 105–21.

58 Etter, 'Cytisine for Smoking Cessation', 1555–6. Current marketing website for Tabex claims a 57 per cent success rate with 21-day tablet course: https://www.tabex.net/ Accessed 24 October 2017.
59 Etter, 'Cytisine for Smoking Cessation', 1558.
60 Natalie Walker, et al., 'Cytisine versus Nicotine for Smoking Cessation', *The New England Journal of Medicine* 371.25 (2014): 2353–62.

Part Three

Artefacts

8

Illuminating microbes: Preventing infectious diseases with bactericidal lamps in Soviet medicine, 1917–53

Johanna Conterio

In 1937, A.P. Omeliants, the director of the department of mud therapy and thalassotherapy of the I.N. Sechenov Institute for Physical Medicine in Sevastopol, described methods to augment the power of nature with the use of technology. He discussed a glass lens technology that could 'concentrate' the rays of the sun to more than six times sun radiation.[1] As he wrote, the first experiments with this type of therapeutic technology had been made by Niels Ryberg Finsen in Denmark. But as Omeliants noted, a Soviet researcher in Crimea, affiliated with the Feodosiia institute of physical methods of therapy, P.I. Nanii, had created an original technology to augment the power of the sun: a glass reflector. The reflector was made using common window glass, which was covered on one side with a silver amalgam, reflecting sunlight onto the body. Because they had by design a long focus length, these reflectors could be used to treat patients at a distance, creating the possibility of situating them in the shade, thus avoiding their 'overheating and exhaustion', or situating them indoors, protecting them from cold weather.[2] The Nanii reflector was used to treat disorders of the peripheral nervous system, such as sciatica, plexitis (acute pain, weakness and loss of sensation) and neuralgia (pain caused by damaged or irritated nerves), as well the organs of movement, immune conditions such as eczema and asthma, and tuberculosis of the skin.[3]

The use of such technologies as the Nanii reflector fit into a discipline of medicine called variously physical medicine, physiatry, physical therapy and physiotherapy. Physical therapy included the use of various lamps and other electric therapies and reflectors; vibration therapies; sun, light and air bathing; and massage. It was an area of significant therapeutic innovation in the interwar period throughout Europe, including the Soviet Union. Physical medicine has not been prominent in the history of medicine. But I suggest that physical therapy occupied a role parallel to nature cures in the interwar period, part of a therapeutic complex that was marginalized in scientific medicine in the face of antibiotics.[4] At their broadest, these were therapies that filled a therapeutic gap that bacteriology had as yet failed to fill. While bacteriologists had identified bacteria as disease agents and associated specific bacteria with specific infectious diseases, they had not yet produced effective antibacterial or antibiotic therapies in their laboratories. Historians of medicine argue that contemporary medical researchers within bacteriology expected that such therapies as sun and light baths would be used only until pharmaceutical antibiotics that eliminated infectious disease agents were developed in bacteriology laboratories.[5]

Explanations of how therapeutic lamps worked evolved over time. A common framework for explaining the efficacy of lamp and reflector therapy was to link the sweating that resulted from these therapies to the release of poisons or toxins in the body. In the context of the bacteriological age, physicians working in physiotherapy in Russia, Central and East-Central Europe and Scandinavia attempted to associate physical therapies with scientific medicine by reconceptualizing therapies through the lens of bacteriology. Bacteriology provided the explanatory framework that most closely aligned physical medicine with the vanguard of scientific medicine, in turn placing lamps at the vanguard of modern therapeutics, as a form of bactericidal therapy. A pioneer of this approach was Finsen, who between 1893 and 1896 developed a new type of ultraviolet lamp exclusively for the treatment of an infectious disease, tuberculosis of the skin, drawing on a bactericidal framework.[6] Such a line of thinking had even been suggested by the bacteriologist Robert Koch himself, who argued that electric lamps had a 'germicidal effect', killing pathogenic bacteria.[7] Yet the impact of bacteriology on physical medicine, including lamp therapies, was diverse depending on the setting, as indeed in other branches of medicine.

The historiography at the intersection of environment and health has developed a consensus that bacteriology led to a medical focus on the body in isolation from its ecological surroundings.[8] The historiography on the reception of such therapeutic lamps in Central Europe reflects this argument. The use of therapeutic lamps in Central Europe focused on the individual, clinical treatment of the human body.[9] Yet, as explored in this chapter, the impact of bacteriology on physical therapy had a different outcome in the Soviet Union. This chapter explores this outcome in four aspects. First, in the Soviet context, even initial scientific research on the therapeutic use of lamps focused not only on the human body in isolation, but also on the environmental conditions surrounding the body. Second, in the Soviet context, bacteriological frameworks were shaped by the Soviet emphasis on prevention, or 'prophylaxis'.[10] Lamps were used not only to treat an already infected body showing signs of disease or an environment already known to harbour and cultivate bacteria, but to prevent the infection of body and environment, by making bodies and environments inhospitable to microbial growth. Third, after the mid-1930s, a nervous framework became more prominent in Soviet physical medicine, becoming dominant after the Pavlovian turn of 1948–51, which decentred aetiologies focused on bacteriology in physical medicine. Finally, whereas in Central Europe the use of lamps was limited to therapeutic use in clinical settings, in the Soviet Union, they were adopted for use in the public health disciplines, to treat environments. Hygiene, epidemiology, sanitary medicine, microbiology, bacteriology and other disciplines of prophylaxis in Soviet medicine that focused on the physical environment adopted the use of ultraviolet lamps to prevent the spread of infectious disease agents through the environment, and Soviet industry developed a new type of lamp, the bactericidal lamp, for that purpose. However, such lamps were used to treat environments, with bodies in them.

The study of the use of therapeutic lamps allows this study to reflect on the control of infectious diseases in the Soviet context more broadly. In the Soviet context, I argue, bacterial disease agents would not only be controlled at the threshold of the body, through the skin or lungs, but also in the surrounding environment. Soviet medical researchers within physical medicine and adjacent disciplines did not starkly differentiate between methods for treating the body and its surrounding environment, seeing these as necessarily entangled. A single therapeutic apparatus or method could be used across human and non-human bodies and landscapes, as well as the abiotic world. Anti-microbial interventions swept across the otherwise seemingly bounded bodies of humans, animals, plants, and other living beings and the abiotic world. Moreover, the Soviet approach to the use of ultraviolet lamps in the environment in public health fields diverged from public health practice as it was developing in the interwar period elsewhere. The focus was not on environments in isolation, or indeed, on the study of pathogen behaviours in the laboratory rather than in the field.[11] Rather, Soviet researchers explicitly studied field environments with people in them. They traced the ecological entanglement of microbes, airs, bodies and landscapes. And they studied not 'pure culture' bacteria but bacterial colonies as they were found in the field.

In this chapter, I first explore the use of lamp therapy in Soviet physical medicine. I examine the impact of bacteriology on Soviet physical therapy and examine how bacteriology shaped the clinical use of ultraviolet lamps, treating both bodies and environments, and how this framework was de-centred by a turn to *nervizm*. I then turn to the use of bactericidal lamps in branches of prophylactic medicine that focused on the physical environment, especially hygiene, sanitary medicine, epidemiology and microbiology. Here, the medical focus shifted subtly from the clinical treatment of bodies embedded in environments, to the treatment of environments with bodies entangled within them. A bacteriological framework dominated explanations of their utility, but one marked by systemic difference, rooted in a medical theory that entangled microbes, human bodies and environments.

The impact of bacteriology on Soviet physical medicine, 1917–53

Initially, electric light was thought to be harmful to human health. Many physicians and especially factory workers exposed to electric light expressed concern about its potentially damaging effects.[12] Common lamps used in factory settings could lead to sweating and tears, night blindness, and red and burning pain in the skin, as well as blisters and scaling, and researchers found that factory workers could even experience 'sun stroke' when working under hot electric lights, marked by irritations of the eyes and skin, headaches, fever, or insomnia.[13] Early use of electric light for therapy took place in the United States in the 1890s, led by John Harvey Kellogg, who in his Michigan healing complex built therapeutic light cabinets filled with dozens of light bulbs.[14] This technique was quickly brought to Europe. The 1890s saw widespread experimentation with lamp therapy. This was the decade when Finsen innovated with lamp therapies and had his own lamp constructed. Individual experiments were also made by A.V. Minin in Russia, who developed the infrared Minin Lamp in the 1890s.[15] The use of the lamps increased during the First World War, when patients were disconnected from their usual bath and sanatorium circuit, and took off in the interwar period.

In the 1920s, as electrification swept Europe and electronic technology developed rapidly, electric light therapy became a mass phenomenon. It was at this time that the production and use of electric lamps for mass illumination and mass medical therapy took shape. Light therapy was pushed into mass use in part due to an innovation in therapeutic lamp technology that made it possible to produce less expensive lamps. The first lamp that reached a mass market in Europe was the 'mountain sun' ultraviolet spotlight lamp produced by the Quartz Lamp Association Hanau, in a factory outside Frankfurt am Main, Germany, established in 1906, which dominated the western European market through the 1970s.[16] The Quartz Lamp Association Hanau soon developed a warm, infrared spotlight, the Sollux lamp, as well.[17] These lamps were not only less expensive to produce than Finsen lamps, but also simpler to use, as they did not require specialist nurses to administer the treatments to patients individually, to press the lamps into the skin and to prevent burning. They could be used to treat patients assembled in groups. In the interwar period, they were largely used to treat patients with tuberculosis and rickets.[18]

Therapeutic lamps reached broad medical use in the Soviet Union at the same time as they did so in Central Europe. Indeed, the USSR was at the vanguard of their study and mass use, and researchers were deeply connected to research published abroad on the topic as well. In the Soviet Union, physical medicine was integrated into a discipline of medicine, called *kurortologiia* (health resort medicine), where it was brought together with balneology, climatology, as well as mud, kumys (a drink of fermented mare's milk), and other types of nature therapies. With the discipline of *kurortologiia*, Soviet medical officials aimed to place physical and climate therapy on scientific foundations, creating a new, research-based approach. The growing research enterprise (by 1941, there were eleven institutes of *kurortologiia* in the Soviet Union, all operating under the Main Health Resort Administration of the Commissariat of Public Health) also served to marginalize the role of lay healers in the Soviet Union. Only accredited physicians were admitted to practise medicine in the state research institutions, state sanatoria and state clinics. This eliminated the distinction made between physical medicine and other disciplines under the broad, vague category of 'natural healing' (based on the understanding that physical medicine was a branch of scientific medicine and natural healing was largely non-medical) which characterized the field in Central Europe.

In 1924, S. B. Vermel', the director of the State Institute of Physiatry and Orthopaedics, wrote an article dedicated to the discipline of 'physiatry' in the Soviet Union. He summarized that the study of physiatry was 'the study of the physical characteristics and biological action of the natural and artificial forces of nature (*estestvennykh i iskusstvennykh sil prirody*), from which are derived therapeutic indications and actions'.[19] As Vermel' wrote, physiatrists were particularly interested in the study of the energy of various 'rays' (electric waves, sun rays of the entire spectrum, Roentgen rays and radiation) and mechanical energy (both applied from the outside, as in massage and passive gymnastics, and in the forms of the active use of various machines for exercise, sports and rest). Physical therapies involved treatments to the body, often in its entirety and largely externally, as opposed to surgery or medication.

Medical research and experiments with therapeutic lamps filled the pages of the scientific research journal of the Main Department of Health Resort Affairs of the People's Commissariat of Public Health, *Kurortnoe delo*, in the 1920s and the early 1930s. The use of medical lamps therapeutically reached specialist institutions such as sanatoria in the 1920s. Here therapies were given in a clinical setting, mainly to individuals. However, in the 1930s, there was a turn from a focus on individual, clinical therapy with ultraviolet lamps to mass therapy, and a turn to prophylactic therapy. The first mass illumination hall in the Soviet Union was established for the military. The 'Great Quartz Hall', a mass illumination hall, was established in 1933 in Moscow in the Central House of the Red Army. In Moscow in the Winter of 1933, 356 people (212 men and 144 women) were treated in groups of 12–14 people. As a rule, the patients were grouped according to their hair colour and skin colour.[20] The patients were physical culture practitioners of the sports sector of the Red Army house, organized in the sports section (acrobatics, boxing, etc.)[21] (Figure 8.1). Here, a major point differentiating lamp use in the Soviet context from the Central European context was apparent.

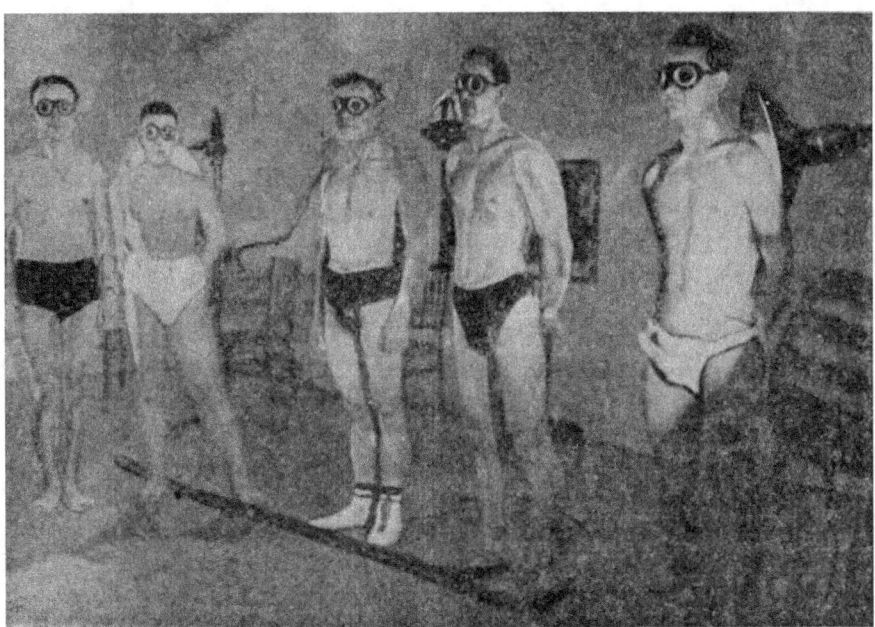

Figure 8.1 Physical culture practitioners in the sports sector of the Central House of the Red Army in Moscow undergoing treatment in the Great Quartz Hall, 1933.

In this, the first instance of mass illumination in the Soviet Union, the patients selected for treatment were patients in good health, and the experiments were for their use prophylactically, to raise working productivity, rather than to treat tuberculosis or rickets. As a researcher on the project wrote, 'We have adopted quartz lamps in the prevention business as one of the main links of apparatus physio-prophylaxis, which have recently won their legitimate right to exist.'[22] Moreover, whereas bacteriology and the treatment of infectious diseases with lamps had been crucial for winning legitimacy for the therapies in scientific medical circles in Central Europe and Scandinavia, as opposed to frameworks prominent among lay natural healers around toxicity and sweating, in the 1930s in the Soviet Union ultraviolet lamps were increasingly viewed as acting on the human body through the central nervous system. Indeed, in the Great Quartz Hall study, the utility of the lamps was explained mainly through the framework of nervous health. Patients sick with infectious diseases were explicitly excluded from the mass treatments in the study. Not allowed in the study were patients with several categories of diseases or ailments, including patients with tuberculosis of the lungs, patients with fevers (suggesting an acute infection), with heart disease, women with heavy periods or in the second half of a pregnancy.[23]

The experiments were made with four Hanau UV quartz lamps, with Bach reflectors, from Germany, four Soviet-made UV quartz lamps from the factory Elektrolampa in Moscow, with the Soviet-made reflector Ieznionek, four infrared Sollux lamps and two projectors.[24] Patients were organized into two different scenarios. Some patients did simple physical culture movements. Other patients laid down on a 'beach': a soft mattress covered in white cloth, surrounded by lamps[25] (Figure 8.2). On the beach, they turned from front to back. After the treatments, rest for 8–10 minutes was recommended.[26] The treatments lasted from 3 minutes at the start of a course to as many as 25 minutes, and the distance of the patients to the lamps shortened over the course of a cycle of treatments from 100 cm to 50 cm.[27] A course of treatment was 14–16 seances.[28] Without elaboration, the author noted that the Elektrolampa lamps were not of good quality.[29]

Due to a lack of laboratory facilities, the researchers were unable to produce findings based on blood and urine samples. But they did find through the analysis of patient charts that the treatments raised appetite, led to gaining weight, improved working ability and the resistance of the organism to infections, particularly that flu infections passed much more quickly.[30] The authors observed that the Sollux lamp was especially good for its painkilling influence. Menstruating women who continued their radiation did not see a diversion from norm, but said they felt better, and premenstrual and menstrual pains were lighter. They also found that local irradiation was not as effective as full body irradiation.

The authors noted that the use of the quartz lamps led to physical development, and because of this, some considered the use of quartz lamps among athletes as a form of doping (indeed, the authors wrote that physicians had banned the use of quartz lamps among swimmers in the German society of swimmers in 1924 as a form of doping).[31] However, they disagreed with categorizing the use of these lamps as a form of doping.

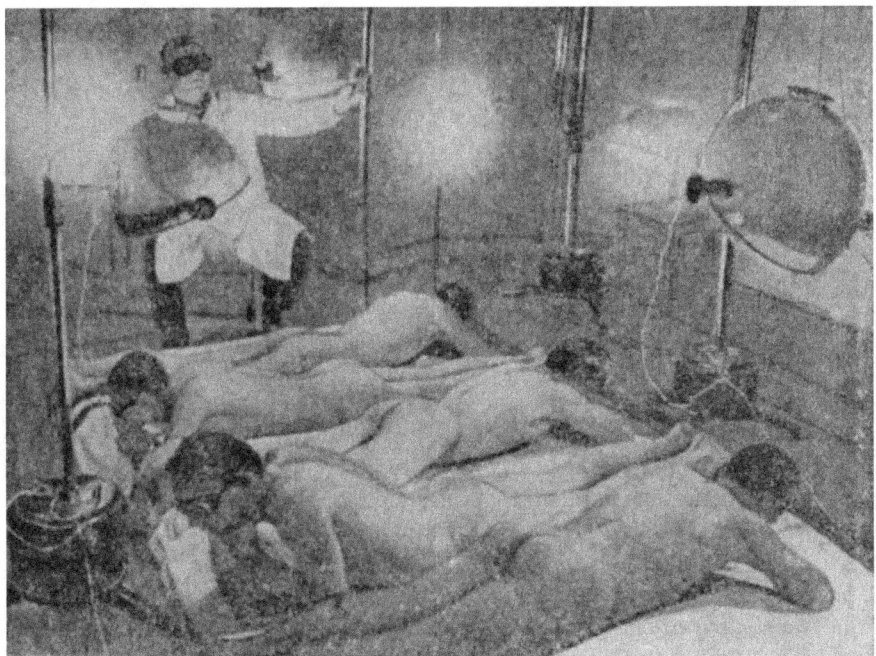

Figure 8.2 Patients on the 'beach' of the Great Quartz Hall, 1933.

The lamps did not have any of the negative effects on human health that defined doping, as they argued, 'there are absolutely no manifestations of harmfulness, which are inherent in the concepts of doping'.[32] Moreover, they claimed that Soviet physicians were not interested in the use of the lamps for individual athletic glory, but for improved health and overall worker productivity, 'We are in no way interested in the question of the use of ultraviolet rays for the pure purposes of sport, with its individual "recordism" (*rekordsmenstvom*)'.[33]

Researchers also examined what they called the 'subjective' data produced in the study, based on eighty-two patient records. Here, the focus was on improvements also in nervous health. One patient allegedly wrote, as cited in the study,

> I can't say anything but positive things about the treatments. Work at the institute used to take away all my energy and when I came home, I couldn't do anything. I fell into bed and fell asleep, often dressed. But today the picture has changed … My energy has become more stable, and after working at the institute, I still have several hours of active existence ahead of me. Physical fatigue caused me flashes of sharp nervous irritation earlier. Now I've forgotten the last time I yelled at someone or threw things across the rooms. I have become calmer, more balanced, both to myself and to others.[34]

Another thirty-year-old female patient wrote that her menstruation became less painful while under treatments, particularly before menstruation, and also reported that there was more blood. Generally, she argued that the treatments reduced pain. The author of the study also admitted that patients for whom the treatment was not effective had left the study. One woman with indications of loss of appetite, strong excitability and weakening of muscle strength simply 'disappeared'.

The researchers also paid attention to how the lamps affected the environment in which patients were treated. They argued that the advantage of the Sollux lamp was that it heated the premises, so had a good effect in mass illumination halls. Heating the room also opened the capillaries of patients, allowing UV rays to penetrate deeper into the body.[35] The Sollux lamp was seen to have a pain killing effect. The author recommended the treatment especially for miners and Moscow Metropolitan workers.[36] He recommended the treatment also for patients with menstrual pain.

As this study demonstrated, by 1933 a nervous paradigm had begun to emerge for explaining the utility of the lamp therapies, rather than a strictly bacteriological one. This fit into a broader shift in *kurortologiia* away from the treatment of infectious diseases, especially tuberculosis (lung tuberculosis patients were removed from admission to health resorts of state significance in 1933), to focus on nervous ailments. A nervous framework for explaining health and disease developed in the discipline, which the Pavlovian turn in medicine of 1948–51 reinforced and made more dominant. Yet, before 1948–51, and indeed afterwards, this nervous paradigm competed with and was at times combined with bacteriological explanations of the utility of therapeutic lamps.

The use of therapeutic lamps was not reserved only for making healthy people stronger, but also found clinical use in hospitals, for preventing the infection of wounds as well as strengthening the bodies of patients in hospitals. In 1935, P.D. Guzikov used ultraviolet irradiation with a mercury-quartz lamp during complex gynaecological operations. The aim was not only to fight 'wound microflora' but also to use them as a means of 'positively influencing the organism of the patient'.[37] In a comparative study of the use of the lamps during caesarean sections, he used the lamp with 742 patients, with a control group of 1,258 patients. He found that mortality among irradiated patients was 5.8 per cent less than among the control group. Moreover, he found that wounds healed more completely with their use, finding 18.5 per cent more primary healings in the irradiated group.[38] He combined explanations for this outcome, engaging the nervous as well as bacteriological paradigms: According to the author, irradiation 'only to a certain extent is connected with the effect on bacteria directly, the main thing is the stimulation of the whole organism'.[39]

Researchers demonstrated an awareness of the effects the lamps had on environments surrounding bodies as well. Indeed, the focus on prevention of infectious diseases reenforced the emphasis in Soviet physiotherapy on the environment as well as the body. In a 1933 study of mass illumination in military barracks, researchers made a connection between the illumination of bodies and the illumination of interiors directly. As this study found, the illumination of barracks had a bactericidal effect. This was particularly important to prevent the reinfection of the sick. Focusing on diphtheria and its treatment with UV lamps, the study found that irradiating barracks was key to preventing reinfection. As the authors wrote, reinfection took place frequently in a 'bacteria-saturated diphtheria barracks'.[40] As the authors found, the radiation not only directly killed bacteria, but prevented their growth by creating unfavourable conditions: 'These changes are not limited to illuminated areas, but spread along the periphery, creating conditions unfavourable for the growth of bacteria.'[41] The authors argued that the radiation acted on the environment as well as the human body:

> The very mechanism of action of UV irradiation, we believe, consists of a number of factors, such as the direct bactericidal effect of UV rays, a large change in the physico-chemical ratios in the environment under the influence of lighting and, thanks to this, the creation of conditions that are not conducive to bacterial growth; the general effect of lighting on the human body, and finally the known influence of ionized air, including ozone, which during the operation of the heater concentrated in a closed casing and abundantly penetrated into the nasopharynx.[42]

Here what was illuminated was not only the body in isolation, but also the environment surrounding the body, in which the body was entangled and which acted on the body.

A nervous framework became dominant in Soviet physical medicine after the Pavlovian turn of 1948–51, which decentred aetiologies focused on bacteriology, focusing instead on the centrality of the central nervous system to understanding the causes of health and disease. By the late Stalinist period, in physical medicine as well as in other branches of clinical medicine, the nervous framework had become central to explaining the mechanism by which UV lamps acted on the human body. As a bacteriologist at the Erisman Central Scientific-Research Sanitary-Hygiene Institute in Moscow, Ia.E. Neishtadt argued typically in a 1955 text on bactericidal ultraviolet irradiation, in a chapter dedicated to the influence of bactericidal lamps on humans, ultraviolet lamps acted on the organism of the human through the nervous system: 'A significant role in the reactions that occur in the human body in response to radiation belongs to the nervous system.'[43] Neishtadt elaborated in detail how radiation acted on various functions of the nervous system, including breathing.[44] It acted, via the nervous system, on infections, because of the sharp stimulating effect of the radiation on the central nervous system: 'Short-term, but high dose use of short-wave ultraviolet radiation (up to 5–7 biodoses) can have a beneficial effect in some infectious diseases characterized by an increased reactivity of the body (A. Ia. Goldfeld).'[45] The nervous framework also justified the use of ultraviolet lamp therapy for the treatment of pain. A 1942 study found that the localized use of ultraviolet treatments was effective at ameliorating causalgia (nerve pain) and lessening rates of partial paralysis.[46] Yet the nervous system was not separate from the surrounding environment, but was deeply influenced by it.

Even in the earliest studies published in the discipline of physical medicine in the Soviet Union, medical research into the uses of therapeutic lamps focused not exclusively on the effects of therapy directly on the human body, but also on the bactericidal effects of the therapies on the environments surrounding the body. Moreover, a focus on prevention meant that the therapies were understood not only to treat the unhealthy body and environment, but also to prevent the spread of microbes through space and inside the human body. The use of lamps to prevent infection of the body was combined with the use of lamps to prevent the cultivation of microbes in the environments in which the body was understood to be entangled. This fit into a broadly preventive approach to the spread of infectious diseases and minor infections overall. In this context, the use of medical lamps spread from physical medicine to broader use in preventive branches of medicine. Even as in physical medicine the bactericidal use of therapeutic lamps competed with their use to treat neurological pain and to act via the central nervous system on the health of the body, in preventive fields they found widespread use in the prevention of the spread of airborne infectious diseases and minor infections in clinical settings as well as in spaces of mass assembly.

Bactericidal lamps and the 'natural microflora of the air' with people in it

After the Second World War, the study and use of UV lamps extended beyond the discipline that had brought the lamps to Russia and the Soviet Union, physical medicine, and entered Soviet preventive medicine more broadly, in such disciplines as hygiene, sanitary medicine, epidemiology and microbiology. A bacteriological framework dominated explanations of the action of the lamps on the environment, but one marked by systemic difference. Soviet researchers traced the influence of human presence on how microbes acted in space. Moreover, they studied how the behaviour of airborne microbes was influenced by a wide range of climatic influences, including humidity, temperature, altitude, and time of day.[47] They studied, in short, airborne microbes in the field, in their ecological context.

As the Moscow bacteriologist Neishtadt wrote, bactericidal lamps found application in surgical clinics, at blood transfusion stations, and in infectious diseases wards of hospitals.[48] Their broad adoption was accelerated by the development of a new type of Soviet-produced lamp, the 'bactericidal lamp of uviol glass' (*bakteritsidanaia lampa iz uviolevogo stekla*) or 'BUV' lamp, commonly called a 'bactericidal lamp'. BUV lamps (coming in 15-watt BUV-15 and 30-watt BUV-30 models) were of lower intensity but more robust and economical to use than mercury-quartz lamps.[49]

The study of the use of bactericidal lamps in these fields of public health focused on the prevention of the spread of airborne infectious diseases. Indeed, studies in epidemiology, sanitary science and microbiology approached the environment largely through the concept of air, and particularly, air in spaces of mass assembly. They worked within a broadly bacteriological framework. To prevent the spread of infectious diseases and reinfection of patients, they studied the use of bactericidal lamps largely with the aim of reducing overall levels of microbial contamination in the air. A smaller group of researchers also examined the effects of ultraviolet radiation on individual bacterial agents of particular interest, such as staphylococcus (a deadly infection often caught in hospitals), to gauge how much radiation would be needed for their elimination, in a competing, specific approach to the study of microbial-rich air.[50] Both types of researchers mainly studied airborne microbes as they occurred authentically, as one study held, the 'natural microflora of the air' (*natural'noi mikroflore vozdukha*), as they interacted with people, surfaces, and objects and changed over time, rather than individually isolated bacilli or viruses cultured in a lab.[51]

This was a consciously made and articulated approach to studying airborne microbes and the spread of infectious diseases, and the use of ultraviolet radiation to prevent their spread from the air to humans. Researchers at the Erisman Institute rejected the study of cultured, isolated microbes in lab settings, because these microbes were easier to destroy than those that existed outside the lab, in life, where individual microbes were rarely if ever present in isolation from each other, and where the environment also influenced the effectiveness of UV treatment. They found that microbes in 'artificially contaminated air' were easier to eliminate than the 'natural microflora of the air' that was found in the field.[52] Neishtadt contrasted this approach of studying 'natural microflora' to research conducted abroad, where ultraviolet radiation was tested on purified bacterial cultures in laboratory settings, even including bacteria that did not frequently occur in the air:

> In a number of studies carried out by different authors, white staphylococcus was used as a test object for characterizing the action of short-wave rays, sprayed in the air of experimental chambers, in boxes, etc. In the works of foreign authors (Lekish et al.), E. coli was used for this purpose, which is not at all a microorganism characteristic of the air environment.[53]

As he wrote, ultraviolet irradiation was significantly more effective in such laboratory settings, with cultured bacterial monocultures: 'Our studies have confirmed the position that microbial culture suspensions are much less stable in relation to short-wave ultraviolet radiation than ordinary microflora in the air of residential and public buildings.'[54]

Because the main agents introducing microbes into the air were humans, the behaviour of humans in space was also included in the studies. As Neishtadt wrote, the main agent of the infection of air was the person. Dust also played a role: 'A number of microbiologists have established that humans are the main source of air pollution by microflora, but soil dust also plays a significant role in microbial contamination of the air.'[55] This approach to studying microbes, air, dust, and bodies together characterized many Soviet studies of air. As N.P. Shastin found in his 1953 dissertation, colonies of microbes increased by 204 times during an operation in a surgical theatre. But he found the contamination of air depended on the number of people and their behaviour during the operation. He presented a table showing contamination levels (measured in quantity of microbes in a cubic meter of air) before and during an operation. Before the operation, the number of people in the theatre ranged from 1 to 4 people, whereas during the operation, they ranged from 12 to 20 people. The table demonstrated a rough correlation between microbial levels in an interior and the number of people in those interiors.[56] As A.I. Shafir found in a study of microbial levels in a dressing room of a polyclinic, before the arrival of patients, there were 13,000–16,000 microorganisms in one cubic meter of air, whereas at midday, the level of contamination had reached 23,500–23,800.[57] Generally speaking, the more people in a space, the more microbes there would be. In another study, the author explicitly wrote that people were allowed to walk through the experimental setting, acting as they usually would in the space. He admitted that this made results variable, but this was not considered problematic.[58] The understanding that human variability and its impact on microbial life in the air was itself an object of study would, indeed, allow for a more effective approach to prophylactic irradiation of environments in practice. In measuring the microbial contamination of the air, no great effort was made to control and make consistent the flow of people through the air. Rather, researchers studied air as conditioned necessarily by the human flux that characterized the spaces they were studying.

The study of air with humans in it came with its own type of sociology. Not all groups of people had the same microbial impact on the air, and so microbial levels were different in different interiors. Contamination levels were dynamic, depending on the health, age, movement and behaviour of people. In a study of naturally occurring microbes in various places, the highest contamination levels were found at the cash register of a pharmacy, in the scarlet fever and birthing wards of a hospital, and in a kindergarten.[59] Researchers measured microbial contamination broadly, examining cinemas and stadiums, auditoriums and classrooms.

Bodies and environments were understood to be so closely entangled that researchers in many cases measured the effect of irradiating the environment with bactericidal lamps through the human bodies circulating through it. A number of studies were conducted where the ultraviolet lamps were used to irradiate hospital wards, with patients in them, and the results of the irradiation were measured in terms of epidemiological outcomes, through the bodies of the patients who occupied the irradiated spaces, rather than through the microbial levels found in the air.

In 1952, V.I. Vashkov and R.M. Ginzburg and their co-workers irradiated a scarlet fever ward with a bactericidal lamp with a shield for 12–13 hours a day, daily, over the course of a month. No mention was made of a strictly curative effect of the irradiation, improving outcomes of primary infections; in this study, rather, the focus was strictly on prevention. They established an epidemiological improvement. In the wards where they carried out irradiation, there were three repeated incidents of scarlet fever, whereas in the control group, with a roughly equal number of patients, thirteen patients were reinfected with scarlet fever in the ward. Moreover, the use of the lamps prevented the spread of flu and catarrh of the upper respiratory tract in the wards, where there were two incidents in the irradiated ward and thirty-five in the control ward.[60] Such studies indicated that the use of bactericidal lamps in the infectious disease wards prevented patients from catching infections at the hospital. The effects of irradiation were also influenced by variations in climate and indoor climate. High humidity rates decreased the effectiveness of radiation. Radiation worked better at lower temperatures.[61]

As the use of ultraviolet radiation lamps broadened, researchers began to reflect on the possible harm systemic irradiation of spaces was having on the humans within them. Overexposure, and establishing thresholds of exposure above which harm to humans would be found, became a research interest for the Erisman Institute. The Erisman Institute set out to reform the use of ultraviolet lamps, to take account for the fact that humans occupied these spaces. It was established that over-radiation with lamps came with risks. One study found that patients in irradiated wards had peeling skin in areas that were exposed to light: 'However, it should be noted that with the indicated air irradiation in the wards, the patients who were in them showed premature peeling of the skin on the exposed surfaces of the body, which should be considered an unfavourable indicator of the action of short-wave ultraviolet radiation.'[62] Eye conditions were also found to be common, including tearing, inflammation of the eye, bloodshot eyes and photophobia (extreme sensitivity to light).[63] The lamps themselves also led to low levels of pollution in the air, producing ozone, which researchers maintained was not harmful to human health (indeed, as seen above, some thought it curative) but produced an unpleasant smell, and trace amounts of toxic nitrogen oxides.[64]

Researchers at the Erisman Institute were challenged by a contradiction in the use of bactericidal lamps to decontaminate the air. The institute established a maximum threshold of exposure that was allowable for systemic ultraviolet exposure to humans, based on experiments on animals such as rabbits and mice. According to this norm, radiation should not exceed 0.8–1 kilogram force per square metre.[65] Yet very high dosages of ultraviolet rays, of several thousand kilogram force per square metre, had been found to be necessary to eliminate bacteria in the field.[66] As the use of lamps was becoming more widespread, researchers, especially at the Erisman Institute, looked for technological approaches to ultraviolet irradiation that would address this contradiction.

Their prize innovation was the development of a bactericidal recirculation installation, for use with standard Soviet bactericidal lamps. This installation consisted of placing bactericidal lamps in a cylinder that blocked the ultraviolet rays. The air was decontaminated by circulating through the cylinder, past the lamps, with the use of fans, while the cylinder itself shielded human bodies from direct ultraviolet exposure. For further protection, large discs were installed at the end of each cylinder, to prevent radiation from reaching people from the side. This system shielded humans in the wards from direct irradiation.

The Erisman Institute also promoted the use of low intensity, fluorescent lights with low levels of ultraviolet radiation for general prevention, 'combined fluorescent light emitters', adding a low dose of ultraviolet to standard lighting.[67] And they developed a type of hand-held ultraviolet cleaner, comparable to a vacuum cleaner, to sanitize objects, which protected their user from exposure,

> To irradiate the surfaces of enclosures, mainly walls, doors, door handles, heating devices, window sills, as well as household items in the room, we made a portable irradiator with bactericidal lamps. The design intended for irradiation of surfaces and objects, should ensure the maximum use of the ultraviolet flux of the emitted lamp, cover the lamps from direct exposure to people, should be easy and convenient to use.[68]

Finally, they promoted simpler solutions. Placing a semi-circular shield covering the bottom half of a standard bactericidal lamp mounted 2–2.5 metres above the ground on a wall protected people located below the lamps, for example, from irradiation.

Another option was to use lamps only when people were not present, for example, in surgical theatres at night. Those working with the lamps were recommended to wear glasses of simple glass.[69]

The Erisman Institute researchers developed technology according to the ideology of Soviet medicine, to accommodate a view to the environment with people in it, making environmental treatments safe for humans. These variations made the use of lamps less economical, however. As one study noted, the use of one type of lamp with a cover would require a norm of one lamp for 8–10 cubic metres of space, whereas their use without a cover, if people were not present, would be one lamp for 12–15 square metres of space.[70] At the same time, this added cost was partly offset by the relative economy of the use of Soviet-made bactericidal lamps as opposed to mercury-quartz lamps, which Soviet researchers calculated were about five times more expensive to use.[71]

While understanding the full scale at which the use of bactericidal lamps entered everyday practice is beyond the scope of this study, there is evidence that the state attempted to push them into broader use. On 25 May 1951, the Presidium of the Scientific Medical Soviet of the Ministry of Health RSFSR issued instructions on how to use bactericidal lamps, approving 'Instructions for the application of bactericidal lamps for decontaminating the air and objects in premises'.[72] The instructions claimed that BUV lamps had entered domestic production. The instructions held that bactericidal lamps could be used for disinfecting the air of interiors of social buildings ('schools, auditoriums, children's institutions, hospitals, various industrial enterprises') and for the disinfection of enclosures in premises (such as walls), furniture, hard and soft inventory and household items.[73] Demonstrating familiarity with concerns about the potential harm of lamps to humans, the instructions held, 'The use of unshielded bactericidal lamps in the presence of humans is not permitted.'[74] For the disinfection of air where people were present, the instructions recommended the use of recirculation installations, at a norm of one lamp for 4 square metres of air, which led, so the instructions claimed, to a reduction of 50–60 per cent of microbial contamination (*mikrobnoi obsemennosti*).[75] Uncovered lamp use was not to exceed 1 MKVT/cm^2 if people were present (a threshold within a norm established by the Erisman Institute).[76] Here, too, the focus was on air with humans moving through it, in flux: 'The purification of the air of microflora requires the long and systematic use of ultraviolet radiation, since the pollution of the premises by microorganisms occurs continuously due to the presence of people and the spread of microbes from neighbouring rooms.'[77] Indeed, the instructions recommended the use of bactericidal lamps especially when human activity was causing dust to be circulated into the air, when sweeping the room, dragging objects through it, with increased movement of people.[78]

In keeping with the Soviet 'combined' approach to the eradication of infectious disease, the instructions also emphasized that the use of UV lamps should be combined with other measures to prevent the spread of infectious disease. These measures included ventilation, preventing unnecessary contact between the healthy and sick, and the systematic care of the nose and hands of medical and service personnel.⁷⁹ No mention of mechanical cleaning or the use of chemical cleaning agents was made.

As the instructions and the development of what could be called the ultraviolet hoover indicated, bactericidal lamps were also increasingly seen as useful for decontaminating domestic objects and interior spaces. One researcher proposed the broad preventive use of ultraviolet lamps in Soviet interiors, particularly in the Far North and other regions that experienced regular 'sun famine'. He argued that the ultraviolet lamp would act as a bactericide on all surfaces: 'In conclusion, we can mention a few more beneficial moments that can accompany the use of daily radiation from combined lamps. One of such moments is the fact that ultraviolet rays have bactericidal power, therefore, sterilization of surfaces under the influence of light should be a very significant fact.'⁸⁰ Indeed, lamps created a 'microclimate' in a room, as another study found, which influenced treatment, including effects on the humidity, relative humidity and the movement of air in a given premises.⁸¹

At the same time, tiny spores of ambivalence about taking a strictly antibiotic approach to microbes in the landscape developed within Soviet medicine. These ideas were raised indirectly, by citing international literature. In his entry on disinfection for the Great Medical Encyclopaedia, A. Sysin argued that Carlos Chagas, a physician in Rio de Janeiro, argued 'radically' that many disinfectant operations were unnecessary and futile. Paraphrasing Chagas, Sysin wrote: 'Parasites are a part of life.' Quoting directly, he argued: 'Parasitism is a foundation necessary for life; outside the organism, where they parasitize, microbes die extremely quickly and do not reproduce.'⁸² At a time when strictly antibiotic approaches to landscapes were unfolding in public health, the makings of a divergence in point of view in the Soviet Union were apparent. Perhaps general bactericide was not what was best for human health, after all? But that is another story for another day.

Conclusion

In the Soviet Union, the use of ultraviolet lamps, as they moved from physical medicine into the fields of public health, was marked by an important continuity across disciplines: ongoing attention to and control of the environmental dimensions of health and disease. Here, the focus of study shifted subtly from the clinical treatment of bodies embedded in environments, as in physical medicine, to the treatment of environments with bodies entangled within them. Soviet researchers studied microbes in the field and traced the influence of the material environment and human movement and behaviour on how microbes acted in space and in bodies. They studied environments with humans in them.

The Soviet approach to public health meant that Soviet researchers were particularly attuned to the unintended, harmful effects of public health interventions in the environment on human health. They were committed to reconciling the effectiveness and economy of measures to intervene in the environment and the competing priority of human health. Those people who actually existed in treated environments and their health were not treated as collateral damage in the grand project of microbial decontamination, but rather, humans remained the focus in these interventions, and their health mattered, too. Indeed, this was an approach that focused on human health outcomes. Reducing microbial contamination did not become a value in itself, but rather remained closely coupled to measurable epidemiological outcomes in really existing populations and environments subject to public health interventions.

Notes

1 A. P. Omeliants, 'Kontsentrirovannoe solntselechenie nekotorykh zabolevanii', *Voprosy kurortologii*, 3 (1937): 19. See also P. I. Nanii, 'Lechenie kontsentrirovannymi luchami solntsa', *Voprosy kurortologii*, 3 (1937): 14–17.
2 Nanii, 'Lechenie kontsentrirovannymi luchami solntsa', 14.
3 Omeliants, 'Kontsentrirovannoe solntselechenie nekotorykh zabolevanii', 22.
4 The writing in the history of medicine on natural healing is vast and is particularly deep in the Central European context. For Central Europe, see especially Uwe Heyll, *Wasser, Fasten, Luft und Licht: Die Geschichte der naturheilkunde in Deutschland* (Frankfurt: Campus, 2006); Wolfgang R. Krabbe, *Gesellschaftsveränderung durch Lebensreform: Strukturmerkmale einer sozialreformerischen Bewegung im Deutschland der Industrialisierungsperiode* (Göttingen: Vandenhoeck und Ruprecht, 1974). See also Kai Buchholz, ed., *Die Lebensreform: Entwürfe zur Neugestaltung von Leben und Kunst um 1900* (Darmstadt: Institut Mathildenhöhe, 2001); Claudia Huerkamp, 'Medizinische Lebensreform im späten 19. Jahrhundert: Die Naturheilbewegung in Deutschland als Protest gegen die naturwissenschaftliche Universitätsmedizin', *Vierteljahrschrift für Sozial – und Wirtschaftsgeschichte*, 73.2 (1986): 158–82; Gunnar Stollberg, 'Die Naturheilvereine im Deutschen Kaiserreich', *Archiv für Sozialgeschichte*, 28 (1998): 287–305; Eberhard Wolff, ed., *Lebendige Kraft: Max Bircher-Benner und sein Sanatorium im historischen Kontext* (Baden: hier + jetzt, 2010); Avi Sharma, 'Medicine from the Margins? Naturheilkunde from Medical Heterodoxy to the University of Berlin, 1889–1920', *Social History of Medicine*, 24.2 (2011): 334–51; John Alexander Williams, *Turning to Nature in Germany: Hiking, Nudism, and Conservation, 1900–1940* (Stanford: Stanford University Press, 2007). On the rise of the Swiss mountain cure, see Felix Graf, ed., *Zauber Berge: Die Schweiz als Kraftraum und Sanatorium* (Baden, Switzerland: hier+jetzt, 2010); Susan Barton, *Healthy Living in the Alps: The Origins of Winter Tourism in Switzerland, 1860–1914* (Manchester: Manchester University Press, 2008); Alison F. Frank, 'The Air Cure Town: Commodifying Mountain Air in Alpine Central Europe', *Central European History* 45.2 (2012): 185–207; Andreas Schwab, *Monte Verita – Sanatorium der Sehnsucht* (Zürich: Orell Füssli Verlag, 2003). On the traditions of thermal medicine (hydrotherapy) in spas in France and the French Empire, see Eric Thomas Jennings, *Curing the Colonizers: Hydrotherapy, Climatology and French Colonial Spas* (Durham: Duke University Press, 2008); Douglas Peter Mackaman, *Leisure Settings: Bourgeois Culture, Medicine and the Spa in Modern France* (Chicago: Chicago University Press, 1998).
5 Heyll, *Wasser, Fasten, Luft und Licht*.

6   Niklaus Ingold, *Lichtduschen: Geschichte einer Gesundheitstechnik, 1890–1975* (Zürich: Chronos Verlag, 2015), 42.
7   Ibid., 25.
8   Linda Nash, *Inescapable Ecologies: A History of Environment, Disease, and Knowledge* (Berkeley: University of California Press, 2006); Gregg Mitman, *Breathing Space: How Allergies Shape Our Lives and Landscapes* (New Haven: Yale University Press, 2007); David Rosner and Gerald Markowitz, *Deadly Dust: Silicosis and the On-Going Struggle to Protect Workers' Health* (Ann Arbor: University of Michigan Press, 2005); Brett Walker, *Toxic Archipelago: A History of Industrial Disease in Japan* (Seattle: University of Washington Press, 2011); Nancy Langston, *Toxic Bodies: Hormone Disruptors and the Legacy of DES* (New Haven: Yale University Press, 2010); Christopher C. Sellers, *Hazards of the Job: From Industrial Disease to Environmental Health Science* (Chapel Hill: University of North Carolina Press, 1997).
9   Ingold, *Lichtduschen*.
10 On mass health education as a form of prevention, see Trisha Starks, *The Body Soviet: Propaganda, Hygiene and the Revolutionary State* (Madison: University of Wisconsin Press, 2008). On sanitary enlightenment texts on sexual affairs, see Frances Lee Bernstein, *The Dictatorship of Sex: Lifestyle Advice for the Soviet Masses* (DeKalb: Northern Illinois University Press, 2007). On social hygiene, see especially Susan Gross Solomon, 'Social Hygiene and Soviet Public Health, 1921–1930', in Susan Gross Solomon and John F. Hutchinson, eds., *Health and Society in Revolutionary Russia* (Bloomington and Indianapolis: Indiana University Press, 1990), 175–99.
11 On the turn in public health to laboratory research in the United States in the interwar period, see especially Sellers, *Hazards of the Job*.
12 Ingold, *Lichtduschen*, 28.
13 Ibid., 28–9.
14 Ibid., 32.
15 'Minina lampa', in A. N. Bakulev, ed., *Bol'shaia meditsinskaia entsiklopediia* (Moscow: Gosudarstvennoe nauchnoe izdatel'stvo Sovetskaia Entsiklopediia, 1960), 18, 629–30.
16 Ingold, *Lichtduschen*, 64.
17 Ibid., 179.
18 Ibid.
19 S. B. Vermel', 'Klassifikatsiia fiziatrii', *Kurortnoe delo (Bal'neologiia, klimatoterapiia i fiziatriia)*, 1 (1924): 28.
20 A. A. Mazel', 'Rtutno-kvartsevaia lampa kak metod apparatnoi fizioprofilaktiki', *Kurortologiia i fizioterapiia*, 3 (1934): 24.
21 Ibid., 23.
22 Ibid.
23 Ibid., 25.
24 Ibid., 23.
25 Ibid., 23–4.
26 Ibid., 24.
27 Ibid.
28 Ibid., 24.
29 Ibid., 30.
30 Ibid., 26.
31 Ibid., 22.
32 Ibid.
33 Ibid.

34 Ibid., 26–7.
35 Ibid., 23.
36 Ibid., 29.
37 Ia. E. Neishtadt, *Bakteritsidnoe ul'trafioletovoe izluchenie (profilaktika vozdushnykh infektsii)* (Moscow: Medgiz, 1955), 106.
38 Ibid., 106.
39 Ibid.
40 N. S. Zimilov, 'Opyt bor'by s batsilonositeliami difterii u.-f. oblucheniem', *Kururtologiia i fizioterapiia*, 7 (1933): 11.
41 Ibid.
42 Ibid.
43 Neishtadt, *Bakteritsidnoe ul'trafioletovoe izluchenie*, 14.
44 Ibid., 44.
45 Ibid., 46.
46 Ibid.
47 Ibid., 59, 63–4, 67.
48 Ibid., 5.
49 Ibid., 5, 133.
50 Ibid., 10.
51 Ibid., 68.
52 Ibid., 67–8.
53 Ibid., 68.
54 Ibid.
55 Ibid., 62.
56 Ibid., 104.
57 A. I. Shafir, *Aerogennye infektsionnye zabolevaniia i sposoby ikh preduprezhdeniia* (Leningrad: Medgiz, 1951), as cited in Neishtadt, *Bakteritsidnoe ul'trafioletovoe izluchenie*, 65.
58 Neishtadt, *Bakteritsidnoe ul'trafioletovoe izluchenie*, 90–1.
59 Ibid., 65.
60 Ibid., 48.
61 Ibid., 63–4.
62 Ibid., 48–9.
63 Ibid., 35.
64 Ibid., 56.
65 Ibid., 85.
66 Ibid., 86.
67 Ibid., 98–9.
68 Ibid., 111.
69 Ibid., 139.
70 Ibid., 137–8.
71 Ibid., 18.
72 Ibid., 140.
73 Ibid.
74 Ibid.
75 Ibid.
76 Ibid., 141.
77 Ibid.
78 Ibid.

79 Ibid.
80 Dots. V. M. Badimov, 'Bor'ba s solnechnym golodaniem v noveishie istochniki ul'trafioletovogo sveta', *Kurortologiia i fizioterapiia*, 3 (1935): 82.
81 Prof. L. I. Veingerov, 'Radiatsionnyi rezhim v mestnykh svetovykh vannakh', *Kururtologiia i fizioterapiia*, 1 (1934): 73.
82 A. Sysin, 'Dezinfektsiia', in N. A. Semashko, ed., *Bol'shaia meditsinskaia entsiklopediia*, 8 (Moscow: Aktsionernoe obshchestvo 'Sovetskaia entsiklopediia', 1929).

9

Embodied technologies: Lilya Brik's *The Glass Eye* (1929) and Esfir Shub's *Today* (1930)

Lilya Kaganovsky

The years 1929–1930 might be thought of as a turning point in the history of Soviet film because they saw the release of such classics of avant-garde silent cinema as Sergei Eisenstein's *General Line*, Oleksandr Dovzhenko's *Earth*, and Dziga Vertov's *Man with a Movie Camera* (though none of these were well received in their own time). Already aware of the coming of sound and the changes brought on by the First Five-Year Plan and Stalin's cultural revolution, these films represented a final push of Soviet montage cinema to assert its visual and ideological superiority over bourgeois forms of entertainment that dominated the world outside (and even inside) its borders. Yet, at the same time that Vertov, Eisenstein, Dovzhenko (as well as Pudovkin, Ermler, Barnet, Kozintsev and Trauberg, and others) were completing what would become their last avant-garde projects, several female directors working in the Soviet film industry were also making breakthrough films. Indeed, by the end of the 1920s, the USSR could boast of a significant number of women working in the film industry, including Olga Preobrazhenskaya, the first well-known Russian female director, who released her feature film, *The Women of Ryazan'* (*Baby riazanskie*) in 1927; the kinok Elizaveta Svilova, assistant director and chief editor on all Vertov films, as well as a documentary director in her own right; and the established editor-director Esfir Shub, who by 1929 had completed three historical documentary features and in the process invented the genre of the 'compilation film' (*montazhnaia fil'ma*).[1]

Joining these 'amazons of the avant-garde', as Maya Turovskaya has dubbed them, was the relative newcomer Lilya Brik, one of the subjects of this chapter.[2] Brik's 1929 *Glass Eye* (*Stekliannyi glaz*) and Shub's 1930 *Today* (*Segodnia*) form part of the larger avant-garde effort to secure the place of the documentary chronicle and the uses of constructivist techniques in cinema before the intrusion of sound, on the one hand, and socialist realist aesthetics, on the other, would make this kind of 'formalist' experimentation impossible. As such, these films add significantly to our understanding of Soviet cinema at the end of the 1920s, but they also do something else: by remediating the documentary images from films by Mikhail Kaufman, Walter Ruttmann, and others, they give us a different perspective on the world and on cinema as an artistic practice. Specifically, they speak to the way cinema is an embodied technology that – to follow Walter Benjamin – fragments and rearranges the world:

> Our bars and city streets, our offices and furnished rooms, our railroad stations and our factories seemed to close relentlessly around us. Then came film and exploded this prison-world with the dynamite of the split second, so that now we can set off calmly on journeys of adventure among its far-flung debris.[3]

For Miriam Hansen, Benjamin's 'prismatic' work of film at once unveils and refracts the everyday, making it available for play – 'for a mimetic appropriation and reconfiguring of its ruined fragments'.[4] In this way, cinema acts 'as a counter to the anaesthetizing effect of the sensory assault of modern life'.[5]

In their two films, Shub and Brik emphasize the textural, material qualities of the screen, its surface and *faktura*, and the tendency of film as a medium towards abstraction – dissolving into non-signifying patterns of dark and light – pointing in an alternate relationship to the visual from similar films shot by male camera operators (and often using the same raw footage as their base) and directed by male directors. This is not cinema used for the purposes of illustration or *agit-prop* (or, not only for this), but film as a handmade, tactile object, a play of shadows and light, interiors and exteriors, reflections, refractions and prismatic reconfigurations. As Emma Widdis has argued, for many members of the Soviet avant-garde, 'the ludic impulse – the imaginative, hands-on quality of play, and its capacity to reshape reality – was the key to the power of art in the revolutionary context'.[6] Brik and Shub are clearly interested in the texture of the material world, in the way cinema can be used to either conceal (through artifice, costuming, fantastical plots or adventures) or reveal (by baring the device, by emphasis on the documentary material – what Viktor Shklovsky, Sergei Tret'iakov and Shub herself called 'ustanovka na material'), the conditions of production that go into making a film, specifically, a montage film, made by the hands of the director-editor.[7] Their films reveal what Widdis has called 'the cinematic pleasure in texture, touch, and embodied experience' and its 'ludic moments': instances of playfulness as a 'material encounter between body and world'.[8] For both Brik and Shub, cinema is a playful, material affair, a coming together of bodies and technologies, of the handmade with the mechanically reproducible. It is a playful, tactile, materialist approach to remaking the world – an embodied encounter between the (female) filmmaker and the film.

Lilya Brik's *The Glass Eye*

For Soviet cinema, Lilya Brik (Figure 9.1) was an amateur. A 'sometime writer and socialite', Brik was very well educated, spoke German natively and French fluently, studied mathematics, and later, painting and sculpture at the Moscow Institute of Architecture.[9] She also danced ballet, drew, composed poetry, sculpted and published memoirs that reveal her talent as a writer.[10] And she wrote scholarly articles, several of which appeared in the journal *Novyi put'* (*New Way*, 1921–2) published in Riga.[11]

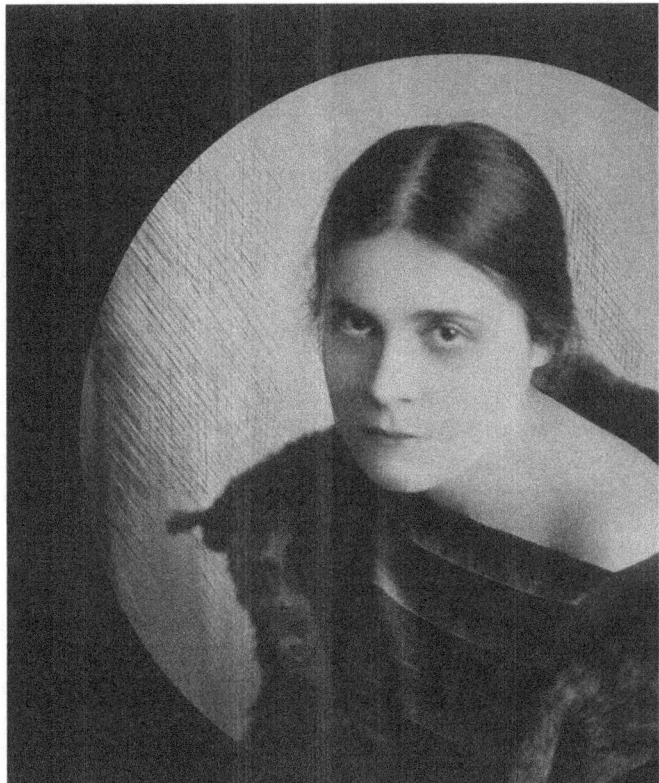

Figure 9.1 Director Lilya Brik, courtesy of Heritage Images/Getty Images.

Her younger sister, Elsa Triolet, became a prominent writer and translator in France, writing in both Russian and French, and the first woman to be awarded the Prix Goncourt, in 1944. But because Brik had talent but no defined profession, her role in the avant-garde community was to serve as its 'muse'. (It was Pablo Neruda who first called her the 'muse of Russian avant-garde'.) As Maya Turovskaya puts it, Brik appeared on the screen, but never became an actress. She made a film, but never became a director. Turovskaya jokes that in those hyper-materialist times, even the artist's muse became a 'concrete thing' (*opredmetilas'*), materialized in the form of Lilya Brik.[12]

In 1918, while Mayakovsky was in Moscow, he wrote screenplays and acted in three silent films made at the Neptun Studios in Petrograd, the third of which, *Shackled by Film* (*Zakovannaia fil'moi*), was written with and starred Lilya Brik in the role of a ballerina who comes off the film screen and into real life.[13] In 1926, Brik worked for OZET (Obshchestvo zemledel'tsev evreev trudiashchikhsia/Society for the Settlement of Jewish Toilers on the Land), and was involved in the making of a documentary, *Jews on the Land* (*Evrei na zemle*, 1927), about Jewish communal farming in Crimea, directed by Abram Room and with a script co-written by Mayakovsky and Shklovsky.[14] In 1927, Brik, together with Lev Kuleshov, wrote a script for Mezhrabpom based on a

Nikolai Nekrasov short story, and a year later, she began work on her half-fiction/half-documentary film, *The Glass Eye*, a parody on 'bourgeois cinematography'.[15]

The little that we know about this film all comes from Brik's own diaries and correspondence: in April 1928, she wrote to Osip Brik from Berlin, asking him about Mezhrabpom funds for purchasing German documentary footage to include in her film; in August 1928, she wrote to Mayakovsky about having successfully shot the camera operator sequence for the film, noting that it came out well and that Vsevolod Pudovkin was a great help; and in October 1928, she wrote to Mayakovsky to say that she had been so busy with editing the film that she hardly missed him.[16] Mayakovsky wrote from Paris that despite not being able to locate Walter Ruttmann, he had been promised documentary footage or even possibly, an 'entire *Kulturfilm*', which arrived on 28 October 1928.[17]

The Glass Eye was co-written with the director Vitaly Zhemchuzhnyi, and was directed and edited by Brik. Osip Brik thought the picture 'elegantly made' and wonderfully edited, while Kuleshov found the montage 'brilliant', and claimed that he could not do better himself. It also received high praise from the film administration, which released the picture in two Moscow theaters, 'Koloss' and 'Ars' on 15 January 1929,[18] and Brik was immediately engaged to work on a new screenplay, 'Love and Debt, or Carmen' for Mezhrabpom, which was supposed to star Mayakovsky and many other members of the Russian avant-garde.[19] The censorship body of the screenwriting section, however, found the idea that 'for 1800 meters people would dress and undress, kiss, strangle, arrest, liberate, and stab Karmen, and not just once but four different times', abhorrent. They concluded that the screenplay was to be banned, without the right for revision.[20] While definitive in its negative opinion of the screenplay, the commission's description nevertheless suggests that the imagined film was meant to be quite experimental, presenting the death of Carmen from multiple angles and perspectives.

Indeed, this type of experimentation – playing with both the content and the form of cinema – is already evident in Brik's only completed film, *The Glass Eye*.[21] Brik opens *The Glass Eye* – itself already a reference to the optical properties of the camera lens as well as a call-back to Vertov's concept of the Cine-Eye (*kinoglaz*) – with the invention of the movie camera by the Lumière Brothers in 1896. This title card is followed by an animated sequence in which a camera lens quickly advances towards the viewer, a roll of film that winds and unwinds, the moving hand-crank of a film camera spinning faster and faster, and finally, the Parvo camera itself: shown first in profile, then *enface*, assembling its different parts right before our eyes, climbing on top of its tripod, etc. If this sequence seems familiar (or perhaps even derivative), we must remember that this film was made *the same year* as Vertov and Svilova's *Man with a Movie Camera* (*Chelovek s kinoapparatom*, 1929); that Vertov, Svilova, the Briks and Shub were all friends; and that both *The Glass Eye* and *Man with a Movie Camera* use documentary footage shot by Mikhail Kaufman (and released as his 1928 film *Moscow/Moskva*), while Brik and Shub's films also borrowed documentary footage from Walter Ruttmann's *Berlin: Symphony of a City* (*Berlin – Die Sinfonie der Großstadt*, 1927). All of these films are products of the LEF group, constructivist methodology, and like-minded ways of thinking about non-played film and the role of cinema in documenting contemporary life. Each tries to showcase the power of the cinematic apparatus to not only photograph, but also to construct our physical reality.

After a prologue displaying the technological aspects of filmmaking, Brik gives us a brief history of the cinema, starting with one of the first films shot in Russia: the coronation of Nicholas II, followed by the coronation of the King of India, and the burning of the Maly Theater in 1915, two women of the 'old world' posing for the camera. The next sequence, however, takes us out of the historical narrative to the present, to the 'glass eye of the contemporary man'. We see a camera operator (Anatoly Golovnya, Figure 9.2) assembling his equipment – dusting off a 35mm movie film canister, checking on lenses, choosing filters, before departing for the day's shoot. We see different cameramen (Golovnya, Kaufman) moving around Moscow, as well as footage from their cameras and excerpts from Kaufman's *Moscow* – some of these will also be used by Vertov in *Man with a Movie Camera*. The editing (done by Brik herself) is not rapid and does not aim for the kind of virtuosity Vertov and Svilova give us in their films, but there is more attention paid to the visual aspects of the shots – to patterns, lines, shadows and geometric shapes – than what was visible in Kaufman's own film that was more concerned with camera movement than with screen-as-canvas. Here, too, we follow a cameraman as he descends into mines, climbs to the roofs of buildings, hangs suspended over construction sites, stands in between passing

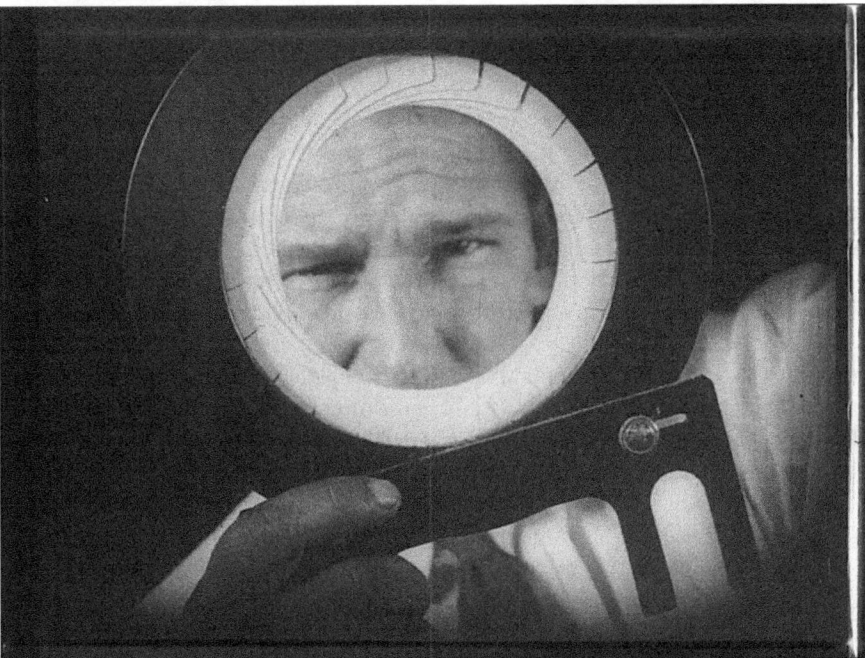

Figure 9.2 Cameraman Anatoly Golovnya with an adjustable iris diaphragm: Film still from *The Glass Eye*, dir. Brik, 1929.

trams, shooting from high above and down below: the privileged view of the world as captured by the movie camera, underscored by the intertitle: 'the glass eye can see into all corners of the world'.

Next, we see newsreel shots of the tropics (African forests and villages, with footage likely shot by colonialist Western explorers, a male-female team we briefly see setting up their camera equipment) and of the Far North (but also: skiing, sledding, ice-skating, boating), before Brik's film takes us under water to watch synchronized swimming, and even further: inside the body. Circular motifs, already evident in the shot of Golovnya looking at us through an adjustable iris diaphragm, are echoed by African women's circular dancing, their grass skirts and circular jewellery, the waltzing ice-skaters, and finally, a female figure-skater doing an upright spin, her skirt flaring around her, caught in slow-motion by the camera. Moreover, the focus on women – from African women at work and play, to Western female athletes, skating, swimming, and diving – suggests that the earlier inclusion of shots of bourgeois women posing for the camera in their finery was not accidental. Brik is telling a story about women's roles, about women's bodies and about how the 'glass eye' sees them. Bourgeois cinema sees women only as objects of the gaze – and they embody that role by preening before the camera – while non-bourgeois (Soviet, documentary, women's) cinema is able to see them as subjects, as 'lived bodies' whose movements are 'intentional', 'a pure fluid action, the continuous calling forth of capacities, which are applied to the world'.[22] Like Vertov's attempt at a 'non-museum' gaze in *A Sixth Part of the World* (*Shestaia chast' mira*, 1926), Brik shows us women not as objects of the male gaze – the camera's, the director's, the spectator's – but as subjects whose bodies are allowed to take up space and whose movements are free and expansive.[23]

The circular motif is picked up again by the 'special camera' (a large compound microscope) used for photographing inside the body. It is this segment that is perhaps visually the most stunning for the way it patterns the screen, removing even the loose narrative support of the earlier 'day in the life of a cameraman' or the ethnographic *Kulturfilm*. As we look at the images captured by the microscope, they become more and more abstract, until they are no longer recognizable as anything but a play of shadow and light. This is the glass eye 'in the service of science', but what it's really doing is reducing cinema to its most basic elements: marks of light left on a dark surface.

As the glass eye takes us around the world, we might similarly note the magnificent patterning of the iron works as we ascend to the top of the Eiffel Tower. Brik is clearly drawn to shots that are by themselves graphically patterned and that represent the random beauty of the world captured by the camera. This is a very different viewpoint from Kaufman or Vertov, who, while they are certainly looking for unusual perspectives, are perhaps less interested in the surface or texture of the screen. For Brik, the manipulation of the filmed material via rapid cutting or montage is not the goal in itself, but rather, forms part of the display of the material's own inherent qualities: patterns, surfaces, visual rhymes, movement within as well as between shots. The camera – and, by extension, the film – is a spectator, embodied (in its cameraman, in its material presence as an apparatus, but also in its active viewing), 'taking up' space, observing the world. As Vivian Sobchack notes, while the film's 'body' is not 'sexed', it is 'sensible and sensual'.[24] It is less a prosthetic device ('the man *with* the movie camera') than a 'cyborg' (in Donna Haraway's formulation): 'an other body that signifies possibilities and liberation from the disfigured bodies some of us presently live'.[25] She writes:

> A film is experienced and understood not as some objective mechanism like a water heater. It is also not experienced and understood as an enabling and extensional prosthetic device like the telephone or microscope. Rather, the film is experienced and understood for what it is: a visible and centered visual activity coming into being in significant relation to the objects, the world, and the others it intentionally takes up and expresses in embodied vision.[26]

Moreover, cinema offers the female filmmaker 'an other body' that, while she remains positioned as both subject and object (or between subject and object), can move freely through the world, as a liberated 'organ of perception'.[27]

This is particularly notable in Brik's repurposing of the footage from Ruttmann's *Symphony of a City* to re-centre our point-of-view from women as objects of the gaze to the female gaze as organ of perception. While Ruttmann's *Symphony* often follows the inhabitants of the city, focusing especially on the young women walking the streets of Berlin (as window shoppers/prostitutes), Brik discards all of the shots that appear staged, voyeuristic and subject to the male gaze, and instead focuses on the objects seen in the shop windows. Mechanical toys and bobble-headed dolls that move ostensibly on their own; female mannequins being taken off trucks, which Brik playfully dresses and undresses through a series of jump cuts; people on stilts dressed in 'African' garb to advertise German Alka-Selzer – together these speak to a playful relationship to the objects on display, to their material and physical properties rather than to their commercial or consumer effects as 'goods' for sale (along with the women who are reflected in the shop windows). A spinning pin-wheel and a rotating Murphy bed bring back the circular motif, reminding us of cinema's illusory nature that produces movement out of still images. But the repurposed sequence also serves as 'play' in the Benjaminian sense – a taking apart and putting back together of a world.

Finally, we get the political message: the glass eye can show us 'real life' in the bourgeois West, including a soldier pillaging a house (removing belongings, a mattress, etc. through the window), women crying, children hiding in corners as items are taken out the house (Jews? Communists? We see the words 'Rotfront' written on the side of the building), workers' demonstrations; dead bodies, washing blood off the pavement – some of these we recognize as shots from Vsevolod Pudovkin's 1932 *Deserter* (*Dezertir*, shot by Golovnya in Germany); then May 1 celebrations in Paris, Prague and Moscow. It is too dangerous, says Brik, to show all of this to the masses, so the West replaces actuality with 'sensationalism' and 'piquant' images. Cinema has been compromised, placed in the service of a ruling ideology that pulls the wool over our eyes and instead of showing us the world *as it really is*, shows us make-believe. What follows is Brik's send up of a typical romantic pot-boiler, complete with beautiful actress (Veronika Polonskaya), a handsome stranger, a villainous count and a ship wreck. Again, here we have the baring of the cinematic device: we first see the preparations for the shoot (a worker dusting a 'bowl of fruit'; a make-up artist brushing out a wig or painting tears on an actress's face; a peasant stuffing a pillow under his tunic to make himself look fat). In this way, the fictional film-within-a-film is contextualized by the larger framework that first shows us how all the 'magic of cinema' is made and the labour that it requires: buckets of water being carried by workers to make the 'ocean' for the sea voyage, an airplane propeller needed to simulate wind, rehearsals of 'the kiss', of the 'panic' aboard the ship, etc., as the intertitles make clear. Throughout this sequence, Brik emphasizes the work of the film crew: the role of the director, the cameraman, the stage hands, the actors. A romantic love story, an attempted rape, a daring rescue, a murder, a shipwreck and a 'happy end' are told entirely through the visual language of cinema: close ups, gesture, facial expression, montage. We can agree with Kuleshov: the film-within-a-film is a brilliant condensation of all of the rules of silent cinema, demonstrating the degree to which Brik has mastered the language of the bourgeois 'kissing' film she is ostensibly making fun of.[28]

But perhaps, there is something else here as well: a cinephile, who watched many films and even starred in one, Brik is conscious of the way film has been used to construct the female subject, both on screen and off. The pot boiler is a female genre (as Vlad Korolevich reminds us), and here, it is used in direct contrast with the more 'masculine' documentary cinema (as exemplified by footage taken from Kaufman and Ruttmann).[29] Yet, through her screenplay, direction and editing, Brik is able to take control of the apparatus for her own purposes, to make it show us a different world not only from the one constructed by bourgeois cinema of the capitalist West, but also from the cinema being actively constructed by Soviet male directors and cinematographers. Her choice of the 'glass eye' as metaphor is itself indicative of a different relationship to the camera and its uses than Vertov's *kino-glaz*. Brik's cinematic apparatus is not a prosthesis or a 'mechanical' eye superior to the human organ, as Vertov imagined it, but rather, a prism: a glass surface that reflects, refracts, and yet, is at the same time transparent – both taking in and reflecting back the physical world outside the cinema.

Esfir Shub's *Today*

In contrast to Lilya Brik, by 1929, Esfir Shub (Figure 9.3) was a full-fledged film director, with three major films behind her and credit for inventing a new cinematic genre, the 'compilation documentary' (*montazhnaya fil'ma*) to her record. She started her career in the theatre working for Vsevolod Meyerhold, but in 1922, she took a new job at the fledgling film studio Goskino, where she was put in charge of re-editing foreign films imported for Soviet distribution. Without any prior training in montage, Shub learned her craft on the job and during evenings spent in Lev Kuleshov's apartment watching him edit pieces of film on his light table.[30] At Goskino's Montage Bureau, Shub re-edited over 200 foreign films and a dozen Soviet films for ideological content, becoming an expert at montage, and experimenting with composition and rearrangement to create new films on the editing table. Sergei Eisenstein learned

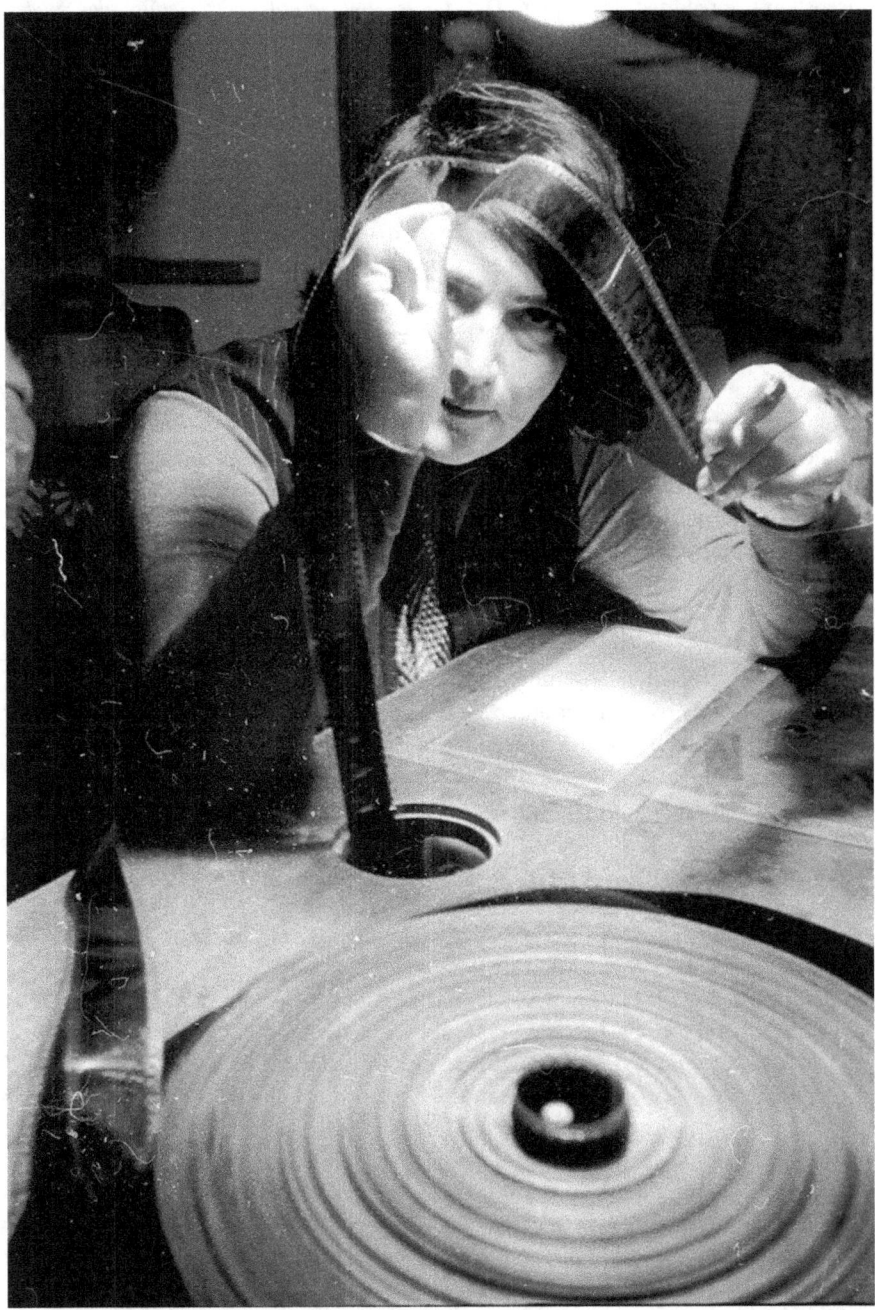

Figure 9.3 Director Esfir Shub at flatbed with celluloid-strip, 1931.

montage from Shub. The 'Brothers' Vasil'iev were her students.[31] Together with Eisenstein she reedited Fritz Lang's *Dr. Mabuse, the Gambler* (*Dr Mabuse, der Spieler*, 1922, Germany), in which, according to Shub, they 'changed the narrative structure of the film as well as the intertitles. Even the film's title was changed; it became *Gilded Rot* (*Pozolochennaia gnil'*)'.[32]

As Shub notes in her memoirs, *Cinema Is My Life* (*Zhizn' moia – kinematograf*), the editing table and the screening room taught her the proper construction and composition of a shot, forced her to develop a memory for different shots, their internal structure, content and movement, as well as to determine the rhythm and tempo of the work as a whole. She learned when to cut from a long shot to a medium one, from a medium to a close up, and the reverse. Re-editing films made it possible for her to understand the 'magnetic power' of scissors in the hands of someone who is literate in the art of montage, and to begin to work towards a form of invisible or continuity editing, cutting in such a way that the shots would replace each other smoothly with a match on both movement and content within the shot (*'stremit'sia, chto by perekhody byli ne zametny'*).[33] Re-editing both foreign and domestic films – including Westerns, detective films, films with Mary Pickford and Douglas Fairbanks, Pola Negri, Asta Nielsen, Lillian Gish and others – Shub learned the way pieces of celluloid are not merely glued together, but need to be organized in order to produce both rhythmic and dramatic effects.[34] She saw that film required a different kind of acting from the theatre, and that montage was a way to bring out the 'emotional' quality of both the actor and the film.

In 1925 she moved to Goskino's Third Film Factory to edit new Soviet films, where she worked closely with Viktor Shklovsky, Yuri Tarich, Sergei Yutkevich, and others.[35] As part of her belief in the artistic responsibility of the editor, Shub spent a lot of time on set, on location, on storyboarding (*raskadrovka*), attending rehearsals. Eisenstein invited her to join his film crew on his first film, *Strike* (*Stachka*, 1925), and had that worked out, it is possible Shub would have become a director of 'played' films. It is also possible, she would have remained 'Assistant Director' for her entire career, as happened to so many others.

Instead, Shub met Dziga Vertov. And while they did not necessarily agree on the task of documentary – according to Shub, for example, Vertov did not like using pre-existing footage because of the low artistic quality of the material (both form and content), and believed, 'wrongly', in the primacy of montage – Shub calls Vertov her close friend and 'teacher'.[36] Shub notes that Vertov was the first to understand the significance of cinematography and the importance of the camera operator for documentary films, as well as the need for a newsreel chronicle to be a 'complete film', not just different segments arranged together under a title.[37] In 1927, Shub moved to Goskino's First Film Factory on Zhitnaya St., and began to campaign to be allowed to make her own films (despite the studio director's rejections), and where she eventually produced her first three compilation documentaries: *The Fall of the Romanov Dynasty* (*Padenie dinastii Romanovykh*, 1927), *The Great Way* (*Velikii put'*, 1927) and *The Russia of Nicholas II and Lev Tolstoy* (*Rossiia Nikolaia II i Lev Tolstoi*, 1928).[38]

In 1929, Shub travelled to Berlin (along with Vertov, Dovzhenko, Ilya Trainin, and others) to acquire materials for her new film on contemporary events, a co-production with the Weltfilm studio, initially called 'Two Worlds', and which was released in Germany in 1930 under the title, *Tractors and Cannons*, and in the USSR as *Today* (*Segodnia*).[39] For this new film, Shub made selections from documentary materials held at the film archive in Neubabelsberg, home to the UFA studio. She also shot new segments in Berlin and arranged for archival documentary footage to be bought from the United States. Not all of this selected material made it into the final film (Shub notes at a certain point that Soiuzkino refused to buy the footage she actually wanted because it was too expensive, and cut her funding for her travel around the USSR), but the overall structure of the film, comparing the two worlds of 'decaying' capital and 'developing' socialism, remained intact.[40]

This was the first film Shub made using mainly new footage directed by her. Together with her assistant Leonid Felonov, and the camera operators Stepanov and Stilianudis, Shub travelled all over the Soviet Union, including Karelia, Lake Kivach, tea plantations in Chakva and Baku. This was also her last silent film. Indeed, while in Berlin, Shub had the opportunity to watch the first sound films (both German and American, including the *Singing Fool*, 1928), and the credits to *Today* include the 'musical montage' of D.S. Blok. Her next film, *KShE* (*Komsomol: shef elektrofikatsii / Komsomol: Patron of Electrification*, 1932) was a sound film that included both sync sound and a musical score; her documentary and yet at the same time playful approach to its sound design in *KShE* was partially a response to the unsatisfactory early sound films she had seen in Berlin. I stress this last point because I think that like Vertov's films, *Today* has a musical sensibility; it is organized by a musical rhythm we cannot hear, but can sense through its visual montage. As one of the German reviewers noted, this is a silent film that 'speaks'.[41]

Today opens with a quotation from Molotov about 'two worlds' – the world of developing socialism and the world of decaying capitalism – facing off against each other. Shub's film is structured around similarity and contrast, with the same kinds of shots found in the West as what we first see in the USSR. But while this is very much a political picture – we come back again and again to the main slogans of the day ('Five-Year Plan in Four Years', 'Plan of Great Works', 'Liquidate the Kulaks as a Class') – this is also a picture about texture, *faktura*, and the surface patterning of the screen that moves us beyond 'content' and into 'form' – an appreciation for the materiality of the world as captured on film. From the beginning, Shub is interested in patterns and the handmade, and we see this most clearly in early shots of a Karelian village, with elaborately decorated wooden houses covered in lacy woodwork. While we are certainly supposed to understand that this old way of living (with no running water, with roofs made from straw, with everything carved by hand) will be replaced by mechanization, factories, urban grids, high rises and trams, we are nevertheless asked to pause for a minute on the beauty of the handmade and hand carved. The same thing happens in a bathhouse in Baku: while ostensibly, we are looking at the 'old ways' of being – men washing and massaging other men's bodies – there is a physicality (and even eroticism) to this sequence that speaks to something else as well: the power of hands, of bodily contact, of a profound sense of touch.

These are the haptic elements of cinema that foreground materiality (of the human body, of the world, but also of the film body) and speak to cinema's engagement with the haptic, where 'the eyes themselves begin to function like organs of touch'.[42] It reminds us that cinema is a technology that not only captures the human body (preferentially making people its object of study), or relies on the human body for its production (the screenwriter for the idea, the actor for the performance, the cameraman for the recording, the editor for the shaping, the projectionist for the viewing and finally, the spectator for the reception), but the way film is itself a *body*, with 'skin', 'musculature' and 'viscera'.[43] Film, as Laura Marks suggests, signifies through its materiality, 'through a contact between perceiver and object represented'.[44] It suggests that vision itself can be tactile, as though one were touching a film with one's eyes. It is, as Jennifer Barker has argued, a 'literal, tangible, physical contact between two bodies': we and the film are 'adjacent to one another', she writes, 'pressed against each other, in contact'.[45]

Unlike her earlier films that were constructed from historical archival footage, *Today* gives Shub a chance to film the world as she sees it (or, as she can direct her cinematographer to see it) and what we get is a densely material, textural screen-space. Familiar shots of Soviet construction sites are here filled with steam and smoke; the camera glides along the water, over rails, is suspended from cranes. And while individual shots do not as readily dissolve into abstraction as the ones chosen by Brik for her film, there is a painterly quality to these industrial images particularly, with light, shadows, smoke, steam and water combining to create a diffused effect, deepening our perception. Patterning shows up in unexpected places: women's hats, women's veils, attention paid to mirrors, reflections and reflective surfaces. Moreover, there is a 'lightness of being' to the images taken from the bourgeois world (mostly New York) that is clearly part of Shub's fascination with movement and dynamism: workers high above the ground building sky scrapers; couples dancing on rooftops; church goers performing the St Vitus dance; figure roller skating captured in slow motion; an underwater wedding with floating, suspended bodies; giant balloon animals released on Broadway (Macy's Day Parade?) – Shub is clearly fascinated by height, space, air, things that fly or swim, bodies that are ungrounded, and the ability of the camera to float freely among these suspended, liberated objects. The last segment of the film returns us to Dneprostoi (the Dnipro Hydroelectric Dam – one of the major sites of Stalin's industrialization campaign), but to Dneprostroi filmed at night and contrasted with nightlife in the West, where electricity is used to advertise products, to illuminate the dancefloor, a waste of energy. In the Dneprostoi section instead, as they will again in *KShE*, dancing lights form patterns on screen, the fully electrified Palace of Culture is an abstract image of white squares on a black ground; fireworks light up the sky in lacy, decorative patterns.

I am not trying to make Shub's film something exclusively 'feminine' – there is plenty of 'masculine' Vertovian/Kaufman-esque industrial footage here as well, plenty of marches, demonstrations, speeches, factories billowing smoke, tractors, tanks, cars, trams, and other forms of light and heavy industry, as well as the overall message of socialist competition and readiness for war. Rather, I am trying to draw attention to the way Shub, like Brik, conceives of the screen-space in terms of pattern and design. A shot is just as often selected for its visual, graphic or textural aspects, as it is for its political import. A sequence is given its full length in order to demonstrate the power of cinema to reveal the world in unexpected ways. There is a 'freedom' to the camera movement, as there is a freedom to the editing that puts them together (sometimes, with humour, as in the shot of Catholic priests cut together with waddling penguins, or two 'ladies who lunch' who are made to look up the skirt of a woman washing windows). Shub returns again and again to certain themes – dirigibles, balloons, toys, tractors and tanks, mechanized labour – and it is this, perhaps, that gives her film musicality and an internal rhythm, moving us beyond the visual register to an embodied perception of the physical world. The haptic is used as a strategy to create an alternative visual tradition to the aggressively masculinist cinemas of Vertov, Kaufman and Ruttman (such as Vertov's domination of space by vision in *A Sixth Part of the World*), to offer instead a new tactile sensibility. Following Marks, we can see this alternative visual tradition (to which Brik's *The Glass Eye* also belongs) as indicative of 'women's and feminist practices, rather than a feminine quality in particular'.[46] It supplants 'phallocentric models of vision' with a vision that is more 'ambient and intimate' – and, I would add: playful.

Women's work and children's play

The final segment of *Today* takes us to a 'children's corner' in the Palace of Culture – a daycare centre for children of Dneprostroi workers who have come to attend a lecture on collectivization. We watch happy children of different ages playing with toys, sliding down ramps, constructing buildings out of wooden blocks, assembling Matryoshka dolls, engaging in pretend play with toy animals and the like (Figures 9.4a and 9.4b). From here, an overhead shot pans over a room full of adults playing dominos – with emphasis again placed on the interaction of hands and rectangular-shaped game pieces, close-ups of faces animated with pleasure or brows furrowed in concentration. We then see a lecture hall filling with audience members to listen to Yemelyan Yaroslavsky speaking about the goals of collectivization (the banner behind him reads: 'Liquidate the kulaks as a class') before a Red Putilov tractor drives across the stage, bearing the sign: '5000 Soviet tractors as a valuable contribution to national industrialization'. Thus, Stalinist policies and ideological slogans of the day are all on display here, but how to understand the emphasis on the ludic that preceded them? How best to read the element of 'play' that we see in both films – from the animated film camera and mannequins in *The Glass Eye* to the children's corner in *Today*?

As Emma Widdis has suggested, 'play and playfulness, were at the center of the modernist project', both in pre- and post-revolutionary Russia, as well as in a wider international context.[47] For members of the pre-revolutionary artistic and literary avant-garde, children's art – and children's language – had provided a powerful stimulus for experiment. Futurist Aleksei Kruchenykh published an anthology of works (written and drawn) by children in 1916. Andrei Belyi's *Kotik Letaev* (1920) was explicitly concerned with the creativity of children's language and imagination. VKhUTEMAS had its own studio of children's drawings. Alexander Rodchenko and Varvara Stepanova collaborated on illustrations to Sergei Tret'iakov's children's

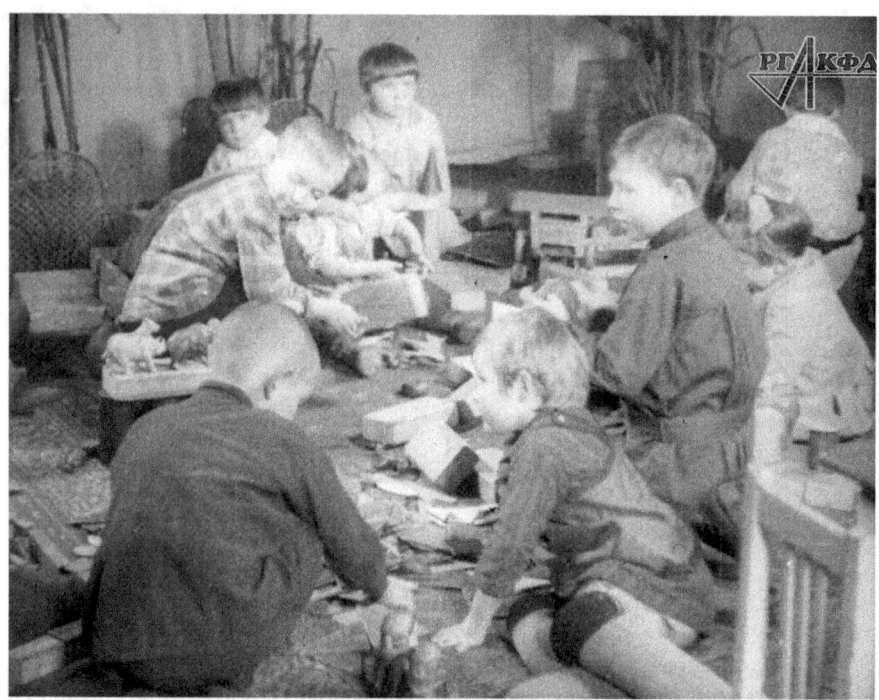

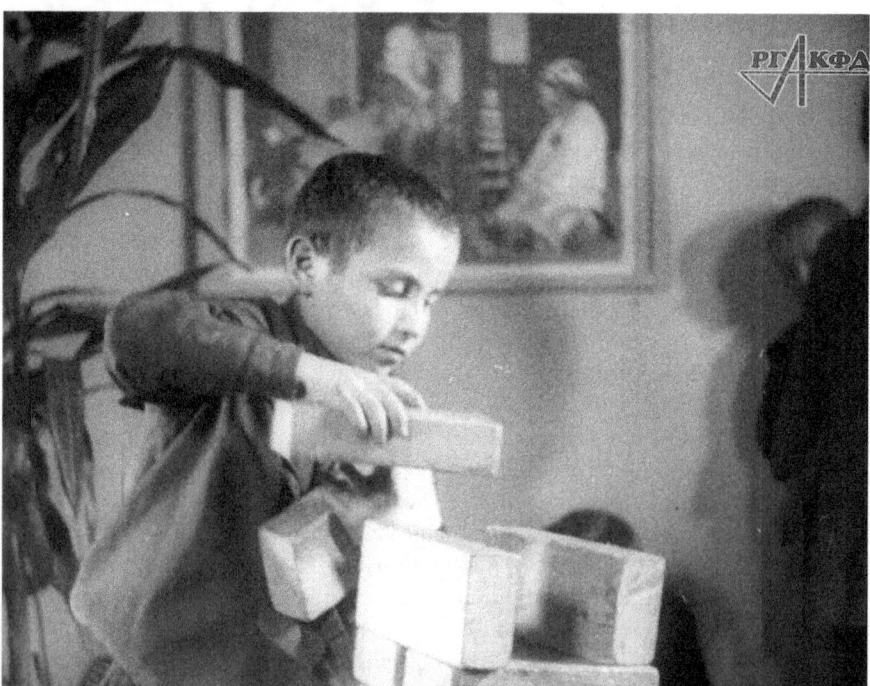

Figures 9.4a and 9.4b Children at play: Film still from *Today*, dir. Shub, 1930.

poems, *Autoanimals* (*Samozveri*) envisaging pop-out cardboard models that could be shaped and manipulated by child readers.[48] And in the context of the international revolutionary avant-garde, such as Bauhaus, play was likewise linked to the intuitive, hands-on relationship with the world that was central to the concept of 'making'.[49]

For Widdis, this hands-on play also underlay filmmakers' interest in toys during the 1920s – part of the broader exploration of cinema's capacity to reveal the *faktura* of the material world.[50] The first *Kino-Nedelia* episode (20 May 1918, likely not yet edited by Vertov[51]), for example, featured a brief sequence of 'Handmade Toys', focusing on the moving shapes of the wooden toys, their white silhouettes standing out against the disparate textures of the crowds in a market. The use of toys, suggests Widdis, 'was linked to an interest in the material properties of objects and their relation to the human body', noting the focus specifically on traditional, handmade, wooden toys: 'These are not mechanized objects, providing access to a fantastical realm of the imagination; they are simple products of craft. They speak not to the relationship between cinema and technology, but rather to a relationship with material and making.'[52]

I would argue that for Brik and Shub, who show us *both* mechanized objects *and* hand-made wooden toys, the two aspects of filmmaking – as technology, emphasizing the act of filming as captured by the camera and as handcraft, emphasizing editing – are on display. The emphasis on mechanization and technology is clear watching Brik's film, which – playfully – animates the film camera, dresses and undresses mannequins through the use of jump cuts, lingers over the bobblehead dolls, spinning pinwheels, mechanized toys and physical objects galvanized by means of electricity. Yet, we must recall that Brik, like Shub, is not only the director of this film, but also its editor; and that a film's construction into a film-*thing* from building blocks (raw footage) is the process of piecing together of different bits of film – a haptic, material, hands-on enterprise. Viktor Shklovsky complained about his brief time working at the Third Film Factory as an editor, claiming that the film strip, when he handled it, cut his hands: 'As you wind [the film] you have to be careful not to cut your hands on the edges of the film. Wounds from films heal very slowly.'[53] But for Shub, editing was a form of 'play': her favourite task was to splice together partial and unmarked rolls of film, without intertitles or libretto, into a coherent narrative – or, as she put it, 'to create a scenario for an already existing film'.[54]

Writing about 'played' and 'non-played' film (*neigrovaia fil'ma*) in 1929, Shub noted that most of Soviet cinema's resources were being spent on fiction films in which people 'played at life', and then transferred this 'played life' (*igrovuiu zhizn'*) onto celluloid, using this 'speculative material' to 'emotionally move the viewer' ('*emotsional'no vozdeistvovat' i zariazhat' zritelia*'[55]). The distinction between the played and non-played rests on the former's reliance on actors, sets, scripts, costuming and narrative to represent fictitious life on screen, while the non-played cinemas of Shub, Vertov and others is built from concrete 'facts' captured by the camera.[56] But this does not mean that there is no element of 'play' in the non-played film. Rather, the element of play is transferred from staging a fictional world to a hands-on remaking the world through editing.

The children's corner sequence in *Today* works similarly to the Chinese magician sequence in Vertov's *Man with a Movie Camera* as a metaphor for filmmaking as a whole.⁵⁷ But for Vertov, the point of the magician sequence is both to reveal and to conceal the operations of the cinematic apparatus: the magic trick is left unexplained, the editing is potentially deceitful (the magician and the children never appear in the same frame, for example); instead we witness the wonderment of children captivated by the play of illusion. In contrast, children's play in Shub's film and even her choice of dominos for the adult's play are not about illusion, but touch: they signal the constructed/Constructivist enterprise that is cinema for someone trained not only to see the world but also to touch it. Black and white game pieces, both different and similar to one another, are assembled together into a pattern; they are the building blocks, the material objects with which the game is played. As Widdis puts it (in a different context), 'the spectator is brought into a sensory encounter with toys as *things* – handled, animated, textured'.⁵⁸ This is not just a cinema of the 'ready-made' (as Mikhail Yampolsky has described Shub's historical films) but of the hand-made: a focus on the haptic, material nature of the world as captured by the film camera and transformed by the hands of its (female) director.⁵⁹

Notes

1. While it is true that Vertov made his *History of the Civil War (Istoriia grazhdanskoi voiny*, 1921, USSR; long considered lost, this film has been reconstructed by film historian Nikoali Izvolov), and Svilova had edited the *Goskinokalendar' (State-CineCalendar*, May 1923–April 1925), Shub's *Fall of the Romanov Dynasty (Padenie dinastii Romanovykh)* was a breakthrough film in terms of work with archival materials and is widely considered the first compilation film ever made. Lev Kuleshov wrote that she 'created a new stage in the development of the non-fiction film' (see: Yuri Tsivian, ed., *Lines of Resistance: Dziga Vertov in the Twenties* (Pordenone, 2004), 274); and Varvara Stepanova noted in her diary from 1927, Sergei Tret'iakov railing against 'Shubism' in favour of Vertov's methods of making documentary films (Tsivian, *Lines of Resistance*, 280); Vlada Petrić states that 'Shub established a specific cinematic genre, the so-called compilation film, movies made exclusively from existing documents, mainly newsreel footage taken by many, often unknown, cameramen. Working with newsreel material, Shub discovered some crucial principles of editing and intertitling, which were further developed by Eisenstein, Vertov, and Pudovkin' (Vlada Petric, 'Esther Shub: Cinema is My Life', *Quarterly Review of Film & Video*, 3.4 (1978): 429–48; here 429); and Annette Michelson refers to Shub as 'one of the earliest and most innovative of Soviet documentary filmmakers' and 'the inventor of the compilation film' (Annette Michelson, 'An Interview with Mikhail Kaufman', *October* 11 (1979): 54–76; fn. 8).
2. Maia Turovskaia, 'Amazonki russkogo avangarda', *Kinovedcheskie zapiski* 62 (2003): 56–63.
3. Walter Benjamin, *Selected Writings*, vol. 3, ed. Jennings et al. (Cambridge, MA: Harvard University Press, 2002), 117. Quoted in Miriam Bratu Hansen, 'Room-for-Play: Benjamin's Gamble with Cinema', *October* 109 (Summer, 2004): 3–45; here: 38.
4. Hansen, 'Room-for-Play', 38.

5 Emma Widdis, *Socialist Senses: Film, Feeling and the Soviet Subject* (Bloomington: Indiana University Press, 2017), 301.
6 Ibid., 301.
7 Sergei Tretiakov, 'Igrovaia i neigrovaia', LEF i kino. Stenogramma soveshchaniia, *Novyi LEF*, 11–12 (1927): https://chapaev.media/articles/7391. This is different from Shklovsky's 'ustanovka na material' that Widdis discusses in *Socialist Senses*, 128–9, 145 (and elsewhere), which emphasizes the new relationship to the object, a new 'tuning' of the human body towards the material world.
8 Widdis, *Socialist Senses*, 298.
9 As the English-language entry on her Wikipedia page describes her. Documents held at the Russian State Archive of Literature and Art (RGALI) include a note from Moscow RABIS to central RABIS defending Brik's status as film director on *Stekliannyi glaz* and providing a detailed biography of her involvement in cinema, literary translation and all cultural activities of LEF (Left Front of the Arts) from 1916 to 1927. The document specifically protests against accusations of Brik's 'lack of qualifications' which led to her temporary firing from the set of *Stekliannyi glaz*. The unsigned and undated document demands her immediate restoration to the post of director on her film. RGALI, f. 2577, op. 1, d. 597 (fond: Brik and Katanian), l. 7.
10 Lilya Brik kept a detailed diary most of her life, and most of what we know of the Briks and Mayakovsky comes from excerpts from that diary and her many letters, most of which have not been published. (There are over 600 letters to her sister, Elsa Triolet, for example.) The diary was revised many times, and in particular, after the arrest of her third husband Vitaly Primakov, and her full archive has not yet been made available to scholars. As a result, much of what has been written on Brik is made up, extrapolated from the few known facts and largely based on rumour. Here, I have mainly consulted: *V.V. Maikovskii and L. Iu. Brik: perepiska 1915–1930/Vladimir Majakovskij and Lili Brik: Correspondence 1915–1930*, ed. Bengt Jangfeldt (Stockholm: Amlqvist & Wiksell International, 1982), which was extensively researched by Jangfeldt while Brik was still alive and includes first time publications of letters and telegrams; and *Lilya Brik: Pristrastnye rasskazy*, eds. Ia. I. Groisman and I. Iu. Genis (Nizhnii Novgorod: DEKOM, 2003), based on archival materials held by Brik and her fourth and last husband, Vasily Katanian.
11 See: Jangfeldt, *Correspondence*, 45, n11. See also: http://www.emigrantica.ru/item/novyi-put-riga-1921-1922.
12 Turovskaia, 'Amazonki', 61.
13 The only surviving one, *The Lady and the Hooligan* (*Baryshnia i khuligan*, 1918) was based on the *La maestrina degli operai* (*The Workers' Young Schoolmistress*) published in 1895 by Edmondo De Amicis, and directed by Evgeny Slavinsky. The other two, *Born Not for the Money* and *Shackled by Film* were directed by Nikandr Turkin and are presumed lost. Gianni Toti used the few remaining frames from *Shackled by Film* in his *La trilogia majakovskijana* (Rai, Settore Ricerca e Sperimentazione Programmi, 1983–1984). Among other things, Moscow RABIS's review of Brik's film qualifications mentions that she co-wrote the screenplay for *Shackled by Film*. RGALI, f. 2577, op. 1, d. 597, l. 7.
14 Produced by VUFKU (Ukrainian Photo and Cinema Administration) (Yalta) for OZET in 1926. Screenplay by Vladimir Mayakovsky and Viktor Shklovsky, titles by Vladimir Mayakovsky, director: Abram Room, cameraman: Avgust Kiun, assistant director: Lilya Brik. The film was first shown on 15 November 1926 to delegates of the First All-Union Congress of OZET.

15 Nikolai Nekrasov, 'Novoizobretennaia privilegirovannaia kraska brat'ev Dirling i K*', 1850. The film was never made. L. Brik to V. Mayakovsky, 17 August 1927, in Jangfeldt, *Correspondence*, 166.
16 Brik, *Pristrastnye rasskazy*, 183; Jangfeldt, *Correspondence*, 176.
17 L. Brik to V. Mayakovsky and O. Brik, 22 April 1928; L. Brik to V. Mayakovsky, 14 October 1928; V. Mayakovsky to L. Brik, 20 October 1928; L. Brik to V. Mayakovsky, 2 November 1928, in Jangfeldt, *Correspondence*, 178–9. The '*Kulturfilm*' in question was Ruttmann's *Berlin: Symphony of a City*, parts of which Brik included in her film.
18 As opposed to 'Artes', which was the original, less prestigious venue. See L. Brik to V. Mayakovsky, 2 November 1928, in Jangfeldt, Correspondence, 178–9.
19 RGALI, f. 2577, op. 1, d. 597. Archival documents include signed contracts from Mezhrabpom acquiring Brik's screenplays for the Nikolai Nekrasov story, *Stekliannyi glaz*, *Liubov' i dolg*, and *Zelennyi chelovek* – a colour and sound film, originally conceived in three parts and 1200m in length, to be completed by October 1934; as well as a second document asking for substantial revisions and cuts that would turn the film into a two-part short.
20 V. Bosenko, 'Lilya Brik: "Liubov' i dolg"', *Iskusstvo kino*, 10 (1998).
21 RGALI, f. 2577, op. 1, d. 39 holds a partial shooting script for *Stekliannyi glaz* (the film is listed as being in six parts, with the fictional segment occurring earlier on as a 'film within a film' shown to movie goers in the West).
22 Iris M. Young, 'Throwing Like a Girl: A Phenomenology of Feminine Body Comportment, Motility, and Spatiality', in Jeffner Allen and Iris M. Young, eds., *The Thinking Muse: Feminism and Modern French Philosophy* (Bloomington: Indiana University Press, 1989), 59; as quoted in Vivian Sobchak, *The Address of the Eye: A Phenomenology of Film Experience* (Princeton: Princeton University Press, 1992), 153.
23 The idea that film – in contrast to the museum – could present 'real' ethnographic material by exploring the vast reaches of the USSR, and when properly used would be able to escape the fetishized, implicitly colonial vision of ethnic particularity and provide a more 'genuine' understanding of the real life of the national republics. See: Widdis, *Visions of a New Land: Soviet Film from the Revolution to the Second World War* (New Haven: Yale University Press, 2003), 111–12.
24 Sobchack, *The Address of the Eye*, 162.
25 Ibid., 163.
26 Ibid., 171.
27 Ibid., 159.
28 In the shooting script, intertitles stress that bourgeois society has ruined cinema by putting it in the service of eroticism and violence («Ежевечерне буржуазные кино-предприниматели одурманивают сознание … миллионов людей показом бесконечных убийств и поцелуев»/'Every night bourgeois film entrepreneurs stupefy the minds of … millions of people by showing endless murders and kisses'); elsewhere she refers to the these as 'kissing films' (*potseluinye kartiny*). RGALI, f. 2577, op. 1, d. 39.
29 Vladimir Korolevich, *Zhenshchina v kino* (Moscow: Tea-kino-pechat', 1926).
30 Shub's memoirs and writings on cinema are collected in Esfir Shub, *Zhizn' moia – kinematograf* (Moscow: Iskusstvo, 1972); partially translated in 'Esfir Shub: Selected Writings', trans. Anastasia Kostina, *Feminist Media Histories* 2.3: 11–28. Unless otherwise noted, all translations from the Russian are my own.

31 I am quoting Sergei Yutkevich here, though, as Yuri Tsivian points out, only Georgii Vasil'iev worked at Goskino's Montage Bureau, while Sergei Vasil'iev was a re-editor at Sevzapkino (Yutkevich in Shub *Zhizn' moia*, 9; Yuri Tsivian, 'The Wise and Wicked Game: Re-Editing and Soviet Film Culture of the 1920s', *Film History*, 8.3 (1996): 327–43; here: 333).
32 Shub, *Zhizn' moia*, 75; See also Vlada Petric, 'Esther Shub: Film as a Historical Discourse', in Thomas Waugh, ed., *Show Us Life! Toward a History and Aesthetics of the Committed Documentary* (London: Petric, 1984), 21–46.
33 Shub, *Zhizn' moia*, 76.
34 Ibid., 8.
35 Martin Stollery notes that unlike the typical editorial experience, Shub's original post in Goskino's Montage Bureau enabled her to exercise and develop her creativity, without being overshadowed by a director (Martin Stollery, 'Eisenstein, Shub and the Gender of the Author as Producer', *Film History*, 14.1 (2002): 87–99; here: 95). Shub is the only woman recorded as having worked at what Yuri Tsivian describes as this 'professional elite club', which acquired a 'certain reputation within the film industry' (Tsivian, 'The Wise and Wicked Game', 336).
36 Shub, *Zhizn' moia*, 83. Recall that Shub is writing her memoirs in the 1950s, after Vertov's consistent marginalization and exclusion from the Soviet cinema industry finally culminated in the 'Open Party Session of the Central Studio of Documentary Films' on 14–15 March 1949, with 200 people attending, where, as part of the anti-Semitic campaign of the late 1940s–1950s, Vertov was charged with 'cosmopolitanism' and accused of continuing to undermine Soviet documentary cinematography with his formalist tricks and his 'love' of the machine. See: 'Protokol N. 11 otkrytogo partiinogo sobraniia Tsentral'noi studii dokumental'nykh fil'mov ot 14–15 marta 1949 goda' (Record #11: Minutes of the Open Party Meeting of the Central Studio of Documentary Films, from 14–15 March 1949), published in *Iskusstvo kino* 12 (1997): 128–33. We might note, for example, that despite Fadeev's suggestion, Shub says almost nothing in her memoirs about Meyerhold, who was rehabilitated in 1955, shortly before she completed her book. A. A. Fadeev to E. I. Shub, letter dated 24 November 1955 (Shub, *Zhizn' moia*, 413–16; here 415–16.)
37 Shub, *Zhizn' moia*, 83–5.
38 'Trainin says "no" to all my proposals', she noted in her memoirs (Shub, *Zhizn' moia*, 100).
39 The company was founded in 1928 by International Labor Assistance and was closely associated with Prometheus Film. Weltfilm produced mainly short communist documentary and propaganda films, mostly with Albrecht Viktor Blum or Phil Jutzi as a director. In addition to production work, Weltfilm also acted as a non-commercial distributor for productions of the Prometheus Film, selected socially critical films of bourgeois production companies, as well as for Soviet feature and documentary films.
40 She had intended for the film to include segments on Donbass and Sel'mashstroi, as well as night-time footage of Moscow. The film was released in Germany to good reviews (see Shub, *Zhizn' moia*, 95), and had a response at the initial public screening in Moscow at the Ars theater. Nevertheless, the film then spent five months on the shelf, which meant that by the time it was released, it wasn't so much *Today* as 'yesterday' (Shub, *Zhizn' moia*, 278). In a letter to Eisenstein, Shub notes that the GRK gave the film a first rating (meaning, for wide release), but that the battle between played and non-played film continues ('fil'me dali pervuiu kategoriiu, no boi

idet – i ne zdorovyi'). E.I. Shub to S.M Eisenstein, letter dated 2 August 1930 (Shub, *Zhizn' moia*, 384).
41 Shub, *Zhizn' moia*, 95.
42 Laura U. Marks, *The Skin of the Film: Intercultural Cinema, Embodiment, and The Senses* (Durham: Duke University Press, 2002), 162.
43 'Skin', 'Musculature', and 'Viscera' form the three body chapters of Jennifer M. Barker's *The Tactile Eye: Touch and the Cinematic Experience* (Berkeley: University of California Press, 2009).
44 Marks, *The Skin of the Film*, xi.
45 Barker, *The Tactile Eye*, 31.
46 Marks, *The Skin of the Film*, 170.
47 Widdis, *Socialist Senses*, 299. See specifically, Chapter 9: 'Socialist Pleasures', 297–336.
48 Aleksandr Rodchenko and Varvara Stepanova, 'Fotomul'tiplikasionnye illiustratsii k detskoi knizhke "Samozveri" S. Tret'iakova', *Novyi LEF*, 1 (1927): 14–15. See Widdis, *Socialist Senses*, 307.
49 Widdis, *Socialist Senses*, 301.
50 Ibid., 307.
51 As John MacKay argues, Vertov likely got involved with editing and reediting *Kino-Nedelia* (Film-Week, forty-three instalments between May 1918 and June 1919) sometime after 1 September 1918: 'that is, certainly not before *Kino-Nedelia* 14 (released September 3) and probably not until around the time *Kino-Nedelia* 22 (released October 29) was produced'. John MacKay, *Dziga Vertov: Life and Work, Vol. 1 (1896–1921)* (Boston: Academic Studies Press, 2018), 194.
52 Widdis, *Socialist Senses*, 303.
53 Viktor Shklovskii, *Kak pisat' stsenarii: posobie dlia nachinaiushchikh stsenaristov s obraztsami stsenariev raznogo tipa* (Moscow-Leningrad: Gosudarstvennoe izdatel'stvo khudozhestvennoi literatury, 1931), 31. In Russian: 'При перемотке нужно следить, чтобы не обрезать руки краями лент. Раны от ленты не заживают очень долго.' In *Third Factory*, Shklovsky also comments on the 'unhealthy' work of splicing film: 'The cutting room at the factory smells of lozenges. […] The smell […] comes from pear oil, which is used to splice the film. Female assistants do the splicing. An unhealthy line of work'. Viktor Shklovskii, *Third Factory*, trans. Richard Sheldon (Chicago and Normal, IL: Dalkey Archive P, 2002), 59.
54 Shub, *Zhizn' moia*, 76.
55 Ibid., 263.
56 Ibid., 264.
57 See Annette Michaelson, 'Man with a Movie Camera: From Magician to Epistemologist', *Artforum*, 10.7 (1972): 60–72; and Elizabeth Astrid Papazian, *Manufacturing Truth: The Documentary Moment in Early Soviet Culture* (DeKalb: Northern Illinois Press, 2009), 91–6.
58 Widdis, *Socialist Senses*, 321.
59 Mikhail Yampolsky, 'Reality at Second Hand', *Historical Journal of Film, Radio and Television*, 11.2 (1991): 161–71.

10

Arm race: The Cold War story of a bionic arm

Frances Bernstein

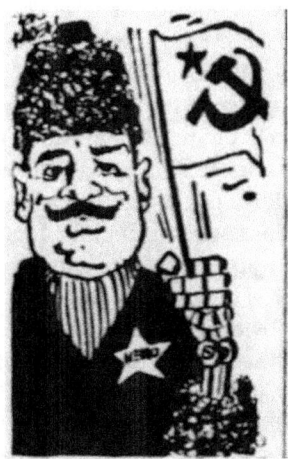

Figure 10.1 'Electronic hand made by Reds for amputees': Illustration, *Tribune News Service*, 1965.

> *In this small area of the cold war, we feel it important for the American system to compete on a scientific and economic basis. The world has ceded to the Russian hand, and the Yugoslavian hand, a position of technical eminence which rightly belongs to an American hand.[1]*

Introduction

On 17 April 1958, the world's eyes were trained on Brussels, where Expo 58, more commonly known as the Brussels World's Fair, opened to great fanfare. The first held after the war, the Fair's theme was 'A World View: A New Humanism,' and its intent was to celebrate peace, understanding and the common good.[2] Those objectives would explain the planners' idealistic decision to locate the Soviet and American pavilions adjacent to one another, especially when there were so many other countries whose buildings could have been situated between them.[3] To the surprise of no one, the Expo served as a proxy battleground for Cold-War ideological conflict, with the proximity of the US and Soviet exhibition halls facilitating each side's efforts to track its rival in the planning and construction stages as well as during the Expo itself.[4]

Both the American and Soviet pavilions, along with those of fifteen other states, received the Expo's highest honour, the Grand Prize. In addition to this recognition for the building's design, the USSR more than held its own, garnering 527 awards for its more than 700 entries from the fields of science, technology and the arts.[5] Spy dramas and the nightly news would lead us to expect the contest between superpowers to be on view during the fair, and the Soviet pavilion did not disappoint. Unsurprisingly, its biggest attractions were the Grand Prize-winning models of Sputnik One and Two, displayed prominently, near an oversized statue of Lenin. (Sputnik Three was launched during the Expo itself.)[6] But competition played itself out not only in the race for space.

Introduced at the Soviet pavilion was another recipient of the Grand Prize: the world's first functional bionic arm (Figure 10.2). Developed in collaboration by the Central Scientific-Research Institute of Prosthetics and Prosthetics Manufacturing and the Institute of Machine Technology of the Academy of Sciences, the apparatus performed the same propaganda function as did many of the other pavilion exhibits, underlining the value the country placed on science and its claim to technological superiority.[7]

This is the story of the Russia arm. An emblem of international prestige, an avenue for hard currency, a domesticating tool for adult male amputees, a short-cut response to the Thalidomide tragedy[8]: before the invention was eclipsed in the early 1970s, it would live a number of different public lives, both within the Soviet Union and without. Overseas, the Soviet achievement was cause for both celebration and alarm. On the one hand, as 'the most sensational development of the period, ... it raised expectations about what could be done for amputees and provided fuel for scholarly and popular science articles on the future of the interface and the field of cybernetics'.[9] On the other, as *Popular Electronics* put it: 'As with the first Sputnik, Russia has stolen a march on the rest of the world in the field of myoelectric control of artificial limbs.'[10]

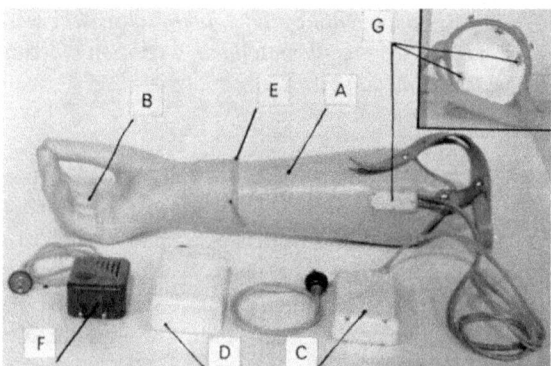

Figure 10.2 The Russia Arm prosthesis: Photograph, 1965.

This article focuses on three lives of the bioarm: as depicted at home, purchased abroad and imagined by ideological opponents. Ultimately, as an aid to people with disabilities, the arm was a failure; its greatest success by far was the anxiety it generated among cold warriors. As I show, these differing responses to the appliance were reflected in how its functions and uses were understood. Even the same words and terms had different meanings, depending upon the language and geopolitical arena in which they appeared. Conceived as a replacement, in the Soviet context and that of its clients, the action of the invention was understood in terms of the body. Although some Americans likewise regarded it as a replacement, others viewed the arm as an enhancement, especially threatening because it was controlled by the mind. 'Mind control' meant something very different in Washington, DC and Moscow.

While this article also discusses scientific and technical developments, the emphasis here is on the public lives of the device, as presented to a non-specialist, general audience: readers of mainstream newspapers, of amateur engineering and popular science publications, moviegoers, and even members of the US Congress. It only addresses the ongoing, steady work conducted in labs and clinics when findings reached beyond those exclusive, scientific spaces.

The bioarm domesticated

Patented in the USSR as a 'forearm prosthesis with electric servodrive, controlled by biocurrents, with a mechanism for sensing grip strength',[11] that the device would have multiple identities might have been predicted, owing to the wide variety of names by which it was known, even within the same country, language or publication. Russian examples include: bionic upper limb prosthesis controlled by myoelectric signals, bioelectric control system in the form of a human hand, and forearm prosthesis with bioelectric control. These competed with simpler names such as bionic arm and bioelectric prosthesis. Perhaps the most user-friendly, bioarm, was never employed consistently or widely, either in the USSR or elsewhere. As in Russian, in English the words bioelectric and myoelectric were used interchangeably, with the term 'bionic' appearing only in the popular press. Additional confusion had to do with the Russian word *ruka*, which could refer to either the arm or just the hand. Names were complicated further, depending upon the action being described: emphasis might be on the mechanical hand (motorized to open and close), the forearm (where the currents were tapped and the components stored), or the entire limb, but each of these likewise was used interchangeably to refer to the entire prosthesis. Most in the Anglophone world called the invention some combination of Russia or Russian, and hand or arm.[12]

The idea of employing an external power source to operate an artificial hand was first proposed in 1919 in Germany but remained theoretical, and a 1948 effort by Samuel Alderson in the United States also proved unfeasible. That same year, in a development that went largely overlooked at the time, a German physicist named Reinhold Reitner produced a working model but was likewise constrained by the limitations of the existing technology, with the size and weight (initially as much as 500 lbs.) of the power unit and amplifier needed to drive such a device one of the biggest hindrances.[13] As often happens with scientific breakthroughs, many labs around the world were working on similar questions at the same time.[14] The team that would develop the Russia arm (A.E. Kobrinskii, M.G. Breido, V.S. Gurfinkel', A. Ia. Sysin, M.L. Tsetlin, and Ia.S. Iakobson) first came together in late 1956 to test the possibility of using the electric pulses generated by the muscles for control purposes, and in 1957 presented a stationary hand, with fingers that could open and close, to the Academy of Sciences.[15] A modified version of this device, its amplifier reduced to the size of a large box, debuted at the Brussels Expo the following year.[16] Meanwhile, the scientists worked steadily to make all of the device's components (amplifier, power source, tapping device, motor) as small and light as possible.[17]

Enthusiasm for the invention is understandable. This was an active prosthesis (rather than a purely cosmetic one) that did not rely on the wearer's own muscular strength to function, a process that was often too taxing for amputees (using movements of the shoulder, via harness and cable, to open and close a hand). The Russia arm was powered externally, drawing upon the muscles' bioelectricity. Any action of the body is the result of a command sent from the brain via the nerve to the muscle; this process is accompanied by weak electrical signals, known as biocurrents. Even after amputation, muscles at the stump site continue to generate these pulses. To operate the arm, surface electrodes on the skin tapped and amplified the currents, which were then relayed to a feed unit powering the electric motor in the hand to open and close. In later models, the strength of the grasp could be regulated by the wearer.

'Biocurrents Control a Machine': what might be the first article on the invention written for a popular Soviet audience appeared in *Izvestiia* on 6 September 1958, alongside the image depicted in Figure 10.3, which was reproduced in numerous domestic and international publications during this time period. In it, the reporter described his experience directing the bioarm to make a fist, shake hands and hold a box of matches, merely by thinking about these actions. Its creators theorized about possible future uses, once they'd successfully constructed a model with the sense of touch (an achievement accomplished only a few years ago, somewhere around 2019), allowing one to operate in unsafe environments such as atomic laboratories, regulate the oxygen of pilots and divers, or alleviate pain during surgery. They talked about one day replacing the connecting wires with radio waves, enabling its use in space. Another promising application would return lost function to people with polio or other types of paralysis, and perhaps even restore nerve cells.[18]

The Soviet explanation of the arm's operation was quite distinct from that of the Americans, as we will see below. Key to this difference is the relationship of 'mind' and 'control'. In Soviet usage, control happens *by means of* the mind (*upravliat' mysl'iu, upravliat' umom*). In the American case, it is control *of* the mind. As the title of the *Izvestiia* article makes clear, in Soviet coverage the starring role was played by the currents, situated squarely in the body. If mind, thought or brain (used interchangeably) is mentioned at all, it is as the regulator or coordinator of the actions of the body.[19] In effect, Russians turn the mind into a part of the body, interesting only to the extent that it could be used to support the entire system's functioning; this is about electrical

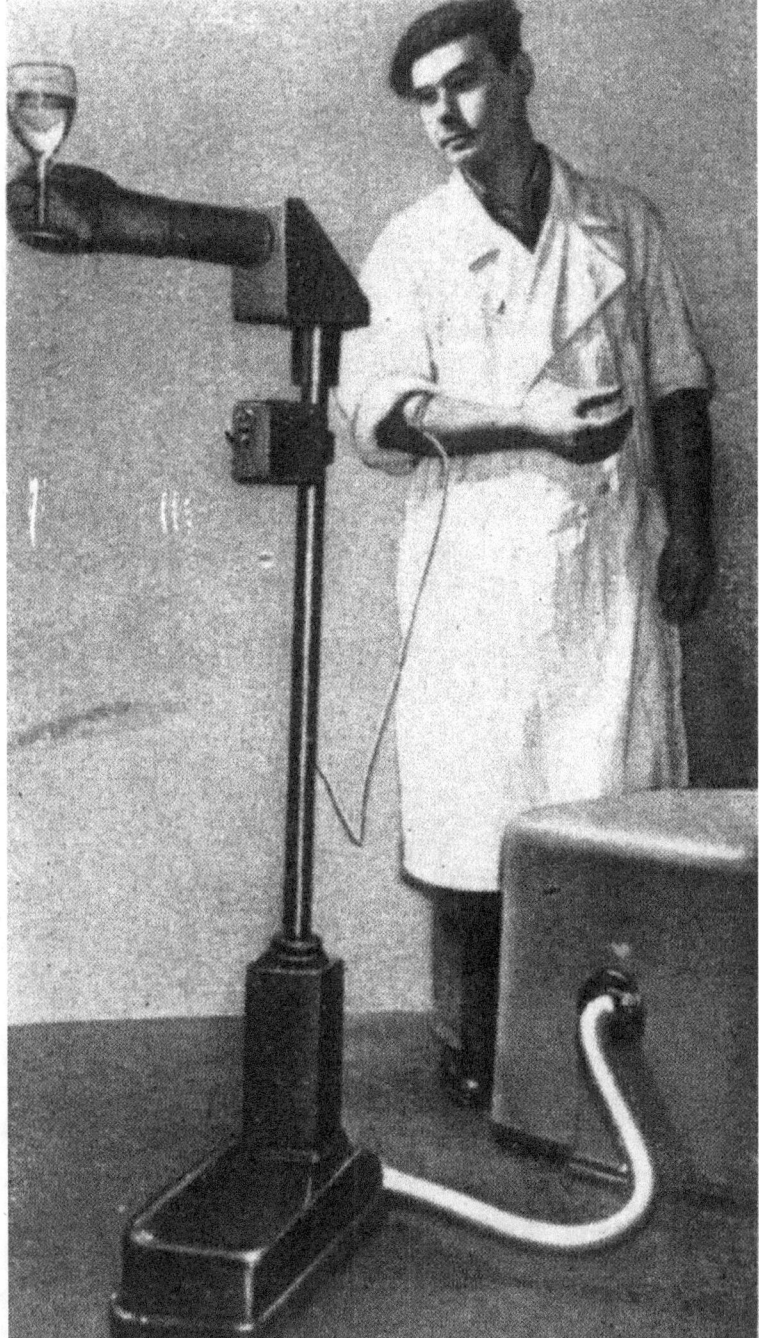

Figure 10.3 The second model of the bioelectric control system: Photograph, Institute of Machine Research and Central Scientific-Research Institute of Prosthetics and Prosthetics Manufacturing, 1960.

impulses, not consciousness. At home, the Russia arm never had a mind of its own; mind control or brain-washing, so frightening to Cold-War America, did not have a Soviet equivalent.[20]

In keeping with its emphasis upon the body, for the Soviets (as well as those who would buy licencing rights), the arm serves as a substitute for a lost or missing appendage, with the goal a return to 'normalcy'. But this normalcy was of a very particular kind: only produced in one size and skin tone, the arm was intended exclusively for a (light-skinned) adult man. Just who this person is meant to be is made clear in 'Bioelectric Arm', a 1961 short from the documentary film journal *Nauka i Tekhnika*, which was shown in movie theaters before the main feature (Figure 10.4).

The scene opens on a man shaving with an electric razor, then taking off his pajama top. Only then is his artificial arm revealed. In the next scene, he sits at a well-appointed table with his family, using the artificial limb to butter toast and hold and eat a soft-boiled egg without crushing the shell. The next scene shows him repairing a delicate piece of machinery. In addition to the actions demonstrated in the film, a MEDEXPORT catalogue advertised a number of additional uses for the invention:

Hold a soldering iron, a screwdriver, a prick punch or a pair of forceps;
Hold a watch in the artificial hand, winding it with his healthy hand;
Hold and light cigarettes and matches;
Trim the finer nails on the fingers of the healthy hand with scissors or a spring
    nail-trimmer;

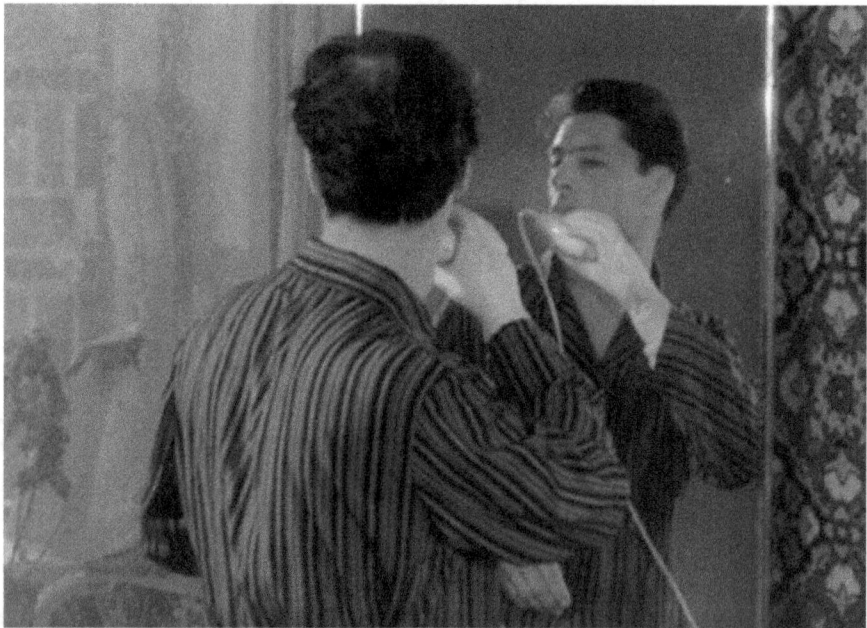

Figure 10.4 'Morning Shave': Film still from 'Bioelectricheskaia ruka', 1961.

Pull off the sleeve of an over-coat;
Hold a comb and comb his hair;
Clean clothes and shoes with a brush, etc.[21]

The bioarm presented to the home audience and to potential purchasers was one of technology domesticated, an implement of everyday (*bytovoi*) life. In the brief glimpse of work-related functions, the action is that of a skilled worker. In fact, the arm was contraindicated for amputees engaged in heavy, manual labour. 'Experience' had shown that this device was best suited for mechanics, electricians, radio technicians and intellectual labourers. Chronic and heavy drinkers were ineligible, as were those with 'imbalanced nerves' or intellectual disability.[22]

Equally significant in the Soviet representation of the arm's user is what is missing: reference to the hundreds of thousands of men who lost their limbs fighting in the Second World War. Just how the man in 'Bioelectric Arm' became disabled is vague; all we learn about the loss of the limb was that it was a 'misfortune'.[23] In discussions of the bioarm, there are almost no allusions to the Invalids of the Patriotic War, as they were known. Because the prosthetics industry was so closely aligned with disabled veterans' treatment and rehabilitation, such an oversight seems intentional. Perhaps the association would get in the way of the device's presentation as a tool with only peaceful, unthreatening applications. The domestic idyll presented in the film: a huge kitchen, a breakfast table laden with food – much more than a three-person family could consume – is worlds away from the living conditions of most Soviet people at war's end.

By the time the Fair opened, criticism in the United States of the Brussels undertaking had become something of a national past time. From the planning stage, the American contribution had been hampered by financial constraints imposed by Congress, especially as compared to the fortune being spent by the Soviets.[24] For many, the launching of Sputnik 1 in October 1957 and Sputnik 2 the following month made this imbalance even starker, a response more urgent: 'We Again Eat Crow,' bemoaned the *Austin American Statesman*, of the limited funds available to showcase America's scientific achievements.[25]

In the lead-up to the Fair, the Soviet wire service introduced the arm in an item that was carried by numerous foreign newspapers, both big and small. It was brief and straightforward, describing the appliance and advertising its appearance at the upcoming Expo. While some articles in the US press discussed the development in neutral terms, like 'Russians Develop New Type of Artificial Arms',[26] others immediately generated alarm with such screaming headlines as 'Red "Thoughts" Control Iron Arm'.[27] In his column in the *Daily News*, eleven days after the Fair opened, Ed Sullivan urged Congress to grant $150,000 to Howard Rusk, the New York physician and founder of rehabilitation medicine, to highlight American achievements in this new field at the Fair. Not only was Sullivan's suggestion ignored, but he learned that 'Russia is rushing to Brussels a model of a brain-controlled artificial arm!' Wrote Rusk: 'This makes it all the more tragic that we will have nothing of this kind at Brussels.'[28]

Rusk's article became a supporting document in Congressman John E. Fogarty's second appeal to the House appropriations committee (the first, in February, was approved by the House but rejected by the Senate) for a Public Health exhibit at the Fair, substantially upping Rusk's original request to 1 million. Fogarty argued that 'our failure to provide a health exhibit would present us to the world as a second-rate power'. He represented the Soviet Pavilion, in contrast, as jammed-full of technological innovations, including 'the artificial arm controlled entirely by impulses from the brain'.[29]

Ultimately, the alarm generated by the invention had little to do with the arm that eventually turned up; in fact, it barely even made it. As Rusk relates, when he attended the fair in late April, the arm had still not appeared and every time someone asked about it they were told it would be arriving the following week. According to the *Izvestiia* article from 6 September, the arm would be leaving for Brussels 'any day', missing most of the fair – which closed on 19 October – but still arriving early enough to win a prize.[30] This would explain why the invention goes almost completely unmentioned in accounts of visits to the Fair, even in Soviet publications, though its award would be mentioned afterwards in almost every domestic story on the limb, as well as accounts written elsewhere. Thus, even at this early date, a distinction was emerging between what the arm represented and the object itself, with the dominant American version mostly a projection of the cold warriors' imagination, encapsulated in an arm-size package.

Curiously, what goes unmentioned in the *Izvestiia* article is the possibility of using the technology for amputees, despite its creation at the Prosthetics Institute.[31] This would have to wait until the following year, when the same group of scientists produced a successful working prosthesis. In earlier models, including the one demonstrated at the Expo, the currents used to power the arm were those of an able-bodied controller, who wore an electronic bracelet on the forearm to tap them. The arm was a supernumerary appendage, affixed to a pole and attached by cables to a large box containing all its components. With the introduction of a transistor battery (invented in 1947) and miniaturized motor, the arm became portable, its small power pack worn under the shirt or on the belt. Now the amputee would be directing his own actions: finally, a limb that could leave the lab.[32]

The arm's next big international moment came in the summer of 1960, when the USSR hosted the First International Congress on Automatic and Remote Control in Moscow, an enormous undertaking with over 2,000 participants from twenty-nine countries delivering 285 papers, including one by the Russia arm team.[33] The group opened its talk with a demonstration. Attendees watched as a fifteen-year-old boy picked up a piece of chalk and wrote on the blackboard, in clear and precise letters, 'Hello to congress participants!' It was then revealed that this was accomplished using the prosthesis.[34]

Writing about this sensational episode, and more generally the enthusiasm for automation and robotics of which it was a forerunner, the eminent mechanical engineer Vladimir Babitskii, who worked under Kobrinskii at the Institute of Machine Studies, would say: 'It was the sort of success story that was easy to talk about publicly: visible, theatrical, emotional, anthropomorphic. It was a showy science, one that could be easily manipulated for the purposes of propaganda.'[35] The same could be said about Norbert Wiener, the originator of cybernetics, who was revered in the Soviet Union, and who participated in the conference and witnessed the performance firsthand.[36] Wiener had raised the idea of using automated principles in the operation of artificial limbs in 1948, noting that existing technology was not yet advanced enough to make this feasible.[37] In his final book, he wrote about the success achieved in this area, singling out the Russia device in particular.[38]

A much less optimistic account of the presentation comes from Dr. J.B. Reswick, another American at the Moscow meeting, who reported that 'The Russians were careful not to divulge any design or operation details', and whose repeated attempts to speak to the inventors or closely examine the device were rebuffed; European efforts to learn more about the technology were also unsuccessful. The correspondent attributed this reticence to the 'general secrecy' which governed so many of the USSR's interactions with the West.[39] In Reswick's own opinion, his Soviet hosts' unwillingness to grant closer access to the hand or its creators indicated that the prosthesis failed to live up to the claims being made about its capabilities.[40] According to a later Russian account of the proceedings, a number of foreign scholars not at the meeting did not believe such a feat possible; the author quotes an American scientist who wrote, 'Russians claim to have an apparatus capable of controlling the movement of an artificial arm with their minds. It's science fiction.'[41]

The bioarm commodified

In the following years, research teams from several countries visited the Soviet Union to examine the invention firsthand.[42] A recent interpretation argues that the incentive to pursue research in myoelectric prostheses was 'somewhat forced upon the Western Bloc by their nemesis, the Russians'. It was embarrassment at the Soviet achievement that compelled these countries, 'to their chagrin', 'to send delegations to Russia to learn about it'.[43] Even so, much of the interest was motivated by the Thalidomide tragedy, as countries sought to adapt the device, designed for an adult male, for children born with shortened or missing limbs. Neither the Soviet Union nor the United States approved the drug's use for morning sickness. As a result, the Soviet Union was spared entirely and in the United States the number was limited to a small group of infants affected as a result of trials of the medication.[44] Ultimately, only Britain and Canada purchased licences for clinical use and manufacturing.[45] (As with mentions of the Brussels prize, the two countries' purchase of the licence was worked into almost every non-specialist Soviet piece on the arm that followed.) In keeping with the Soviet interpretation, in both Britain and Canada the prosthesis was intended as a replacement for a missing limb.[46]

Whatever political motives might be ascribed to the arm, the licensing experience reveals a Soviet Union hungry not for world domination but capital.[47] Visiting the invention early, presumably before any price had been quoted, a Canadian orthopaedic surgeon reported that the cost would be nominal, as '[the Soviets] are not interested in making profits on it'.[48] With a licensing fee of $30,000/£10,000, many disagreed.[49] That the Soviets were mercenary is evident from the high cost extended to consumers as well: the Soviets were willing to sell the prosthesis directly for $700, as opposed to the $300 price tag quoted by the Canadians.[50]

To raise the substantial sum for the licence, the Research and Development teams in both Canada and Britain turned to the public for support.[51] The UK reached its goal in two days, with a donation from an anonymous benefactor.[52] Fundraising was far less successful in Canada. When contributions fell short, the Montreal Rehabilitation Institute made the decision to borrow the money, since the arm was 'so badly needed'.[53] As an article appearing in the Montreal *Gazette*, entitled 'Do You Have $30,000 for a Good Cause?' explained, while the Canadian group could have created its own given more time, the urgency of the problem dictated the shortcut of adapting (and paying for) an already-viable model.[54]

In addition to the expense, a few other factors motivated a negative reaction. In response to an article about the British purchase, a researcher from the Medical Electronics Department at St. Thomas's Hospital was concerned readers might get the impression that Britain lagged behind Russia in such developments, and that the Soviet invention represented a breakthrough, when his own hospital had produced a prototype the previous year.[55] He concluded, 'It is a sad fact that although this country has the technical and scientific capability to manufacture a more sophisticated prosthesis, £10,000 was paid to the Russians in order that their arm might be made in this country under licen[s]e.'[56] Similarly, at least one of the scientists involved in the Canadian effort was unhappy about the continued association of the group's work with that of the Soviets. Two years after beginning the project, the Canadian team rejected the Russian model as being too difficult for young children to operate and developed a hydraulic limb, the 'Northern Arm', in a joint effort of the Montreal Rehabilitation Institute and the Northern Electric Company in 1966. According to Dr. B.P. Nicholls, manager of Northern Electric's cable transmission laboratory, 'The only connection between the Russian hand and our arm is that both are artificial[.]' 'Unfortunately, people keep referring to it as the Russian arm. And this hurts our pride since many features of our arm are novel and we exploited several new engineering materials and techniques.'[57]

What bothered Dr. Gustave Gingras, the executive director of the Montreal Rehabilitation Institute, was neither the limb's foreign origin nor the high cost; he considered it to be a fair price, given the effort. Rather, it was the Soviets' unwillingness to share the technology on humanitarian grounds or as a professional courtesy. Unlike the original, the Canadian device would be available to anyone who wished to examine or modify it.[58] True to his word, the Institute provided a number of the prostheses to research and treatment facilities in the United States and Canada.[59]

The bioarm weaponized

At the same time its peaceful uses were being highlighted at home, the Soviets also pointed to the technology's rather more hawkish applications elsewhere, specifically by the United States. In a 1963 popular work on bionics, author P.T. Astashenkov attributed the American 'imperialist' interest in bionics as owing to its aggressive course of war preparation.[60] Likewise, I.B. Litinetskii described research on myoelectricity being conducted at the Pentagon, where 'apologists for world war' had developed an 'atomic soldier', an iron-plated monster intended for use during a thermonuclear attack.[61] We can assume that the Soviet military was engaged in similar 'imperialist' ventures, including applying myoelectric principles to weapon systems, though little of this documentation is accessible. But both sides were eager and vocal about using this technology for space travel, enabling astronauts to manoeuver under heavy loads, conduct experiments, or make flight corrections during re-entry. In testimony to Congress, Dr. Eugene B. Konecci, Director of Biotechnology and Human Research at NASA, reported in 1964 that the agency looked to the Russian prosthesis as a model for its work.[62]

Others in the United States were more apprehensive about the technology and the system controlling it. Whereas in Russian descriptions, the action of the arm was dependent upon the body, key to the American representation was the mind. The cartoon Communist from the *Daily News* story with which this article begins (Figure 10.1) is a lighthearted representation of a much more broadly held anxiety: that the Russia arm was a mechanical enhancement, capable of doing the mind's bidding. As the *Wausau Daily Herald* put it, 'An artificial arm that can be manipulated by thought has been developed by Russians.'[63] While some coverage identified the arm as iron (it was plastic), its composition was not often specified; in a reverse from the Russian model, the body was far less important than the mind that would be commanding it. Brain waves, not biocurrents, were the real concern.

The distinction between the Soviet and American conceptions of the bionic arm can be seen clearly in a confidential intelligence report for the CIA – the source for which is the very same *Izvestiia* article cited above (!):

> Photographic evidence [meaning the photograph accompanying the *Izvestiia* story, reproduced in Figure 10.3] does not indicate that this specific device operates as the result of brain-wave transmissions. The described technical advance is probably the mechanical translation of electric pulses generated by the operator's forearm and hand muscles, thereby imitating human hand motion.[64]

Needless to say, there are no 'brain-waves' mentioned in the original article, but that the author of the report was looking for them suggests that this nonetheless was a concern already on the part of the intelligence service.

The different lens through which Russians and Americans processed the same information can be seen in a 1958 item appearing in *The Bristol Daily Courier* (Bristol, Pa), entitled 'Reds Claim Another First'. The article first describes the invention as 'An artificial hand that is controlled by "thought waves"'. It then quotes A.J. Kobrinski [sic], 'leader of the "Bio-Hand" project', as saying, the 'mere thought of bunching a first, for example, is fully sufficient to set a series of minute electrical impulses traveling through the muscle of the hand or arm'.[65]

Conclusion

Ultimately, the Russia arm was at its most effective not as a material object but as an idea: the idea of Soviet technological superiority, whether that meant celebrating or fearing it. Lost in most coverage was the question of quality, or the experience of the amputees who would be using it. What information is available about its users is vague; very few speak for themselves. It is unlikely that any Americans used the arm (though it was consulted by scientists, engineers and physicians pursuing their own research in myoelectricity)[66] and access to the British and Canadian children would have been restricted and their impressions mediated by others. As for the Soviets, multiple sources claim that the arm went into mass production starting in 1961 but that information has been difficult to corroborate. The number of Soviet men actually employing it regularly differs substantially, depending upon the source, and ranges from twenty-three, to hundreds, to one thousand, to tens of thousands.[67] Given the barrage of criticism levelled at far simpler domestic prostheses and at Soviet consumer technology more generally, conclusions about the arm's effectiveness and the number of units in actual use must be taken with a grain of salt.[68] Nowhere did the Russia arm ever enjoy commercial success or broad use. It was costly (for Russians as well), heavy, noisy, hard to master, slow and easily damaged, with a weak grasp. Most crucially, its operation was limited to opening and closing the hand.[69] In Britain and Canada, after a few years' efforts at modifying the invention, scientists turned their attention elsewhere. As one scholar concluded, 'Expectations were greater than realities.'[70]

Eventually the bioarm's international moment passed, and with it the status that came from being first. Multiple countries developed devices utilizing similar principles, or rejected myoelectric limbs altogether in favour of lighter, less expensive, and more versatile models. Many of the most far-reaching ambitions for the technology were unrealizable for the time being.[71]

Nonetheless, domestic pride in the Russia arm continued even after the collapse of the USSR. For instance, in 2007, the newspaper *Nezavisimaia gazeta* featured a piece entitled 'Soviet scientists invented prototype of bionic hand in the 1970s', in response to England's claim to have invented the world's first, the i-LIMB. The article quotes Valentin Morzhov, a department head at the very same Prosthetics Institute which produced the Russia arm, 'The report on the bionic hand is not some hot news for us … [W]e were the first to come up with the basic principles of using mental activity to control the muscles.'[72] Just as in 1958, the idea of the arm, rather than the actual arm, was more threatening to Cold Warriors abroad, its reputation as first has remained much more valuable at home than the arm itself ever was.

Notes

1   Dr. Frank H. Krusen, Chairman, Expert Medical Committee of the American Rehabilitation Foundation, Departments of Labor and Health, Education, and Welfare, Appropriations for 1967. *Hearings before a Subcommittee of the Committee on Appropriations of the House of Representatives. 89th Congress, Second Session*, Department of Health, Education, and Welfare, Public Health Service (Washington, DC: US Government Printing Office, 1966), Part 3, 734.

2   Expo (International Exhibitions Bureau), *The Brussels World's Fair, 1958* (S.l.: s.n., 1958); Expo (International Exhibitions Bureau), *Catalogue général/Exposition universelle et Internationale de Bruxelles 1958* (Brussels: Impr. Puvrez, 1958).

3   The number of participating states varies depending upon the source, with some listing as few as thirty-nine or as many as fifty-two. A map of the fairgrounds can be found at 'Expo 1958 Brussels', Bureau International des Expositions, accessed 27 February 2018, https://www.bie-paris.org/site/en/1958-brussels. The USSR and US pavilions are located at numbers 138 and 102, respectively. Robert W. Rydell, *World of Fairs: The Century of Progress Expositions* (Chicago: University of Chicago Press, 1993), 201. Whatever idealism may have motivated the hosts' intentions, they were not above using behind-the-scenes manipulation to encourage both sides' participation. Lewis Siegelbaum, 'Sputnik Goes to Brussels', *Journal of Contemporary History*, 47.1 (January, 2012): 122. See also Rika Devos, 'A Cold War Sketch: The Visual Antagonism of the USA vs. the USSR at Expo 58', *Revue belge de philologie et d'histoire*, 87.3–4 (2009): 723–42; Robert Haddow, *Pavilions of Plenty: Exhibiting American Culture Abroad in the 1950s* (Washington: Smithsonian Institution Press, 1997), 95–6.

4   Susan E. Reid, 'Cold War Cultural Transactions: Designing the USSR for the West at Brussels Expo '58', *Design and Culture*, 9.2 (2017): 129; Robert W. Rydell, *World of Fairs: The Century of Progress Expositions* (Chicago: University of Chicago Press, 1993), 194, 206, 208–9.

5   V. K. Mezenin, *Parad vsemirnykh vystavok* (Moscow: izd. Znanie, 1990), 128; *Pavil'ony SSSR na mezhdunarodnykh vystavkakh*, eds. Anna Petrova, Nelli Podgorskaia and Ekaterina Usova (Moscow: N. O. Podgorskaia, 2013), 167–8; Anthony Swift, 'The Soviet Union at the 20th-Century World's Fairs', *World History Connected*, October 2016, accessed 28 April 2019, http://worldhistoryconnected.press.uillinois.edu/13.3/forum_01_swift.html. Rydell, *World of Fairs*, 211; Reid, 'Cold War Cultural Transactions', 133. Contemporary Soviet accounts include: Iurii Lomko, 'USSR at the Brussels World Fair', *Moscow News*, 2 October 1957, 1–2; Andrei Novikov, 'S utra i do vechera', *Ogonek*, 24 (8 June 1958): 24; Ivan Grigor'evich Bol'shakov, *Vsemirnyi smotr: uspekh SSSR na vsemirnoi vystavke v Briussele* (Moscow: Izvestiia, 1959), 59; *USSR Section at the Universal and International Exhibition of Brussels* (Moscow: Vneshtorgizdat, 1958); *USSR Section at the Universal and International Exhibition of Brussels. Blazers of New Trails. The Soviet Union's Scientists and Technicians* (Moscow: Vneshtorgizdat, 1958).

6   Mezenin, *Parad*, 124–5; Bol'shakov, *Vsemirnyi*, 59, 82; G. V. Deinichenko and I. F. Kharlanov, *Glazami reportera. Zametki o vsemirnoi vystavke v Briussele* (Moscow: Sovetskaia Rossiia, 1959), 23–6. As Siegelbaum writes, 'The expedition enabled the USSR to bask in the glow of its technological achievement before an international audience in excess of 40 million while the United States was still scrambling to catch up. Indeed, the period from the launching of Sputnik-1 on 4 October 1957 to the close of Expo '58 almost exactly a year later arguably coincided with the peak of the Soviet Union's international prestige': 'Sputnik', 120–1.

7   The device was patented (No. 120300) in 1959, with a modified version (No. 163718) following in 1964. A. E. Kobrinskii, E. P. Polian, B. P. Popov, Ia. L. Slavutskii, A. Ia. Sysin and Ia. S. Iakobson, 'Protez predplech'ia s elektricheskim servoprivodom, upravliaemyi biotokami myshts, s ustroistvom dlia oshchushcheniia sily skhvata', Baza patentov SSSR, accessed 19 September 2018, http://patents.su/2-120300-protez-predplechya-s-ehlektricheskim-servoprivodom-upravlyaemyj-biotokami-myshc-s-ustrojjstvom-dlya-oshhushheniya-sily-skhvata.html. Wolf Schweitzer, 'Technical Below Elbow Amputee Issues – Russian Prosthetic Arm (About the History of Myoelectric Arms)', Technical Right Below Elbow Amputee Issues, 23 November 2013, https://www.swisswuff.ch/tech/?p=2366.

8   Prescribed to pregnant women worldwide in the late 1950s and early 1960s for morning sickness and as a sleeping aid, Thalidomide was responsible for causing miscarriages, newborn fatalities and severe birth defects in thousands of children before it was pulled from the market.
9   David J. A. Foord, 'Making Hands: A History of Scientific Research and Technological Innovation in the Development of Myoelectric Upper Limb Prostheses, 1945–2010' (PhD diss., University of New Brunswick, 2013), 107–8.
10 D. S. Halacy, Jr., 'The "Transistorized" Man', *Popular Electronics* (February 1965): 44.
11 'Protez predplech'ia s elektricheskim servoprivodom'.
12 Unless I am referring specifically to the hand, I will use the term 'arm' to refer to the prosthesis. For consistency's sake I use 'Russia' rather than 'Russian'. Quotations will employ whatever name appears in the original.
13 Roy W. Wirta, Donald R. Taylor and F. Ray Finley, 'Pattern-Recognition Arm Prosthesis: A Historical Perspective – A Final Report', *Bulletin of Prosthetics Research* (Fall 1978): 8–9; Kevin J. Zuo and Jaret L. Olson, 'The Evolution of Functional Hand Replacement: From Iron Prostheses to Hand Transplantation', *Plastic Surgery*, 22.1 (2014): 47. In Reitner's estimation, further work was hindered also by Germany's troubled post-war economy.
14 These included a prototype myoelectric hook designed by a British team in 1955. Battye et al., 'The Use of Myo-Electric Currents', 506–10; A. H. Bottomley and T. K. Cowell, 'An Artificial Hand Controlled by the Nerves', *New Scientist*, March 12 (1964): 668–71; Alter, *Bioelectric*, 506–10; R. N. Scott, 'Myoelectric Control of Prostheses: A Brief History'. Proceedings of the 1992 Myoelectric Controls/Powered Prosthetics Symposium, Fredericton, New Brunswick, Canada: August, 1992. Copyright University of New Brunswick, 1.
15 A. E. Kobrinskii, M. G. Breido, V. S. Gurfinkel', A. Ia. Sysin, M. L. Tsetlin and Ia. S. Iakobson, 'Bioelektricheskaia sistema upravleniia', *Doklady AN SSSR*, 117.1 (1957): 78–80; see also Ia. L. Slavutskii, *Fiziologicheskie aspekty bioelektricheskogo upravleniia protezami* (Moscow: Meditsina, 1982); V. S. Gurfinkel', V. B. Malkin, M. L. Tsetlin and A. Iu. Shneider, *Bioelektricheskoe upravlenie* (Moscow: Nauka, 1972).
16 Office of Technology Utilization, National Aeronautics and Space Administration, *Applications of Space Teleoperator Technology to the Problems of the Handicapped* (1973), 20–1.
17 A. E. Kobrinskii, 'Bioelektricheskii kontrol' protezirovaniia', *Vestnik akademii nauk SSSR*, 30 (1960): 58–61; A. E. Kobrinskii, 'Bioelektricheskie sistemy upravleniia', *Radio*, 11 (1960): 37–39; Dudley S. Childress, 'Historical Aspects', 4.
18 A. Evseev, 'Biotok upravliaet mashinoi', *Izvestiia*, 6 September 1958, 4.
19 E. Levnovskii, 'Pul't upravleniia – mozg!' *Iunyi tekhnik*, 5 (1959): 25–6.
20 As Eliot Borenstein shows, the American brand of 'mind control' only comes to Russia in the 1990s. See *Plots against Russia: Conspiracy and Fantasy after Socialism* (Ithaca: Cornell University Press, 2019).
21 *Instruktsiia po naznacheniiu i izgotovleniiu proteza predplech'ia s bioelektricheskim upravleniem* (Moskva: Medexport, 1969), 31.
22 Ibid., 37; *Snabzhenie invalidov protezom predplech'ia s bioelektricheskim upravleniem* (Khar'kov: Prapor, 1967), 7.
23 See, similarly, V. Alekseev, *Iunyi technik* 10 (1964): 62.

24 By one account, the United States spent 12 and the USSR 60 million: Howard Taubman, 'Cold War on the Cultural Front', *New York Times*, 13 April 1958, 107. See also n. 28 and 29.
25 'We Again Eat Crow', *Austin American Statesman* (Austin, Texas), 21 February 1958, 4.
26 'Russians Develop New Type of Artificial Arm', *Wausau Daily Record-herald* (Wausau, Wisconsin), 7 August 1958, 30.
27 'Red "Thoughts" Control Iron Arm', *The Circleville Herald* (Circleville, Ohio), 14 April 1958.
28 Ed Sullivan, 'Little Old New York: "Men and Maids," and Stuff', *The Daily News* (New York), 28 April 1958, 40; Howard A. Rusk, M.D., 'Sold Short (Softly): An Analysis of the Nation's Failure to Tell Its Health Story at the Brussels Fair', *New York Times* (New York), 22 June 1958, 46.
29 'Health Story at Brussels Fair. Extension of Remarks of Hon. John E. Fogarty of Rhode Island in the House of Representatives, Tuesday, 24 June 1958', *Congressional Record: Proceedings and Debates*, 12142–12143. The appropriation request was denied.
30 Evseev, 'Biotok'.
31 See, similarly, N. Posylaev, 'Biotoki upravliaiut mashinami', *Pod znamenem Lenina*, 8 October 1958, 3.
32 A. E. Kobrinskii, 'Bioelektricheskii kontrol' protezirovaniia', *Vestnik akademii nauk SSSR*, 30 (1960): 58–61; A. E. Kobrinskii, 'Bioelektricheskie sistemy upravleniia', *Radio*, 11 (1960): 37–9; Dudley S. Childress, 'Historical Aspects', 4.
33 A. Kobrinskii, S. Bolkovitin, L. Voskoboinikova, D. Ioffe, E. Polyan, B. Popov, Y. Slavutski, A. Sysin and Y. Yakobson, 'Problems of Bioelectric Control', *1st International IFAC Congress on Automatic and Remote Control*, Moscow, USSR 1.1 (August 1960): 629–33. For the technical details of the device, see B. Popov, 'The Bio-electrically Controlled Prosthesis', *Journal of Bone and Joint Surgery* August, 47 (1965): 421–4.
34 Izot Borisovich Litinetskii, 'Beseda tret'ia. Biotiki v upriazhke', *Besedy o bionike* (Moscow: Nauka, 1968), retrieved from http://biologylib.ru/books/item/f00/s00/z0000017/. A. E. Kobrinskii, *Vot oni-roboty* (Moscow: Nauka, 1972), 62; D. M. Komskii and A. B. Gordin, *Uvlekatel'naia kibernetika* (Sverdlovsk: Sredne-Ural'skoe knizhnoe izdatel'stvo, 1969), 193; 'Reds Display Electric Arm', *Pottsville Republican* (Pottsville, Pennsylvania), 15 July 1960, 10.
35 Vladimir Babitsky, *On the Waves of a Pulsating World: An Engineer's Adventures in Innovation, Education and Politics. From Russia to the West* (Cham, Switzerland: Springer, 2019), 60.
36 Ia. I. Fet, *Rasskazy o kibernetike* (Novosibirsk: Izd. SO RAN, 2007), 23–7; and B. Widrow, 'Recollections of Norbert Wiener and the first IFAC World Congress', *IEEE Control Systems Magazine*, June 2001, 65–70.
37 Norbert Wiener, *Cybernetics or Control and Communication in the Animal and the Machine* (Cambridge: MIT Press, 2nd edition 1948 4th printing, 1985), 25–6; Ralph Alter, *Bioelectric Control of Prosthesis*, Massachusetts Institute of Technology Research Laboratory of Electronics Technical report 446 (1 December 1966), v; M. Stewart et al., *The University of Michigan College of Engineering. Department of Electrical Engineering Student Design Project: Electromyographically Controlled Orthotic Hand*, Ann Arbor, April 1968, 5. On the 'cybernetic boom' of the time, see

Irina Sirotkina, 'Ot kontrolia sverkhu k samoorganizatsii: ottepel' i teoriia upravleniia dvizheniiami', *Logos*, t. 30.2 (2020): 129–56.

38 Norbert Wiener, *God and Golem, Inc. A Comment on Certain Points Where Cybernetics Impinges on Religion* (Cambridge: MIT Press, 1964), 73–6; Robert W. Mann, 'Commentary on the Prostheses-Oriented Papers of Norbert Wiener', in P. Mesani, ed., *Norbert Wiener: Collected Works*, vol. IV (Cambridge, MA: MIT Press, 1985), 432–40.

39 National Research Council Committee on Prosthetic Research and Development, *The Application of External Power in Prosthetics and Orthotics* (Washington, DC: Academy of Sciences – National Research Council Printing and Publishing Office, 1961), 30, 141–2.

40 Ibid., 30.

41 Litinetskii, *Besedy*.

42 Regardless of Reswick's experience, clearly access was granted to those who expressed interest in purchasing licensing rights. F. Brohmke, 'Reported Abroad: German Delegation's Report on Russian Arm', *Veterans Administration Bulletin of Prosthetic Research* (1965): 193–201; E. David Sherman, 'Report of a Research Team from the Rehabilitation Institute of Montreal', *Canadian Medical Association Journal*, 91.24 (1964): 1268; Robert Roaf, 'Power Operated Prostheses', *British Medical Journal*, 2 (1964): 242.

43 Dr. Wolf Schweitzer, Prof. Dr. med. Michael Thali, Dipl. Ing. Robert Breitbeck, Dr. Garyfalia Ampanozi, 'Virtopsy', *Health Management*, 14.2 (2014) https://healthmanagement.org/c/healthmanagement/issuearticle/virtopsy; see also Office of Technology Utilization, *Applications of Space Teleoperator Technology*, 72.

44 E. D. Sherman, A.L. Lippay, B. Eng and G. Gingras, 'Prosthesis Given New Perspectives by External Power', *ICIB*, 5.10 (1966): 10–12; David J. A. Foord and Peter Kyberd, 'Ideas and Networks: The Rise and Fall of Research Bodies for Powered Artificial Arms in America and Canada, 1945–1977', *Scientia Canadensis*, 38.2 (2015): 54; G. Gingras et al., 'Bioelectric Upper Extremity Prosthesis Developed in Soviet Union: Preliminary Report', *Archives of Physical Medicine and Rehabilitation*, 47 (1996): 232–7; Ashok Muzumdar, *Powered Upper Limb Prostheses: Control, Implementation and Clinical Application* (Berlin and Heidelberg: Springer, 2004), 11, 14.

45 *Below-Elbow Prosthesis with Bioelectric Control*. Brochure, All-Union Export-Import Corporation (Moscow: LICENSINTORG, 1963); D. S. McKenzie, 'The Russian Myoelectric Arm', *Journal of Bone and Joint Surgery*, 47-B(3) (August, 1965): 418–20; C. K. Battye, A. Nightingale and J. Whillis, 'The Use of Myoelectric Currents in the Operation of Prostheses', *Journal of Bone and Joint Surgery*, 37.3 (1955): 506–10; A. H. Bottomley, 'Myo-Electric Control of Powered Prostheses', *Journal of Bone and Joint Surgery*, 47-B(3) (August 1965): 411–15; Gustave Gingras, 'Canadian Experience with the Soviet Myoelectric Upper-Extremity Prosthesis', *Orthopedic & Prosthetic Appliance Journal*, 20.4 (1966): 294–7. Later, firms in Germany and Austria sold modified versions (without paying the Soviets) under different names. The most successful of these, which continues to produce myoelectric devices to this day, is the German company Otto Bock: https://www.ottobockus.com/about/history/milestones.html; Foord, 'Making Hands', 109, fn 224.

46 Given their age, few if any of these children were given a choice about participating in these limb studies, or indeed, using a prosthesis at all. For the history of Thalidomide in Canada, including a useful discussion of the distinct Canadian and British government responses regarding prosthetics, see Christine Anna Chisholm, 'Life after the Scandal: Thalidomide, Family, and Rehabilitation in Modern Canada, 1958–1990', Unpublished dissertation, Carleton University, 2019. Unfortunately, it does not address the episode of the Russia arm.

47 In this article on the nuances of buying and selling foreign and Soviet licenses, the Russia arm is singled out as an example of an invention which has received great interest from foreign and especially capitalist countries. See M. M. Boguslavskiy [sic], 'Legal Questions of Buying and Selling Licenses', *Sovetskoe gosudarstvo i pravo*, 5 (1968): 53, as reprinted in *USSR International Economic Relations*, Issue 145 (Washington, DC: US Government Printing Office, 1968), 23.

48 'Electronic Hand a Possibility Here', *The Vancouver Sun* (Vancouver, British Columbia, Canada), 28 April 1964, 12.

49 The sum provided a seven-year manufacture option and access to any future modifications. I assume the price quoted was in Canadian dollars, although American coverage reported the same amount. 'Do You Have $30,000?', 3.

50 'Appeals for Funds: Canadian Doctor Seeks Artificial Arm', *The Ottawa Citizen* (Ottawa, Ontario, Canada), 20 August 1964, 47. David Serlin has characterized American motives for the pursuit of myoelectric technology as being prompted by financial interests, as compared to the altruistic motives of the Soviets. As this chapter shows, this distinction cannot be made. *Replaceable You: Engineering the Body in Postwar America* (Chicago: University of Chicago Press, 2004), 49.

51 Donations were solicited because the state would be assuming all costs after the initial outlay.

52 'Hand Obeys Brain', *The Sydney Morning Herald* (Sydney, New South Wales), 10 May 1964, 37. Lady Norah Mary Hoare, Chairwoman of the British Thalidomide Trust Fund, personally travelled to Moscow to collect the arm.

53 It eventually raised the sum thanks to a grant from the Province of Quebec. 'Group to Buy Motorized Arm from Russia', *The Ottawa Citizen* (Ottawa, Ontario, Canada), 2 September 1964, 5; 'Institute Determined to Buy Artificial Arm', *Calgary Herald* (Calgary, Alberta, Canada), 20 August 1964, 28; 'Funds for Soviet Arm', *The Windsor Star* (Windsor, Ontario, Canada), 20 August 1964, 16; 'New Type Artificial Arm Here', *The Gazette* (Montreal, Quebec, Canada), 2 September 1964, 37.

54 'Do You Have $30,000 for a Good Cause?' *The Gazette* (Montreal, Canada), 25 July 1964, 3. See, similarly, the letter to the editor in *The Guardian*, 12 September 1964, 8, in response to 'The Effectiveness of the British Prosthetic Arm'. The same point was made by M. Carr-Jones, Chairman of the UK Society for the Aid of Thalidomide Children.

55 Eventually known as the 'English hand', it was still in the testing stage at the time the letter was written. A. H. Bottomley, A. B. K. Wilson and A. Nightingale, 'Muscle Substitutes and Myo-electric Control', *The Radio and Electronic Engineer*, 26.6 (1963): 439–48; A. H. Bottomley and T. K. Cowell, 'An Artificial Hand Controlled by the Nerves', *New Scientist*, 21.382 (1964): 668–71; 'British Electronic Arm "Copies" Muscles', *The Observer* (London, Greater London, England), 5 January 1964, 4.

56 T. K. Cowell, 'British Prosthetic Arm', *The Guardian* (London, England), 2 September 1964, 8.
57 Art Mantell, 'Nothing We've Ever Done Has Given Us Such Satisfaction', *The Ottawa Journal* (Ottawa, Ontario, Canada), 29 October 1966, 37.
58 David Tafler, 'Arm Brings Hope to Thalidomide Children', *The Gazette* (Montreal, Quebec, Canada), 17 June 1966, 3. See, similarly Scott, 'Myoelectric Control of Prostheses: A Brief History', 3.
59 R. N. Scott, 'Myoelectric Control of Prostheses and Orthoses', *Bulletin of Prosthetics Research* Spring, 1967, 100–1.
60 P. T. Astashenkov, *Chto takoe bionika* (Moscow: Voennoe izdatel'stvo ministerstva oborony SSSR, 1963), retrieved from https://www.perunica.ru/nauka/9908-chto-takoe-bionika.html.
61 Litinetskii, *Besedy*. In fact, The Navy *had* funded research into what were referred to as 'amplified men'. See Kline, *The Cybernetic Moment*, 168, fn 66 and 67; 'Electricity from muscles', *Space World Magazine*, February 1964, 41. For similar projects, see Sharon Weinberger, *The Imagineers of War: The Untold History of DARPA, the Pentagon Agency that Changed the World* (New York: Alfred A. Knopf, 2017), 204.
62 Jack Jones, 'Eyes Have It for Landing Future Rockets', *Dayton Daily News* (Dayton, Ohio), 5 April 1964, 3-C; 'On a Hostile Planet', *The Morning Call* (Paterson, New Jersey), 31 March 1964, 4.
63 'Russians Develop New Type of Artificial Arm', *Wausau Daily Herald* (Wausau, Wisconsin) 7 August 1958, 30.
64 Central Intelligence Agency Office of Scientific Intelligence, *The Soviet Space Research Program, Monograph IX: Space Medicine* CIA/Si 33–59, 21 August 1959, 14–15.
65 'Reds Claim Another First', *The Bristol Daily Courier* (Bristol, PA), 13 November 1958, 10. It is quoting from *Product Engineering: The Magazine of Design Engineering* (New York: McGraw-Hill, 1958).
66 It is unlikely that any Americans used the arm (although, as the notes in this article demonstrate, it was consulted extensively by scientists, engineers and physicians pursuing their own research in myoelectricity), and access to the British and Canadian children would have been restricted and their impressions mediated by others.
67 Scott, 'Myoelectric Control of Prostheses and Orthoses', 95–6; Lidiia Lykova, *Social Security* (Moscow: Novosti Press Agency Publishing House, 1968), 33.
68 Frances Bernstein, 'Prosthetic Promise and Potemkin Limbs in Late-Stalinist Russia', in Michael Rasell and Elena Iarskaia, eds., *Disability in Eastern Europe and the Former Soviet Union* (London: Routledge, 2013), 42–66.
69 Childress, 'Historical Aspects', 4; Foord, 'Making Hands', 105; P. Herberts, 'Myoelectric Signals in Control of Prostheses', *Acta Orthopaedica Scandinavica*, (Suppl.) 124 (1969): 11.
70 David J. A. Foord and Peter Kyberd, 'From Design to Research: Upper Limb Prosthetic Research and Development in Canada, 1960–2000', *Scientia Canadensis*, 38.1 (2015): https://gala.gre.ac.uk/id/eprint/16189/1/16189%20KYBERD_From_Design_to_Research_2015.pdf; R. V. Artemenko, 'Kuia i perekovyvaia sovetskoe kibertelo,' unpublished paper, presented at Ezhegodnaia mezhdunarodnaia nauchno-prakticheskaia konferentsiia, 'Istoriia nauki i tekhniki. Muzeinoe delo', 15 December 2020. Moscow. https://polytech.timepad.ru/event/1497319//; L. V. Bobrov, *V poiskakh chuda* (M: Molodaia gvardiia, 1968), 67.

71 Kobrinskii, *Vot oni-roboty*, chapter 3; Gurfinkel' et al., *Bioelektricheskoe upravlenie*, chapter 2. Many of these devices are discussed in Muzumdar, *Powered Upper Limb Prostheses*, chapter 1; Wirta et al., 'Pattern Recognition'; L. McLean and R. N. Scott, 'The Early History of Myoelectric Control of Prosthetic Limbs (1945–1970).'
72 Alex Naumov, 'Soviet Scientists Invented Prototype of Bionic Hand in the 1970s', Pravda.ru, originally published in *Nezavisimaia Gazeta*, translated by Guerman Grachev, 20 September 2007, https://www.pravdareport.com/science/97404-bionic_hand/. On the i-LIMB, see 'Prosthetics for the 21st Century', European Patent Office, accessed 3 January 2020, https://www.epo.org/learning-events/european-inventor/finalists/2013/gow/feature.html; Foord, 'Making Hands', 127.

11

Dreams of a synaesthetic future: Technologies of deafness in late Soviet socialism

Claire Shaw

In 1960, *Life of the Deaf*, the magazine of the Soviet deaf community, devoted the inside cover of its January issue to a visionary new technology: a synaesthetic device that could transform music into coloured light.[1] The article took readers through the long history of attempts to create such a device, including by the composer Aleksandr Skriabin, himself reportedly a synaesthete, who composed two symphonies in the early 1900s to feature a *clavier à lumières*, a keyboard that would project coloured lights that corresponded to the notes ('do' was red, 're' was a sunny yellow). None of these attempts had been fully successful. But now, on the cusp of a new technological age, the time for such a device had come. The article pointed to the work of the young engineer Konstantin Leont'ev, who had developed and tested an advanced prototype of such a machine in the spring of 1959. It described its workings: 'a microphone perceives the sound of the music, electronic devices analyse it and transform it into a series of commands, which are transmitted to the light apparatus. Streams of light, varying in colour and strength depending on the music, pour on to the walls of the hall or onto the screen. The public not only hears but sees the music!'[2] This prototype had the potential to be adapted into new devices that would help deaf people, including a 'hearing television' that could transform oral speech into a form that could be read on screen. These devices, long dreamed of by the deaf community, were suddenly made possible. 'It's only codes, after all,' the article noted.[3]

While the article stressed the visionary nature of these devices, its publication heralded the start of a boom in very real technological devices for deaf people. This so-called *surdotekhnika*, or 'deaf technology', sought to harness the interface between senses and use advanced electronics to imagine new ways of being in the world. In 1964, under the auspices of the Scientific Research Institute of Defectology in Moscow (part of the Academy of Pedagogical Sciences), a Laboratory of *Surdoktehnika* was established.[4] In 1967, the Laboratory was merged with the Special Technological Planning and Design Bureau of the All-Russian Society of the Deaf (VOG), which oversaw the activities of the Society's deaf-run industrial workshops and designed and built new devices for deaf people. These organizations made a wide variety of apparatuses – from light-based alarms and baby monitors to adapted telephones and 'visible speech' machines – which magnified hearing or harnessed other senses to compensate for its lack.[5] At the same time, articles in the popular press imagined futuristic technological interventions that had the potential to radically reconceptualize understandings of disability and the senses.

This boom in deaf technologies – both real and imagined – exploited the increased investment in scientific research by the late Soviet state, alongside a growing policy focus on the needs of deaf and disabled citizens. Yet it also reflected a pivotal moment in the history of the USSR, one characterized by technological advances and a renewed sense of the potential of science to remake the very foundations of human life. The notion of human plasticity had been integral to Soviet ideology since the revolution, with concepts such as synaesthesia providing imaginative frameworks for scientists, ideologues and artists to reconceive the nature of the physical, and to reimagine the sensory interface between the body and the world. This thinking also encompassed attitudes to disability, which were underpinned by a hope that bodily imperfections might, with the advent of communism, finally and definitively be 'overcome'.[6] In the early decades of the USSR, much of this had remained at the level of utopian imagining. Yet the rapid technological developments of the Cold-War era, on both sides of the Iron Curtain, held out the promise that many of these visions might finally be achieved through microchips, transistors and computer monitors. Such new technological devices in turn birthed their own utopian imaginings, opening up new horizons not yet envisioned.

Drawing on popular science literature and the Soviet deaf press, this chapter argues that the advent of *surdotekhnika* represented a particularly utopian moment, when science was seen to provide unique solutions to problems of the body, of senses and of language. These solutions were not necessarily envisaged as curative: while some of these devices were framed as rehabilitative, seeking to use alternative senses in order to compensate for the 'tragedy' of hearing loss, others revealed more complex utopian dreams of the potential of technology to fundamentally rework the sensory interface between the deaf self and the world, through devices that replaced hearing with the visual and the haptic, and which thus drew on alternative modes of being foregrounded by the deaf community.[7] Not all of these assistive devices were successful; the story of *surdotekhnika* was often one of dreams forestalled. Yet by exploring how these devices were imagined, designed and experienced, this chapter uncovers the particular utopian horizons of late Soviet technologies, and traces their enduring impact on the lives and identities of deaf people.

Foundations of *surdotekhnika*

According to a 1975 article, the term *surdotekhnika* referred to a 'branch of instrument manufacture, the task of which is the perfection of existing apparatuses, and the creation of new ones, to aid in the communication of deaf people'.[8] The term was popularized by two of the founding members of the Laboratory of *Surdotekhnika*, Veniamin Aronovich Tsukerman and his daughter, Irina (Figure 11.1). Veniamin Tsukerman (1913–93) was

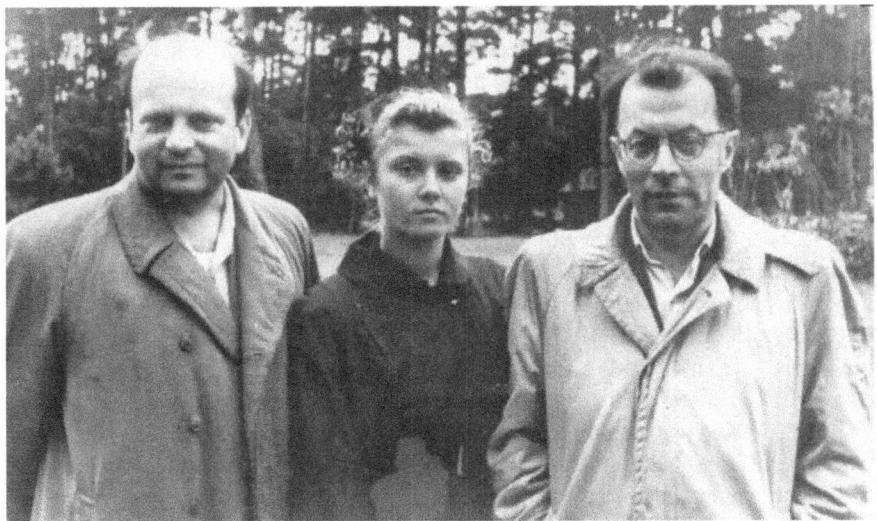

Figure 11.1 Veniamin Tsukerman, Irina Tsukerman and Leonid Galynker, Moscow, 1956.

a physicist whose work in the closed city of Arzamas-16 (now Sarov) contributed to the creation of the first Soviet atomic bomb.[9] He suffered from retinitis pigmentosa, which ultimately caused him to lose his sight, and he was helped in his research by his wife, Zinaida Matveevna Azarkh (1917–2004), who served as his eyes and his co-author in numerous publications. Their daughter, Irina (1937–2018), fell ill at the age of nine with tuberculous meningitis, a disease that at the time in the USSR was inevitably fatal. Thanks to her father's scientific connections, however, the family was able to acquire the newly discovered antibiotic Streptomycin and give the young girl an experimental course of the drug, which cured the disease but took her hearing.[10] The young Irina studied in a mainstream school in Arzamas-16 until the fifth grade, when she travelled to Moscow with her mother to study at Special School for the Deaf No. 337. After graduation, she entered the Moscow Higher Technical College, where she learned sign language and trained to become an engineer. She joined the Institute of Defectology as a researcher in 1958 and, following the foundation of the Laboratory of *Surdotekhnika*, defended her dissertation there in 1968.[11] Alongside their engineering work, the Tsukermans were prolific writers and produced many popular works in the deaf and mainstream press, including several books, that introduced *surdotekhnika* to the deaf and hearing public.

The Tsukermans' work reflected the Soviet state's growing focus on the production of deaf technologies. The Soviet of Ministers of the USSR had produced two major decrees on services for deaf people, in 1951 and 1962. While the 1951 decree focused mainly on community engagement and work placement, and included only a brief mention of 'increased production of films with subtitles for the deaf and deaf mutes', point 9 of the 1962 decree specified a particularly visionary new line of research: 'the creation of equipment for translating audio speech into visible text'.[12] Alongside this exploratory technological work, a decree of the Ministry of Social Welfare of the RSFSR on 18 April 1959 promised for the first time to make hearing aids freely accessible to the vast majority of Soviet deaf people.[13] In the context of the early Cold War, this moment was seen to mark a fundamental difference between US and Soviet approaches to deaf technology; while hearing aids were marketed as a consumer product in the United States, in the USSR, their availability to all was framed as a fundamental right.[14] The foundation of the Laboratory of *Surdotekhnika*, which employed specialists in deaf education, electronics, physics and radio engineering, thus captured a particular historical and technological moment.[15]

As a research field, *surdotekhnika* explored the potential of new technological innovations to make sound and speech accessible to deaf people. Its proponents acknowledged the long history of these attempts, including traditions as far back as ancient Rome of using sticks and other devices to sense speech through touch and vibration.[16] They also pointed to the use of an ear trumpet to magnify hearing by the celebrated 'father of space travel' Konstantin Tsiolkovskii.[17] Yet the development of new technologies meant that the transformation of sound into other senses was now possible in potentially groundbreaking ways. The breakthrough, Irina Tsukerman explained in a book of lectures on technologies for deaf people, came with the advent of the microphone: 'Only after its invention did it become possible to turn sound into waves of electrical current'.[18] These currents, depending on their frequency and the nature of the device, could become outputs of either amplified sound, light or vibration. A diagram included in the book (Figure 11.2) illustrated the variety of devices produced by Soviet laboratories that amplified sound or transformed it into visual or tactile stimuli.[19] Each of these sensory adaptations had the potential to enable deaf people to access the 'joy of human communication [...] to return deaf people to the world of sound'.[20]

The most established of these types of devices – the hearing aid – sought to increase the accessibility of sounds to the hard of hearing (those whose hearing loss did not exceed 70 decibels).[21] Hearing aids had been produced in the USSR since the early 1930s, when the Commissariat of Health had raised the question of the domestic production of 'special medical instruments, apparatuses and prostheses for the deaf and hard of hearing'.[22] As a result, a 'surdoacoustic laboratory' was set up under the Central Institute of the Labour of Invalids (TsITIN), and the first domestic hearing aid factory, named after the Commissar of Health, Nikolai Semashko, was opened in 1934.[23] While these early devices were notoriously unreliable – a situation not unique to the USSR, but compounded by the vagaries of the Soviet command economy, which made batteries and other components hard to come by – considerable advances in hearing aid technology were made possible in the 1950s with the invention of the transistor, and then later the microchip.[24] Yet for proponents of *surdotekhnika*, the hearing aid – and the amplification of sound more broadly – did not hold particular interest. This was partly a practical issue, according to Irina Tsukerman: 'for a large group of people, the loss of hearing [...] is so significant that existing technologies are not capable of compensating for it'.[25] In those cases, she argued, the role of technology was not to attempt to return hearing, but to engage other senses to compensate: 'the

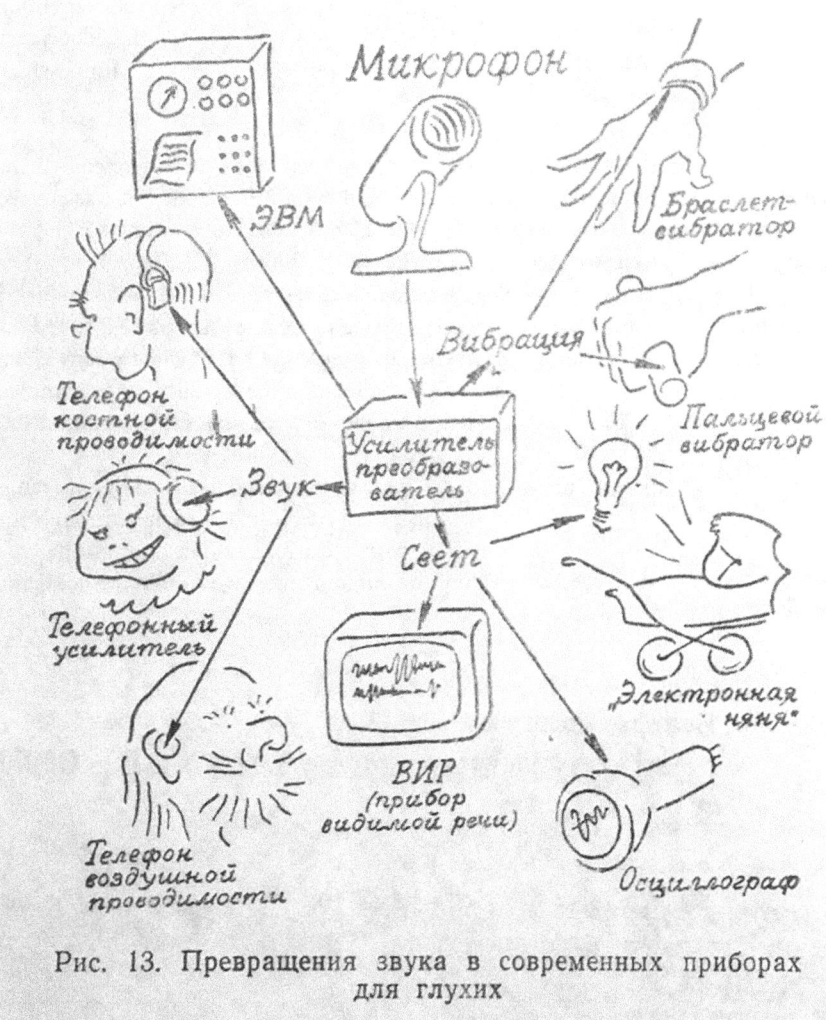

Figure 11.2 Sensory devices for deaf people: Illustration by Irina Tsukerman, 1973.

greatest help to a deaf person is sight and partly touch. In the most severe cases, with loss of hearing and sight at the same time, information about the surrounding world comes with the help of touch'.[26]

This turn to alternative senses was driven in part by the experiences of the Soviet deaf community, which had developed a strongly visual community identity in the first half of the twentieth century.[27] It was also rooted in the theories of defectologists Lev Vygotskii and Aleksandr Luriia, who referred to the type of sensory swapping by deaf and blind people that would be explored by the Laboratory of *Surdotekhnika* as 'compensation' for sensory lack.[28] Deaf technologists thus turned their attention to the transformation of sound into tactile and visual stimuli. While the Laboratory produced a wide variety of popular gadgets, including the 'electronic nanny', which used a light to alert parents if a child's cries reached a certain decibel level, two devices received particular attention: the Morse Code telephone and the 'visible speech' machine (*vidimaia rech*, or VIR).[29] The Morse Code telephone was developed by Irina Tsukerman and formed the basis of her doctoral dissertation in 1968.[30] It was created to meet the demand for a means for deaf people to communicate over long distances, a necessity that had developed in response to the concentration of deaf people in urban centres in the USSR. While accessible videotelephones remained a distant dream, Irina set about finding a means to converse using existing telephone lines. She explained the criteria she used to design her device: 'Above all, it needs to be sufficiently convenient and easy to use. Other fundamental conditions include the legibility of transmitted messages and low cost. The time taken to learn how to operate the machine should also preferably be minimal.'[31]

In response to these demands, Irina Tsukerman created a box-like apparatus, attached to a standard telephone, that transmitted Morse Code signals through the telephone line (Figure 11.3). The telephone user had two 'keys': in the right hand, a transmitter that could be used to spell out the outgoing message, and in the left hand,

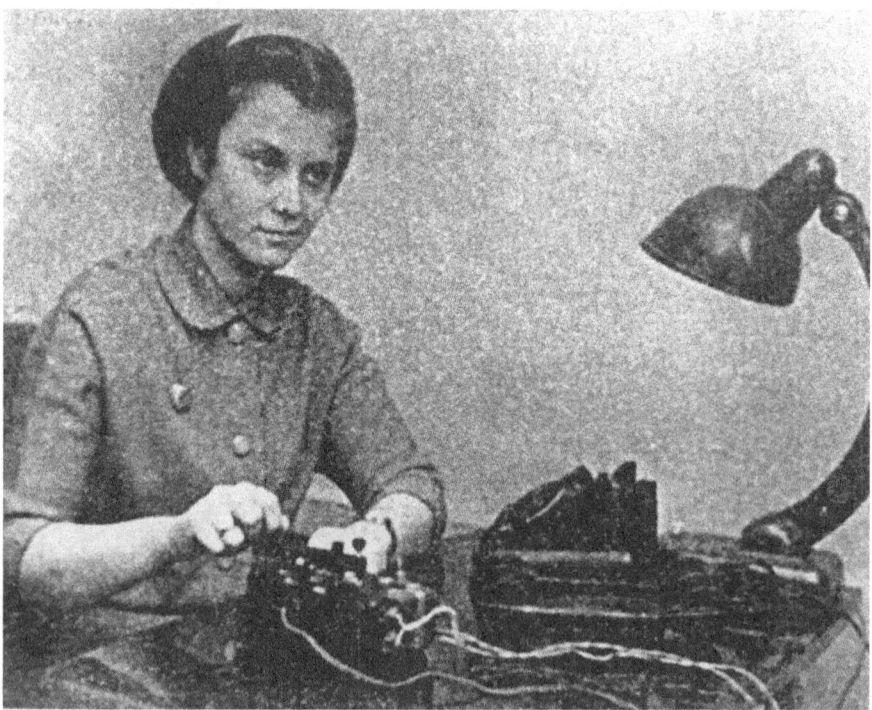

Figure 11.3 Irina Tsukerman with her Morse code telephone adapter, 1967.

a receiver that transformed the incoming dots and dashes into pulses of vibration that could be 'read' through the bones of the fingers. A light attached to the device would illuminate when a new call came in. Users needed to be taught the Russian variant of Morse Code in order to use the device, but as they did not need to learn it to the level of a radio telegrapher, they could pick the skill up in as little as 15–20 hours.[32] While communication via this method was incredibly slow – conversations that would take a minute for hearing people would take about ten to type out – it was certainly better than travelling across town to deliver information, especially in an emergency.[33] By 1967, these devices had been installed in several Moscow flats, and their deaf residents had carried out over 100 telephone conversations.[34]

While the Morse code telephone was acknowledged to be a fairly basic response to the problem of deaf telephone communication, the holy grail of *surdotekhnika* was a device that could transform speech into visual communication, as had been mooted in the 1962 decree.[35] Significant strides in that direction were made with the development of devices for the spectral analysis of speech signals. In 1962, Veniamin Tsukerman, alongside colleagues V.D. Laptev and L.N. Postnikov, designed and built a new device, the VIR, which linked a microphone to a television-like display. When a word was spoken into the microphone, a shape corresponding to the frequency of the sound would be displayed on the screen, moving from left to right. The length of the sound was mapped horizontally, the frequency vertically, and the intensity of the sound was represented by the brightness of the light. The intention of the creators of this device was to teach deaf users to 'read' these characteristic shapes, and thus to be able to understand the words being said visually. While this device was not particularly successful (the deaf users involved in testing the device were able to recognize only a handful of common words, and different speakers inputting the sounds led to confusing variation in the patterns), colleagues at the laboratory continued work on new devices to transform sound into sight. They were particularly interested in new technologies of voice recognition, such as the voice-activated car that was displayed at the Brussels Expo in 1958, and considered how they might be transformed into 'phonetic writing machines'.[36] They also worked on visual forms of communication, including a 'light alphabet' machine that enabled users to type letters and have them light up on a large screen, a device that proved useful both for telephone communication and for simultaneous interpreting of theatre or film presentations.[37]

For deaf technologists, therefore, the advent of advanced electronics created new possibilities to make the world of sound accessible to deaf people through touch and sight. This was not just a Soviet preoccupation. As the popular literature on *surdotekhnika* acknowledged, the boom in electronics, and the resulting focus on sensory transformation technologies, was a global one, and many of the developments in the USSR mirrored those in the West. For example, in 1964, the US deaf inventor Robert H. Weitbrecht designed the 'teletypewriter machine', which enabled deaf people to type communications over the telephone and read the responses on a computer screen. Indeed, a Morse Code telephone known as the Tactophone had been invented by Robert Oaks Jordan of the Illinois Bell Telephone Company in 1958, and had enjoyed some popularity among U.S. deaf-blind users.[38] While the early 1960s represented a period of the intensification of the Cold War, the Tsukermans' scientific contacts with the West – Irina travelled to London to present her research in 1966 – kept them appraised of some of the technological advances there. Yet the particular direction taken by *surdotekhnika*, and the narratives that surrounded it, was driven by much more than just Cold-War competition. These technologies reflected their moment and raised important questions about the interface between technology and the disabled body in the Soviet 1960s.

Soviet deaf futurism

The lives and work of the Tsukermans were testament to the development of the science of the body and deaf identity in the 1960s. In the immediate post-war period, the focus of disability organizations and of wider Soviet society had been on the reconstruction of both infrastructure and bodies in the wake of the traumas of the Second World War.[39] The 1960s, however, heralded what has been referred to as the 'relaunch' of the Soviet utopian project to transform man and society in order to build a bright future in communism.[40] Nikita Khrushchev's new party programme of 1961 placed technology at the centre of this vision: as he explained, 'in our age of rapid scientific and technological progress the development of society and of the individual is inconceivable without planned and all-round utilization of the achievements of science'.[41] This so-called Scientific Technological Revolution (STR) focused particularly on the hard sciences, promoted through the building of new cities of science (*Akademgorodki*) in places such as Novosibirsk, yet recent research has shown the ways in which this turn to science affected visions of the self and body.[42] According to Elana Gomel, the notion of the New Soviet Person in this period was poised between the human and the posthuman, constantly pushing the boundaries of the physical body.[43] As Frances Bernstein shows in her chapter for this volume, the notion of prosthetics and assistive technologies – or 'spare parts' for human bodies, as they were described in one popular science volume of the 1960s – was seen squarely as part of that vision, reanimating the dreams of the revolution and pushing the notion that disability might ultimately be overcome through technological means.[44]

The 1960s were also a moment in which ideas of both deafness and disability were again in flux. Soviet attitudes to disability had always existed in tension between two principles: on the one hand, the visions of the perfectibility of the human body under communism outlined above left little space for disability; on the other, notions of overcoming individual limitation and 'breaking the chains' of oppression and marginality made room for the existence of alterity even within the framework of the New Soviet Person.[45] As Lilya Kaganovsky has shown, even during the height of Stalinist visions of the New Soviet Person, the disabled hero was celebrated.[46] The 1960s saw this latter trend developing further, with an increased awareness of the specifics of the deaf community and their culture. This period has been referred to by the Soviet deaf community as their 'golden age', when a combination of state decrees, infrastructural development and recognition of sign language paved the way for a celebration of deaf culture, community, and an understanding of the self through the visual and the haptic.[47] The presence of deaf people in the laboratories that developed and made these technologies, and their active engagement with the Soviet deaf community (for example, Irina Tsukerman's second husband, Ivan Konstantinovich Danilin, was the chairman of the Moscow branch of VOG, and the couple were very active in the deaf social world) meant that their technological visions fused with broader conversations about how deaf life, and deaf culture, might be envisioned in the future.[48]

In its approach to deaf technologies, *surdotekhnika* set out a particular 'deaf futurist' vision that reflected these wider conversations. Proponents of *surdotekhnika* framed its tasks as, to a certain degree, remedial – to return to those with hearing loss to the 'world of sound' – and thus to enable their active engagement within Soviet society (a process understood, in Marxist terms, to create the necessary conditions for full human development). Yet the utopian nature of the dreams that underpinned these technologies shines through. As the article on the 'light-music' machine concluded, 'Our era, when the boldest dreams of the people are becoming reality, will doubtless give us the opportunity to build, not just "light music" but also the "hearing television"!'[49] Indeed, the notion of engaging alternative senses echoed early revolutionary dreams of the transformation of the mind-body through science – dreams that were being revived in the utopian social climate of the Thaw. As Emma Widdis has argued, early revolutionary thinkers had envisaged a new kind of sensory engagement between the body and the world.[50] At the same time, poets and artists experimented with new ways to bridge the gap between the word, sound and gesture.[51] As Lilya Kaganovsky shows in her chapter for this volume, technologies such as film created new, haptic ways to perceive the world; but the advent of sound cinema had moved away from the haptic towards a more logocentric culture, a move that was particularly disabling for the deaf community. Devices such as the Morse code telephone and the VIR thus held out the opportunity to re-engage alternative senses: 'Deaf people have got used to the fact that they receive almost all information about the world around them through sight. It is not surprising, therefore, that many well-read deaf people dream about a device that can make spoken language visible.'[52] The visions of sensory transformation in *surdotekhnika*, therefore, tapped into an existing revolutionary tradition, albeit in a new technological guise.

As this chapter's opening suggests, synaesthesia in particular represented a conceptual backdrop to this practical sense-swapping that linked deaf technology to wider Soviet imaginaries. Scholars have traced the conversations between Lev Vygotskii, Aleksandr Luriia, and the avant-garde film-maker Sergei Eisenstein in the 1930s and 1940s on how synaesthesia might represent a 'mode of perception that was closer to primitive forms of thought' that would, paradoxically, pave the way for the creation of higher forms of consciousness.'[53] By tapping into this 'sensuous thinking', Eisenstein argued, it would be possible to shape perceptions and transform the human through art.[54] This discussion of synaesthesia is reminiscent of debates during the Thaw over sign language, a form of communication which was often dismissed by defectologists as 'primitive', but whose connections to mime enabled it to be reframed by the deaf community as a 'sensuous' form of communication that would pave the way for new ways of being in the world.[55] Synaesthesia was not a direct object of enquiry for deaf technologists, and theorists such as Luriia (the author of a seminal work on synaesthesia published in 1968) avoided the term when discussing the use of alternative senses by the deaf and blind.[56] It is clear, however, that the imaginative frameworks of synaesthesia underpinned some of the visionary technologies of *surdotekhnika*: 'researchers lost themselves in the question "Is there anything in common between sounds and colour?" It provoked arguments and birthed surprising projects.'[57]

These visions of new sensory alignments also made room for the cultural traditions of the deaf community. The reluctance of deaf technologists to focus on hearing aids, and their choice instead to foreground sight and touch as compensatory means of engagement with the world, is a case in point. Accounts of new deaf technologies stressed their capacity to transform inaccessible cultural forms, such as the telephone, into a new kind of deaf cultural experience. Irina Tsukerman explains that telephones, historically a disabling technology for deaf people, were not initially comfortable to use: 'deaf people using the [Morse code] telephone independently for the first time find themselves completely confused. They feel a kind of panicked fear in front of the telephone apparatus.'[58] However, this 'psychological barrier' was soon overcome, and these deaf telephone users became quickly accustomed to communicating with friends, arranging meetings, and conveying urgent information to peers in far-flung corners of the city. They also rapidly developed new cultural practices for telephone use, including 'call signs' (codes to announce who was speaking, a practice analogous to the use of 'sign names' in sign-language communication), shortcuts to speed up communication (one dot for 'no', two for 'yes-yes'), and signature phraseology in the use of the code, including 'characteristic pauses between elements of a letter, the duration of dots and dashes, etc. These specificities allow users to be identified in telephone conversation, just as people with normal hearing identify each other's voices.'[59] The technology was also widely used by deafblind people, particularly Ol'ga Skorokhodova, the Soviet 'Helen Keller' and a fellow researcher at the Institute of Defectology, who had the device installed in her flat (a puff of air, rather than a light, informed her of an incoming call). Indeed, Skorokhodova and Irina Tsukerman talked nightly on the telephone in Morse code for many years.[60]

While *surdotekhnika* focused chiefly on technological devices, this turn to technology also re-framed existing traditions of communication in the deaf and blind communities. Irina Tsukerman, in particular, engaged with the language of cybernetics, defined by Slava Gerovich as 'an assortment of analogies between humans and self-regulating machines', which had become fashionable in Soviet scientific circles in the late 1950s.[61] Looking at the various forms of communication open to deaf, blind and deaf-blind people, Tsukerman used computer terminology to establish a hierarchy of communication forms, focusing particularly on speeds of information transfer (measured in letters per minute). While lip reading, finger spelling and tactile signing on the hands were all significantly slower than oral speech, she explained, the addition of sign language saw speeds of comprehension increase greatly. As such, sign could be reconceptualized as a modern means of information transfer, rather than a remedial form of basic communication: 'sign and gesture language, in which one gesture represents an entire word or phrase, is transmitted at much greater speed […] In this, evidently, lies the reason for the widespread use of sign and gesture codes in deaf communication.'[62] The use of the term 'codes' aligns Tsukerman's work with Soviet cybernetics-inspired linguists such as Roman Jakobson who, as Gerovich has shown, 'viewed natural language as a code, and therefore included linguistics under the umbrella of information theory'.[63] *Surdotekhnika* thus represented, not just gadgets, but a set of practices and knowledges that enabled new ways of thinking about forms of communication among disabled people, understood for the first time as information technologies in their own right.

In its foregrounding of cybernetic technologies, this strain of Soviet deaf futurism is not dissimilar to the vision of techno-socialism that would be put forward a decade later by Donna Haraway. Her 'Cyborg Manifesto' set out an 'ironic dream' of a networked world in which existing, biologically determined hierarchies are broken down by the productive coupling of man and machine.[64] Although Haraway does not mention disability in her list of identities disrupted by the man-machine interface, more recently scholars such as Mara Mills have pointed to the particular type of cyborg discourse surrounding deaf people developed in the West, especially after the popularization of the cochlear implant in the 1980s; the idea of a deaf person as half-human, half-machine, able to perceive things beyond the bounds of the human senses, made them a resonant image in science fiction.[65] In many ways, the ideas put forward by deaf technologists foreshadowed Haraway: the notion that technology and socialism could together overcome the limitations and boundaries of physical impairment represented a potent vision and an argument for the place of deaf people within the Soviet body politic. Yet the particular frameworks through which technology and the body were viewed in the USSR also placed limitations on this deaf futurist dream, and shaped the ways in which technologies developed.

The limits of *surdotekhnika*

While *surdotekhnika* was engaged with cutting-edge discoveries in physics and electronics, the experiments it pursued followed particular ideological lines, and engaged with certain ways of thinking about the body, self and disability, that directed and sometimes constrained their development. The devices produced by Soviet deaf technologists were 'encoded' with the attitudes and assumptions of their creators. While these attitudes were underpinned by the utopianism of the moment, and of the horizons of opportunity that these new technologies opened up for deaf people, they were also limited by questions of accessibility and collectivism, of funding, and of debates over speech and bodily integrity that persisted throughout the late Soviet period.

The complexities and limits of the Soviet deaf futurist vision can be seen particularly in early reactions to the cochlear implant. Cochlear implants, which involve the transplanting of electrodes into the inner ear to deliver sound signals directly to the auditory nerve, have historically been a contested technology in the West, torn between narratives of medical triumph, and of the oppression of deaf people by a medical establishment which considers lack of hearing to be a problem needing to be 'fixed'.[66] The Soviet response to cochlear implants was shaped by rather different concerns. While experiments with electrode implantation tentatively began in the USSR in 1957, Veniamin Tsukerman in particular remained doubtful of their success, and the number of people receiving such an operation was very low.[67] The general public was made aware of this technology: the Tsukermans' 1975 article in *Nauka i zhizn* included a translated piece from East Germany, which discussed American attempts to create an 'electronic ear' by inserting electrodes directly into the auditory nerve.[68] Yet they made it clear that these experiments were unpromising: 'One of those who had the operation did in fact hear sounds. In his opinion, it was similar to an unknown foreign language, but had no relationship to his native English. [...] The author of these experiments is himself sceptical of their practical use.'[69] In particular, the narratives surrounding the 'artificial ear' stressed its unsuitability for 'deaf-mutes', or those deaf from early childhood who had not developed spoken language: like hearing aids, the possibility of returning deaf people to the world of sound was a 'pipe dream' that remained out of reach.[70]

Scepticism surrounding the cochlear implant focused particularly on two lines of criticism. While the 'science fiction' potential of the technology was clear, the lack of a theoretical understanding of how these implants worked was seen to prevent a strong case being made for their use. At the same time, the prohibitive cost of implantation for one individual, with little knowledge of how long such a device would last, made it very difficult to advocate for in a culture saturated with concepts of collectivism.[71] The latter argument was particularly compelling to those working in the Laboratory of *Surdotekhnika*. All the technologies developed were considered not just for their utility, but for their cost and accessibility to ordinary Soviet citizens. The most effective (and popular) of the technologies were either very cheap to produce, like the Morse code telephone, or had the potential to be used collectively, such as film subtitling devices, text transmitting machines, or the synaesthetic music device discussed in the introduction; according to a 1963 brochure, a similar device had been installed in Moscow deaf clubs and used for dance parties.[72] Collectivism was the watchword of these technologies; as such, the notion of an individual solution to deafness took some time to receive significant attention in the Soviet scientific community.[73] The first successful implantation, of a late-deafened, thirty-two-year-old woman named Nadia, only took place in the early 1980s.[74]

Discussion of the cochlear implant did not follow the lines of argument pursued in the West, therefore, where the development of a particular form of civil-rights inflected deaf identity and 'pride' enabled the cochlear to be framed as an oppressive technology: a form of 'cultural genocide', as one newspaper article controversially argued.[75] Indeed, the debates about *surdotekhnika*, even as they put forward exciting new prospects to broaden the sensory capacities of those without hearing, persisted in viewing deafness as a tragedy that required will and determination, and some expert intervention, in order to overcome. This view was bound up with a wider focus on issues of speech communication. From the early revolutionary period, deaf activists had contended with the Marxist view of oral communication as foundational to human development.[76] In 1950, in a discussion of linguistics in the newspaper *Pravda*, Stalin argued that spoken language had enabled human beings to 'reach the level of progress we have today', and suggested by relying on the 'impressions, sensations and perceptions' that are gleaned through sight, touch, taste and smell, deaf-mutes were left unable to develop higher thought and consciousness.[77]

As I have traced elsewhere, the backlash to this argument in the Soviet deaf community led to a more widespread recognition of sign as a language in its own right by the 1960s, capable, as the Tsukermans explained, of transmitting the 'classics of Shakespeare, Schiller and Ostrovskii' with its 'expressiveness and emotionality'.[78] The discussion of sign-language 'codes' thus engaged with existing linguistic trends which reframed sign as a valuable means of communication. However, in the *surdotekhnika* literature, the belief in spoken language as superior remains tangible. For example, Irina Tsukerman's discussion of the communicative value of various sensory forms of communication, even as it praises the expressiveness of sign, views it only in the context of sign-language interpretation of spoken lectures and speeches.[79] She thus valorizes sign as a means of information transfer, and as a contemporary mode of being, but only in terms of the transfer of existing knowledge to deaf people through the translation of oral speech. There is no real suggestion that sign might be valuable in its own right, or that knowledges might themselves be produced within the deaf world. Indeed, the epilogue to her 1975 set of lectures channels the voice of an imagined deaf reader, asking: 'Is this it? [...] Can contemporary science and technology really offer nothing more to deaf people? When will we be able to hear natural human speech?'[80] In the era of space flight, she suggests, the fact that sensory compensation was the only help on offer represented something of a failure.

The focus on speech knowledge had the result, therefore, of perpetuating the Stalinist privileging of the spoken word, and framed deafness in ways that appear, to a Western eye, to be both medicalized and audist.[81] Publications on *surdotekhnika* also reflect the transition from the utopianism of the 1960s to the 'stagnation' of the Brezhnev years, as they frame utopian 1960s technologies through the lens of a series of 1970s and early 1980s publications. Indeed, many of the technologies discussed in these sources are as narratives of failure: hypotheses that did not pan out, or technologies that failed to achieve what had been predicted. For example, the VIR machine was conceived as a technology that would enable deaf people to create a new form of language, with recognizable word 'shapes' enabling viewers to instantly comprehend what was being said. It soon became clear, however, that this technology did not work as it had been anticipated. The technology was quickly co-opted, however, by colleagues at the Institute of Defectology working in the education department, who saw its potential to help deaf people to perfect their oral pronunciation by working to match the patterns produced on the screen by their hearing teachers. From a visionary synaesthetic technology, the VIR thus became another means to enforce what Anastasia Kayiatos has termed the 'attempts to cure "deaf-mutes" of their silence' that characterized late Soviet deaf education.[82]

Alongside these conceptual constraints, those working to develop deaf technology struggled with some very practical limitations to their activities. Firstly, as the Tsukermans themselves acknowledged, it was very difficult to develop technologies to mimic or replace hearing when much was still unclear about how the biology and neuroscience of hearing functioned. New technological visions, such as a proposal to insert electrodes directly into the hearing centres of the brain, were stymied by 'insufficient knowledge of the processes of encoding and decoding of signals coming from the sight and hearing nerves to the brain'.[83] Another important barrier was financial: despite state interest in deaf technologies, funding remained low (e.g., a proposal to include state funding for the VIR in the 1962 decree was rebuffed by the Council of Ministers).[84] Many of the devices developed by the Laboratory of *Surdotekhnika* would ultimately be funded and produced by the VOG Special Technological Planning and Design Bureau, but accusations of limited productivity and poor quality of devices dogged the organization throughout the 1970s.[85] At the same time, the visionary research of the Laboratory was frequently funded by Veniamin Tsukerman himself:

> [Veniamin Arnoldovich] had a special 'deaf fund'. Today this sounds rather strange – at the time, V. A. was one of the most highly paid specialists, regularly receiving prizes. Other people bought dachas, cars and furniture suites, but he saved money in the so-called 'deaf fund'. With this money, experimental development of devices was paid for, and work on telephone communication for deaf people was carried out.[86]

While the generosity of Veniamin Tsukerman is striking, the lack of consistent funding from central government inevitably stymied certain lines of technological enquiry.

That is not to say, however, that visionary Soviet technologies were not advocated beyond the 1960s. Writing in the mid-1980s, Veniamin Tsukerman and Zinaida Azarkh proposed a new kind of technology to return hearing to deaf people: they pointed to an experiment conducted by Soviet scientists to introduce focused ultrasonic waves directly into the auditory nerve. The waves would be produced by a small generator placed by the head, which the user would orientate so that the waves reached the cochlear.[87] Tsukerman and Azarkh acknowledged the potential dangers of such a technology if ultrasonic waves of too high a frequency were used, but explained that at levels of 1mhz and above, these waves enabled hearing people to clearly comprehend speech, and therefore held the possibility of helping deaf people to hear without the need for costly and painful operations. They also pointed to the potential usefulness of this technology in diagnostics:

> [W]ith electro-implantation prosthetics, it is difficult to predict whether the complex microsurgical operation will truly help the deaf person. Usually, in order to find this out a dangerous operation to introduce electrodes and electrical currents is carried out. If the hypothesis is correct that mechanical, electrical and ultrasonic stimuli have identical effects, then it will be possible to replace tests using surgical intervention with analysis of a deaf person's hearing using focused ultrasonic sounds.[88]

While this technology was clearly in its infancy, its accessibility and universality – and its potential to avoid costly individual surgery – made it an exciting prospect for the deaf technologists, albeit one that moved decisively away from sense-swapping and towards a more conventional focus on the return of sound.

Conclusion

The Laboratory of *Surdotekhnika* closed its doors in 1979.[89] During its years of existence, its members had produced several devices that became ubiquitous in deaf life in the late Soviet period: devices to help deaf children to perfect their pronunciation (the VIR, and the later model I2-M), to assist with communication (the Morse code telephone), and to make everyday tasks easier (the 'electronic nanny'). The birth of these technologies, and of *surdotekhnika* as a discipline, was underpinned by the utopian dreams of body in the 1960s, which envisaged the engagement of alternative senses, and the use of electronics, to shape new ways of mediating between the body and the world. Yet by the time the Laboratory closed, *surdotekhnika* had ceased to be a utopian proposition, and had (within the deaf community, at least) become a symbol of the technological and practical failures of the late Soviet period. According to a 1976 letter sent by Veniamin Tsukerman to the head of the Party Control Commission of the Central Committee, A.Ia. Pel'she, the USSR was 'lagging behind the leading capitalist countries in the sphere of technology for deaf people' by over a decade.[90] Articles in the VOG magazine emphasized the lack of accessibility of these technologies, the poor quality of devices and the failure to provide appropriate batteries or fitting for hearing aids.[91] *Surdotekhnika*'s purpose had also shifted, from a technological facilitator for deaf culture, to a set of broadly remedial devices used in schools to help children to learn to speak.[92] As the state emphasis on facilitating these technologies also faded, the Tsukermans called for amateur inventors to pick up the baton: 'It is not only specialists and professionals who practice *surdotekhnika*, but also representatives of the "people's laboratory" – inventors, ham radio operators – who can do much to resolve such a humane task as to ease the lot of those who live in a world of endless silence.'[93]

The dreams of the deaf technologists were ultimately realized, however; albeit rather later than hoped, and following the eventual collapse of the regime that had fostered them. In her set of lectures in 1973, Irina Tsukerman looked to the future and imagined the new devices that might transform the lives of deaf people. By the year 2000, she predicted, videotelephones would become widely available, enabling deaf people to communicate remotely through sign language.[94] Voice recognition devices presented a particular set of engineering challenges, but she expected them to one day be resolved. Some ideas, such as the implantation of electrodes into the auditory nerve or even directly into the brainstem, were described by her as 'fantastical'.[95] All of these devices are available today.[96] Their adoption in the former USSR still shows traces of ideological and practical frameworks that shaped the early years of *surdotekhnika*, which were poised – as this chapter has argued – between deaf and hearing visions of the technological future. The persistent emphasis on speech has led to the prioritization of cochlear implants as a form of 'miracle cure' for deafness in contemporary Russia, and bypassed many of the cultural debates that frame their use in the West today.[97] At the same time, engagement with alternative sensory frameworks, and the view of technology as a facilitator of new forms of being in the world, remains tangible in Russian deaf culture, with deaf raves and sign-language YouTube representing updated forms of the 'light music' and 'hearing television' devices that animated the dreams of deaf technologists. Yet while the scope of these technologies has been transformed beyond recognition, they continue to demonstrate a 'firm faith in the future of technology', as Irina Tsukerman put it, to transform the nature of deafness and open up new sensory horizons.[98]

Notes

I am very grateful to Mike Gulliver, and to participants of the REES Seminar Series at St Antony's College, Oxford, the History seminar series at the University of Sheffield, and the Women's History Network seminar series, for their comments on earlier versions of this chapter. Thanks, in particular, to Anna Komarova and Irina Makhalova for their generous assistance with my research. Thanks also to Tony Shaw for his guidance on the specifics of hearing aids and other assistive technologies; any remaining errors are my own.

1. N. Nekhamkin, 'Zvuk prevrashchaetsia v tsvet', *Zhizn' glukhikh*, January 1960, inside front cover and 14. This device is also discussed in K. Leont'ev, 'Svetomuzyka', *Tekhnika molodezhi*, October 1959, 22–4.
2. Nekhamkin, 'Zvuk prevrashchaetsia', 14.
3. Ibid, inside front cover.
4. 'Defectology', to use Andy Byford's definition, refers to the Soviet 'discipline and occupation devoted to the study and treatment of child "imperfections"'; this includes deafness, blindness and 'mental backwardness'. As William McCagg has argued, the use of a Latinate term – whatever its later pejorative overtones – was seen to align this new discipline with progressive, international science. In a similar way, the use of the term 'surdotekhnika' (rather than the Russian 'glukhotekhnika') shows the turn to Latin as an attempt to put an international, scientific gloss on a uniquely Soviet discipline. Andy Byford, 'The Imperfect Child in Early Twentieth-Century Russia', *History of Education*, 45.5 (2017): 596; William McCagg, 'The Origins of Defectology', in *The Disabled in the Soviet Union: Past and Present, Theory and Practice* (Pittsburgh, PA.: University of Pittsburgh Press, 1989), 39–62.
5. V. Bicherov, 'Konstruktorskomy biuro VOG – 20', *V edinom stroiu*, 6 (1982): 8–9.
6. For a review of Soviet attitudes to disability, see Elena Iarskaia-Smirnova and Pavel Romanov, 'Heroes and Spongers: The Iconography of Disability in Soviet Posters and Film', in Michael Rasell and Elena Iarskaia-Smirnova, eds., *Disability in Eastern Europe and the Former Soviet Union: History, Policy and Everyday Life* (London: Routledge, 2016), 67–96.
7. This chapter focuses particularly on deafness, but the engagement with synaesthesia and discourses of the senses means that proponents of *surdotekhnika* sometimes also worked on technologies for blind or deafblind people (*tiflotekhnika*). See Vladimir Sergeevich Sverlov, *Tiflotekhnika* (Moscow: Uchpedgiz, 1960).
8. V. Tsukerman and I. Tsukerman, 'Glukhota i surdotekhnika', *Nauka i zhizn'*, no. 6 (1975): 78–85 (hereafter 'Glukhota').
9. For more on the life and work of Veniamin Tsukerman, see Veniamin Tsukerman and Zinaida Azarkh, *Arzamaz 16: Soviet Scientists in the Nuclear Age: A Memoir*, trans. Timothy Sergay and ed. Michael Pursglove (Nottingham: Bramcote Press, 1999).

10 The events that led to Irina's treatment with Streptomycin read like a spy novel: on the day of her diagnosis, her father heard on the radio about experiments using Streptomycin to cure tuberculous meningitis in the United States. One gram of the drug existed in Russia, but it had only been used in animal trials and the correct dosage in humans was unknown. Veniamin Tsukerman, with the help of two friends and some translators, placed an illicit call to the Mayo Clinic in Rochester, Minnesota, from his communal flat in Moscow and was given the necessary information to treat Irina. Weeks later Selman Waksman, the American scientist credited with discovering Streptomycin, smuggled in a further 30 grams of the drug on a visit to the USSR Academy of Sciences. By the end of 1948, 900 children had been saved. For his part in the affair, Tsukerman's friend Leonid Galynker would spend seven years in the Gulag. V. A. Tsukerman and Z. M. Azarkh, 'Zhizn' ili slukh', in Z. M. Azarkh, ed., *Uchenyi, mechtatel', borets: Posviashchaetsia professoru V. A. Tsukermanu* (Sarov: FGUP 'RFIaTs-VNIIEF', 2006), 27–43. See also B. L. Alt'shuler, 'Tri druz'ia: L. V. Alt'shuler, V. L. Ginzburg and V. A. Tsukerman', in B. L. Alt'shuler and V. E. Fortov, eds., *Ekstremalnye sostoianiia L'va Alt'shulera* (Moscow: Fizlatmit, 2011), 314–29. On the controversy over Waksman and the discovery of Streptomycin, see Peter Pringle, *Experiment Eleven: Dark Secrets behind the Discovery of a Wonder Drug* (London: Bloomsbury, 2012).

11 On Irina Tsukerman, see T. A. Basilova and E. A. Malkhasi'ian, 'Vopreki vsem pregradam, vozdvignutym samoi prirodoi', *Klinicheskaia i spetsial'naia psikhologiia*, 8.2 (2019): 185–97.

12 Postanovlenii Soveta Ministrov SSSR ot 27 iiuliia 1962 g. 'Ob uluchshenii obshchego i professional'nogo obrazovaniia, trudovogo ustroistva i obsluzhivaniia glukhikh grazhdan'. See also Gosudarstvennyi Arkhiv Rossiiskoi Federatsii (GARF) f. 5446, op. 96, d. 252, l. 29.

13 Prikaz Ministerstva sotsial'nogo obespechenie RSFSR ot 18 aprelia 1959 goda 'O meropriatiiakh po uluchsheniiu ushnogo protezirovaniia'. See V. G. Ushakov, *Vserossiiskoe obshchestvo glukhikh: Istoriia, razvitie, perspektivy* (Leningrad: Leningradskii vosstanovitel'nyi tsentr VOG, 1985), 200.

14 This right was propagandized widely by the Soviet deaf community in international fora: see, for example, E. Vartan'ian, 'Deviz: "Glukhie sredi slyshashchikh"', *Zhizn' glukhikh*, 11 (1967): 27. On hearing aids as a consumer product in the United States, see Jaipreet Virdi, *Hearing Happiness: Deafness Cures in History* (Chicago: University of Chicago Press, 2020), 207–14.

15 The Laboratory was founded by the deaf education specialist F. F. Rau, the defectologist A. I. D'iachkov, and V. A. Tsukerman, with Irina Tsukerman and the psychologist P. B. Shoshin as researchers. They were later joined by V. I. Antipov, A. L. Lomes and V. D. Laptev; the latter would run the Laboratory from 1965 until its closure in 1979. See Viktor Palennyi, *Istoriia Vserossiiskogo obshchestva glukhikh*, vol. III (Moscow: BAFI-Art, 2011), 258.

16 Irina Tsukerman, *Besedy o glukhote i tekhnike, pomogaiushchei glukhim: Teksty lektsii* (Leningrad: UPP LVTs VOG, 1973), 33 (hereafter *Besedy*).

17 Ibid., 32; Veniamin Tsukerman and Zinaida Azarkh, writing as V. Krainin and Z. Krainina, *Chelovek ne slyshit* (Moscow: Znanie, 1984), 73.

18 Tsukerman, *Besedy*, 37.

19 Ibid., 38.

20 'Glukhota', 78.

21 Ibid., 80.
22 See Ushakov, *Vserossiiskoe obshchestvo*, 199.
23 Ibid.
24 'Glukhota', 81. See also Krainin and Krainina, *Chelovek ne slyshit*, 76. On miniaturization in the development of hearing aids in the United States, see Mara Mills, 'Hearing Aids and the History of Electronics Miniaturisation', *IEEE Annals of the History of Computing*, 33.2 (2011): 24–44.
25 Tsukerman, *Besedy*, 3.
26 Ibid.
27 See Claire Shaw, *Deaf in the USSR: Marginality, Community, and Soviet Identity, 1917–1991* (Ithaca, NY: Cornell University Press, 2017).
28 See L. S. Vygotsky and A. R. Luria, *Studies on the History of Behavior: Ape, Primitive, and Child*, ed. and trans. Victor I. Golod and Jane E. Knox (Hillsdale, NJ: Lawrence Erlbaum Associates, Inc., 1993), 213–18.
29 These two devices were introduced to the hearing public in an article for *Izvestiia* in late 1967: V. Tsukerman, 'Vozvrashchenie k zvukam', *Izvestiia*, 22 December 1967, 5.
30 I. V. Tsukerman, *Priem i peredacha vibratsionnykh signalov azbuki Morze kak sposob sviazi glukhikh i slepoglukhikh po telefonu: Aftoreferat dissertatsii na soiskanie uchenoi stepeni kandidata pedagogicheskikh nauk* (Moscow: APN SSSR, Nauchno-issledovatel'skii institut defektologii, 1968).
31 Tsukerman, *Besedy*, 47.
32 Ibid., 49.
33 Ibid., 53.
34 I. Tsukerman, 'Glukhie razgovarivaiut po telefonu', *Zhizn' glukhikh*, December 1967, 20–1.
35 GARF f. 5446, op. 96, d. 252, l. 29.
36 Tsukerman, *Besedy*, 61.
37 Ibid., 52–8.
38 On the teletypewriter, see Harry G. Lang, *A Phone of Our Own: The Deaf Insurrection against Ma Bell* (Washington, DC: Gallaudet University Press, 2000). On the Tactophone, see Magdalena Zdrodowska, *Telefon, kino i cyborgi. Wzajemne relacje niesłyszenia i techniki* (Krakow: Wydawnictwo Uniwersytetu Jagiellonskiego, 2021), p. 336.
39 See Frances Bernstein, 'Prosthetic Manhood in the Soviet Union at the End of World War II', *Osiris*, 30.1 (2015): 113–33; Robert Dale, 'The Valaam Myth and the Fate of Leningrad's Disabled Veterans', *Russian Review*, 72.2 (2013): 260–84; Beate Fieseler, 'The Soviet Union's "Great Patriotic War" Invalids', *Comparativ*, 20.5 (2010): 34–49; Claire McCallum, 'Scorched by the Fire of War: Masculinity, War Wounds and Disability in Soviet Visual Culture, 1941–65', *Slavonic & East European Review*, 93.2 (2015): 251–85.
40 Susan Morrissey, Juliane Fürst and Polly Jones, introduction to the special issue 'The Relaunch of the Soviet Project, 1945–64', *Slavonic and East European Review*, 89.2 (2008): 201–7.
41 N. S. Khrushchev, *Report on the Program of the Communist Party of the Soviet Union*, 17 October 1961 (New York: Crosscurrents Press, 1961), 127.
42 See, for example, Slava Gerovitch, '"New Soviet Man" Inside Machine: Human Engineering, Spacecraft Design, and the Construction of Communism', *Osiris*, 22.1 (2007): 135–57; Diana Kurkovsky-West, '"Drilled Humans" or Automated Systems? Reconsidering Human-Machine Integration in Late-Soviet Design', in Colleen

McQuillen and Julia Vaingurt, eds., *The Human Reimagined: Posthumanism in Russia* (Boston: Academic Studies Press, 2018), 114–35.
43 Elana Gomel, 'Gods like Men: Soviet Science Fiction and the Utopian Self', *Science Fiction Studies*, 31.3 (2004): 358–77.
44 E. Rudenko, *Segodnia – fantasiia, zavtra – deistvitel'nost'* (Moscow: Meditsina, 1968).
45 See Shaw, *Deaf in the USSR*; Brigid O'Keeffe, *New Soviet Gypsies: Nationality, Performance and Selfhood in the Early Soviet Union* (Toronto: University of Toronto Press, 2013).
46 Lilya Kaganovsky, *How the Soviet Man Was Unmade: Cultural Fantasy and Male Subjectivity under Stalin* (Pittsburgh, PA: University of Pittsburgh Press, 2008), 3.
47 See Shaw, *Deaf in the USSR*, 122–34.
48 Basilova and Malkhasi'ian, 'Vopreki vsem pregradam', 189.
49 Nekhamkin, 'Zvuk prevrashchaetsia', 14.
50 Emma Widdis, *Socialist Senses: Film, Feeling and the Soviet Subject, 1917–1940* (Bloomington: Indiana University Press, 2017), 2.
51 See Ana Hedberg Olenina, *Psychomotor Aesthetics: Movement and Affect in Modern Literature and Film* (Oxford: Oxford University Press, 2020).
52 Tsukerman, *Besedy*, 40.
53 Hannah Proctor, *Psychologies in Revolution: Alexander Luria's 'Romantic Science' and Soviet Social History* (London: Palgrave Macmillan, 2020), 230. See also Julia Vassilieva, 'The Eisenstein-Vygotsky-Luria Collaboration: Triangulation and Third Culture Debates', *Projections*, 13.1 (2019): 23–44; Oksana Bulgakowa, 'From Expressive Movement to the "Basic Problem"': The Vygotsky-Luria-Eisensteinian Theory of Art, in *The Cambridge Handbook of Cultural-Historical Psychology* (Cambridge: Cambridge University Press, 2014), 423–48.
54 Sergei Eisenstein, 'Vertikal'nyi montazh', in *Sergei Eisenstein*, 6 vols (Moscow: Iskusstvo, 1968).
55 See Claire Shaw, 'Speaking in the Language of Art: Soviet Deaf Theatre and the Politics of Identity during Khrushchev's Thaw', *Slavonic and East European Review*, 91.4 (2013): 759–86. On Eisenstein's interest in mime, see Bulgakowa, 'From Expressive Movement', 439.
56 Vygotsky and Luria, *Studies on the History of Behavior*, 213–18; See also A. R. Luria, *The Mind of a Mnemonist: A Little Book about a Vast Memory*, trans. Lynn Solotaroff (New York: Basic Books, 1968).
57 Nekhamkin, 'Zvuk prevrashchaetsia', inside front cover.
58 Tsukerman, *Besedy*, p. 52.
59 Ibid.
60 Ibid. For an account of these nightly telephone conversations, see Anna Komarova, *Soobshchestvo glukhikh i zhestovoi iazyk* (Moscow: VOG, 2020), 42–3.
61 Slava Gerovitch, *From Newspeak to Cyberspeak: A History of Soviet Cybernetics* (Cambridge: MIT Press, 2002), 2.
62 Tsukerman, *Besedy*, 31.
63 Gerovitch, *From Newspeak to Cyberspeak*, 230.
64 Donna Haraway, 'A Manifesto for Cyborgs', in *The Haraway Reader* (London: Routledge, 2004).
65 Mara Mills, 'Do Signals Have Politics? Inscribing Abilities in Cochlear Implants', in *The Oxford Handbook of Sound Studies* (Oxford: Oxford University Press, 2011), 320–46.
66 See Stuart Blume, cited in Ibid., 321.

67 'Glukhota', 79.
68 'Elektronnoe ukho', *Nauka i zhizn'*, 6 (1975): 84–5.
69 'Glukhota', 79.
70 Ibid., 23.
71 See Krainin and Krainina, *Chelovek ne slyshit*, 79.
72 E. Vartan'ian and I. Gitlits, *Of Those Who Cannot Hear* (Stockholm: Vneshtorgizdat, 1963), 22.
73 N. Korshunova, 'Elektronnaia ulitka', *V edinom stroiu*, February 1982, 22–3.
74 Ibid, 22.
75 See Mills, 'Do Signals Have Politics', 324.
76 See Shaw, *Deaf in the USSR*, 70–1. This framing is also used by Tsukerman in his *Izvestiia* article: V. Tsukerman, *Vosvrashchenie k zvukam*, 5.
77 I. V. Stalin, 'Tovarishcham D. Belkinu i S. Fureru', *Pravda*, 2 August 1950, 2.
78 'Glukhota', p. 80. On debates over the theatrical use of sign language, see Shaw, 'Speaking in the Language of Art'.
79 Tsukerman, *Besedy*, 31.
80 Ibid., 63.
81 On audism, see H-Dirksen Bauman, 'Audism: Exploring the Metaphysics of Oppression', *Journal of Deaf Studies and Deaf Education*, 9.2 (2004): 243–5.
82 Anastasia Kayiatos, 'Sooner Speaking Than Silent, Sooner Silent Than Mute: Soviet Deaf Theatre and Pantomime after Stalin', *Theatre Survey*, 51.1 (2010): 7. The article opens with an account of the use of the VIR in a pedagogical setting.
83 Tsukerman, *Besedy*, 64.
84 GARF f. 5446, op. 96, d. 252, l. 29.
85 See, Ushakov, *Vserossiiskoe obshchestvo*, 201.
86 Anna Komarova and Irina Tsukerman, 'Operezhavshii vremia', *V edinom stroiu*, July 2009, 20.
87 Krainin and Krainina, *Chelovek*, 80.
88 Ibid., 80–1.
89 Palennyi, *Istoriia*, vol. III, 258.
90 Quoted in Komarova, *Soobshchestvo glukhikh*, 25–6.
91 See, for example, I. L'vov, 'Pochemu zamolchal slukhovoi apparat?', *Zhizn' glukhikh*, June 1970, 12–13.
92 See I. L'vov, 'Surdotekhnika – zabotlivye ruki', *V edinom stroiu*, March 1972, 10–11.
93 'Glukhota', 85.
94 Tsukerman, *Besedy*, 61.
95 Ibid., 62.
96 See Virdi, *Hearing Happiness*, 260–1.
97 On the use of cochlears, see Vystuplenie vitse-prezidenta VOG S. A. Ivanova na zasedanii plenuma TsP VOG 19 dekabria 2014 goda po voprosu 'Kokhlearnaia implantatsiia: problem i puti ikh resheniia', http://www.voginfo.ru/novosti/newsvog/item/1009-PlenumVOG.html.
98 Tsukerman, *Besedy*, 64.

Index

abortion 8, 40, 43, 67, 72, 74
Academy of Sciences 200, 233 n.10
   Institute of Machine Technology 198
addiction 12, 30, 81 n.54, 129, 139, 141, 147
alcohol 143, 148
   alcoholics 32–4, 65, 129, 203
   alcoholism 69, 140, 143
   and reflexes 32
All-Russian Society of the Deaf (VOG – *Vserossiiskoe obshchestvo glukhikh*) 217, 225, 230
All-Union Conference on Psychotherapy 124
All-Union Congress of the Society for the Settlement of Jewish Toilers on the Land (OZET – *Obshchestvo zemledel'tsev evreev trudiashchikhsia*) 193 n.14
All-Union Scientific Society of Neuropathologists and Psychiatrists (VNMONiP – *Vsesoiuznoe nauchnoe obshchestvo nevropatologov i psikhiatrov*) 124
Aristotle (384–22BCE) Greek philosopher 147
Army, Red 161
   barracks 164–5
   Central House of the Red Army 161
art
   Bulgarian Academy of Art 108
   and consciousness 13
   and folkloric themes 109
   formalism 177
   and neurophysiology 13
   socialist realism 177
   and socialist values 108
   and therapy 13
   and union membership 108–9
artificial limbs 198, 199–200

Astakhov, Sergei Nikolaevich (1900–1962) Soviet psychotherapist
   Patient M. 126
   on psychotherapists as 'teachers of life' 124
   on will to treatment 130
Astashenkov, Pyotr Timofeevich (1920–1980) Soviet colonel-engineer 206
   What is bionics (*Chto takoe bionika*, 1963) 214
asylums
   'moral treatment' 104, 105–6, 122
athletes 5
   doping and light therapy 162–3
   and psychotherapy 131–5
atrophine (anti-smoking chemical) 148
Austro-Hungarian Empire 8, 52
autogenic training 90, 122
   and 'higher nervous activity' 127
autosuggestion 121–2, 129, 130, 132, 137 n.42, 148
avant-garde 177–8, 191
Azarkh, Zinaida Matveevna (1917–2004) Soviet physicist 219, 228, 229, 230

Babitskii, Vladimir (1938–) Soviet mechanical engineer
   on propaganda and bionic arms 204
bacteria, bacteriology 157–8, 164, 169
   bacteriological lamps 159, 166, 168, 169–71
Bakulev, Aleksandr Nikolaevich (1890–1967) Soviet surgeon
   smoking and reflex actions 142, 145
Bakushinskii, A. V. (1883–1939) Soviet art theorist
   Commission for the Study of Aesthetic Production and Reception under the Influence of Hypnosis 41
Bauhaus 191

Bekhterev Vladimir (1857–1927) Russian
    and Soviet neurologist 30
  on associative reflexes 31, 32
  on Bernheim and the Nancy school
      46 n.31
Belyi, Andrei (1880–1934) Russian
    novelist 189
  Kotik Letaev 189
Benjamin, Walter (1892–1940) German
    philosopher
  on film 178, 183
Bernheim, Hippolyte (1840–1919) French
    physician
  hypnosis 30–1
  Nancy School 31
bionics
  bionic arm 15, 199–200, 204, 206, 208,
      209 n.7, 210 n.14
  and consciousness 202
biopolitics, biopower 2, 10
Birman, Boris (1884–1952) Soviet
    physiologist
  'experimental sleep' 31
  lower consciousness 34
body, bodies 5, 6, 7, 110, 132, 139, 164,
    169, 183, 187, 199
  care of 90
  control over 10, 16, 34, 122, 127, 131,
      132, 134, 135
  embedded 158, 159, 164, 167, 168, 171
  and film 183, 188,
  perfection of 7, 16, 87, 131
  reconstruction of 224
  technologies 178
  transcend 1–2, 15, 17
  women's 182
Bondarchick, M. Ia., sports
    psychotherapist
  Project at Laboratory for Medical and
      Biological Scientific Research
      into Technical and Military-
      Applied Sports 131
Brik, Lilya (1891–1978) Russian and
    Soviet artist 177, 178–80, 188,
    191, 193 n.9, 193 n.10
  The Glass Eye (*Stekliannyi glaz*, 1929)
      177, 180, 181–4, 189
  Jews on the Land (*Evrei na zemle*, 1927)
      179

Brik, Osip (1888–1945) Russian and
    Soviet writer 180
Bulgaria People's Republic of 8–9, 11, 13
  Academy of Art 108
  Central Committee of the Union of the
      Deaf 111
  Communist ascension to power 107
  Emergence from Ottoman Empire 107
  health officials and work therapy
      106–7, 111, 112–14
  history of psychiatry in 104–5, 118 n.5
brain 200
  brain inhibition 8, 34, 43
  and consciousness 6
  reflexes 34
  waves 207
Brezhnev, Leonid (1906–1982) Soviet
    leader (1964–1982)
  Brezhnev era 65, 72, 229
Britain 140, 205–6, 208
  English hand 206, 213 n.55

Canada 73, 205–6, 208
capitalism, capitalist
  cinema 181, 182, 183–4, 194 n.28
  deaf technologies 231
  sexual health and fight against 73–4
  society 194 n.28
  sport as battleground against 131
censorship
  Chief Committee for the Control of
      Repertoire (*Glavrepertkom*)
      (GRK) theatre censorship body)
      180, 195 n.40
  Main Directorate for the Protection of
      State Secrets in the Press (*Glavlit*,
      chief censorship body) 40
Central Committee of the USSR, Party
    Control Commission of 231
Central Intelligence Agency (CIA) 207
Central Institute of the Labour of Invalids
    (TsITIN – *Tsentral'nyi institut
    truda invalidov*) 220
Central Scientific-Research Institute of
    Prosthetics and Prosthetics
    Manufacturing 198
Charcot, Jean Martin (1825–1893) French
    neurologist
  on hypnosis 30–1, 37

Chlorpromazine 110
Cicero (106–43 BCE) Roman philosopher 147
cinema, **See** film and cinema
censorship 7, 40, 73, 180
cochlear implant 227–8, 230, 231
Cold War 14, 198, 199, 204, 208, 218, 223–4
    and bionic arms 206–7
    and sexual health 73
    and sport 131
    and stress 86
Communism, Communist 1, 3, 11, 117 n.1, 218, 224
    building Communism 73–4, 91, 102, 105, 108, 114, 224
    morality 66
    The Psychoanalysis of Communism (Psikhoanaliz kommunizma, 1924) 38
    society 54
condoms 66, 71, 72
consciousness 38
    and art 13
    and brain 6
    class consciousness 6, 57
    dream-consciousness 37, 39
    and hypnotism 7, 32, 36–9
    hypoconsciousness 37
    lower-consciousness 38
    norms of 4
    psychophysiology of 123
    question of 6
    secondary consciousness 37
    synaesthesia 225
contamination 167–8
Coue de la Chataignerale, Emile (1857–1926) French psychologist and pharmacist
    suggestion therapy 143
criminal justice
    criminal responsibility 54
    recidivism 57–60
cytisine (anti-smoking chemical, also known as tsititon, Tabex) 11, 146, 148–9
Czechoslovak Socialist Republic 7, 8, 9, 10, 12, 51–60, 83–7, 89, 91
    criminal justice system 53
    Ministry of Health 87
    modernity and stress 86

Danilevskii, Vasilii (1852–1939) Ukrainian and Soviet physiologist
    on hypnosis 34
Darwinism 6
deaf, deafness
    Bulgarian Union of the Deaf 106, 111, 113, 116
    Communities 226
    and consciousness 228
    and labour 104–5
    selves 218, 223–4
    in the Soviet Union 219–20
    technology (*surdotekhnika*) 16, 217, 218–24, 225, 227–31, 232 n.4, 232 n.7
defectology 221, 225, 232 n.4
    Scientific Research Institute of Defectology 217, 218, 226, 229
Departments of Sanitary Enlightenment 65, 68, 69, 71–2, 146, 148
Dessoir, Max (1867–1947) German philosopher
    on 'double-ego' 47 n.59
    on hypnotism 37
Deutsche Demokratische Republik (DDR), **See** German Democratic Republic
disability 104–7, 203, 218, 224, 227
    deaf, deafness
        and labour 104–5
        and technology 16, 218–24
    and masculinity 5, 6–7
    mental disability and institutionalization 106
    veterans 15, 203
disease, diseases
    airborne diseases 166
    asthma 157
    diphtheria 164–5
    lifestyle diseases 84, 140
    neuralgia 157
    neurasthenia 141, 147–8
    plexitis 157
    polio 200
    prevention of 170–1
    psychosomatic disease 86–7
    retinitis pigmentosa 219
    scarlet fever 168
    staphylococcus 166

tuberculosis 144, 157, 160, 164, 219
venereal disease 7, 12
  and capitalism 73
  contact tracing 75–6
  gonorrhoea 69, 70, 71
  increased rates of 68–9, 79 n.29
  laws against transmitting 76
  medical expertise 74–6
  syphilis 65, 71, 76, 140
dispensary, dispensaries 104, 141, 144, 145
  Latvian Republican Skin and VD Dispensary (*Republikāniskais ādas un venerisko slimību dispansers*) 69, 70, 73–7
  Moscow Regional Health Department 144
  Narcological clinics (*narcodispensaries*) 30, 32
divorce
  concern about high rates of 67–8, 71, 133
Dubois, Paul (1848–1918) Swiss neuropathologist
  influence on Soviet psychotherapy 121
  influence on tobacco therapy 143
Dubrovskii, Aleksandr (1899–unknown) Ukrainian and Soviet filmmaker
  To Your Health (*Za vashe zdorov'e*, 1929) 32–4
Dvorianov, Orlin (1951–) Bulgarian artist 103
Dzhurova, Axiniya (1942–) Bulgarian art historian 103

East Germany, **See** German Democratic Republic
education
  of deaf-mutes 229
  pedagogy and psychotherapy 12
  psychotherapists as 'teachers of life' 124–6
  schools 70
  sex education 7, 67–70
Eisenstein, Sergei (1898–1948) Soviet film director 184, 186, 192 n.1, 195 n.40
  General Line (*Staroe i novoe*, 1929) 177
  hypnosis and consciousness 40–1
  Strike (*Stachka*, 1925) 186
electric light therapy 159, 160
electrification 160

Eliasberg, Wladimir G (1887–1969) German psychotherapist
  'targeted therapy' for smoking 143
Engels, Friedrich (1820–1895) German philosopher
  on consciousness 135 n.12
Erisman Central Scientific-Research Sanitary-Hygiene Institute 165, 167, 168–70
Ermler, Fridrich (1898–1967) Latvian and Soviet film director
  Fragment of an Empire (*Oblomok imperii*, 1929) 177
European Court of Human Rights 110
Expo '58, Brussels 197, 204, 209 n.3, 223
  American Pavilion 203
  Soviet Pavilion 204

family
  birth rates 72
  extramarital sex 66
  paternity 72
  and sexual health 71–2
Filatov, Arkadii Timofeevich (1925–1997) sports psychologist 132, 133
film and cinema
  as abstraction 178
  anti-smoking 147
  Berlin: Symphony of a City (*Berlin – Die Sinfonie der Großstadt*, 1927) 180, 183
  Bitter Chronicle (*Gor'kaia khronika*, 1966) 69
  The Cabinet of Dr Caligari (*Das Cabinet des Dr Caligari*, 1920) 42
  Dr Mabus, the Gambler (*Dr Mabus, der Spieler*, 1922) 42, 186
  and ethnography 194 n.23
  The Fall of the Romanov Dynasty (*Padenie dinastii Romanovykh*, 1927) 186, 192 n.1
  formalist experiments 177
  Fragment of an Empire (*Oblomok imperii*, 1929) 177
  General Line (*Staroe i novoe*, 1929) 177
  The Great Way (*Velikii put'*, 1927) 186
  History of the Civil War (*Istoriia grazhdanskoi voiny*, 1921) 192 n.1
  and hypnosis 42

Jews on the Land (*Evrei na zemle*, 1927) 179
Komsomol: Patron of Electrification (*Komsomol: shef elektrofikatsii*, 1932) 187
Kulturfilm 13, 32, 66, 180, 182, 184
A Look into the Depth of the Soul: A Film about the Unconscious (*Ein Blick in die Tiefen der Seele. Der Film vom Unbewussten*, 1923) 32, 37–8, 43
Man with a Movie Camera (*Chelovek s kinoapparatom*, 1929) 177, 180, 191
Miss Mend (1926) 42
The Russia of Nicholas II and Lev Tolstoy (*Rossiia Nikolaia i Lev Tolstoi*, 1928) 186
Science and Technology (*Nauka i tekhnika*, 1961) 202–3
as sensory technology 13, 17
sex education 70, 76–7
Shackled by Film (*Zakovannaia fil'moi*, 1918) 179
A Sixth Part of the World (*Shestaia chast' mira*, 1926) 182, 189
Today (*Segodnia*, 1930) 177, 187–9
and Western ideology 183–4
Finsen, Niels Ryberg (1860–1904) Faroese physician
lamp research 157, 158, 160
First World War, **See** World War One (1914–1918)
Five-Year Plan 14, 187
Forel, Auguste (1848–1931) Swiss psychiatrist 36, 37
Hypnotism (*Der Hypnotismus*, 1924) 37
Foucault, Michel (1926–1984) French philosopher
Foucauldian analysis 2, 4, 51, 119 n.17
on work 105
Freud, Sigmund (1856–1939) Austrian psychoanalyst 37, 43
on hypnotism 37, 38, 39, 49 n.101
unconscious life 37
Freudian psychotherapy 24 n.65, 29, 38, 48 n.72, 122
futurism
deaf futurism 18, 224–7
sensory futurism 16
technofuturism 14

gender 5, 13, 65, 67
and socialist heroism 89
German Democratic Republic (GDR, DDR, East Germany) 3, 7, 10, 12, 149, 228
health risks 84–5
modernity 7, 84
self-optimization 85
stress 86, 89–91
Gertsmark, G. Soviet venereologist 71
Giliarovskii, Vasilii Alekseevich (1876–1959) Soviet psychiatrist
on work therapy 105, 106–7
Gingras, Gustave (1918–1996) Canadian physician 206
Ginzburg, RM., Soviet microbiologist
bactericidal lamp experiments 168
Glavlit (Main Directorate for the Protection of State Secrets in the Press, chief censorship body) 40
Glavrepertkom (GRK – Chief Committee for the Control of Repertoire, theatre censorship body) 180, 195 n.40
Golovnya, Anatoli (1900–1982) Soviet cinematographer 181
Gorky, Maksim (1868–1936) Russian and Soviet writer
'New Man' and 'New Woman' 1
and socialist heroism 88
Goskino (Soviet state-owned film trust, 1922–1924) 184, 186, 192 n.1, 194 n.31, 195 n.35
Grushin, Boris (1927–2001) Soviet sociologist
public opinion survey on love, marriage and sex 68
Gulag 233 n.8
and the reforging of imperfect individuals 7, 118 n.4
Guzikov, P.D., Soviet physician
ultraviolet light therapy 164

haptic 2, 15
elements of cinema 187–8, 189, 191, 192
and subjectivity 218, 224, 225
Haraway, Donna (1944–) American philosopher 17, 183, 227

health
  abortion 72
  against capitalism 73–4
  alcoholism 69
  contract tracing 75–6
  and lifestyle risks 90
  mental health 3, 106–7
  popular health literature 7, 90
  sanitary propaganda 68
  sexual health 69
  women's health 5, 7
health resort medicine (*kurortologiia*) 160, 164
Hegel, Georg Wilhelm Friedrich (1770–1831) German philosopher
  on work 105
Heidegger, Martin (1889–1976) German philosopher 14
Hennecke, Adolf (1905–1975) East German labour hero 88
Higher Art and Technical Studios (VKhUTEMAS – *Vysshie Khudozhestvenno-Tekhnicheskie Masterskie*) 189
historiography
  environment and health 158
  Foucauldian analysis 2, 51, 119 n.17
  material turn 16
  somatic and sensory turns 5
  technology 2, 14–6
history
  in anti-smoking campaigns 147
  history of 30, 36, 37, 157–8
    history of Soviet medicine 29–32, 37, 45 n.16, 122–3, 157–9
  psychiatry in Bulgaria, 104–5, 118 n.5
Home for Men with Mental Disabilities and Idiocy, Pastra, Bulgaria 110–1
Home for the Mentally Retarded Deaf, Tserova Koria, Bulgaria 111
Horvai, Ivan (1926–1970), Czech psychiatrist
  on religion and hysteria 55
humanity
  human nature 2, 6, 10
  human sciences 4–6, 10
  human transformation 3, 10
  humanism 197

New Bulgarian Man 101–2, 107
New Soviet Person 5, 6, 105, 122, 126, 224
  subjectivity 10–1, 118 n.4
  ways of being 217
hygiene 9, 67, 73, 74, 158–9, 165–6
  London School of Hygiene and Tropical Medicine 148
hypnosis 7, 122 **See also** suggestion
  alcoholism, cure of 32
  control over patient 34
  as creative and oratorical technique 41
  in popular culture 42–3
  'hypnoanalysis' 39, 48 n.72
  inhibition theory of, 8, 29, 30, 36, 43
  laboratory study of 30–2
  and reflexology 29, 32, 38
  as tobacco therapy 143, 145, 148
  and unconscious mind 29–30, 36–9
  use in sport 132
  and willpower 128
  Woe from Hypnosis (*Gore ot gipnoza*, 1927) 43

inhibition
  brain inhibition 8, 34, 43
  and hypnosis 8, 29, 30, 36, 43
  mental inhibition 30, 32
  Pavlovian theories of 29, 31
  physiological theories of 31–2
  reflexes 34
insanity defence, 54
Institute of Defectology 217, 218, 226, 229
International Congress on Automatic and Remote Control 204

Jakobson, Roman (1896–1982) Russian linguist 226

Kannabikh, Iurii (1872–1939) Russian and Soviet psychiatrist
  on hypnosis and Pavlov's dogs 44
Kapterev, P.N., Soviet aesthetic theorist
  Commission for the Study of Aesthetic Production and Reception under the Influence of Hypnosis 41
Karpov, Pavel Ivanovich (1873–unknown) Russian and Soviet psychiatrist
  research on hypnosis 41

Kaufman, Mikhail (1897–1980) Soviet
    film director 181, 188, 189
  Moscow (*Moskva*, 1928) 180
Kazakov, Dimitar (1933–1992) Bulgarian
    artist 11, 101, 108, 109
Kazakov, Nikola (1935–2007) Bulgarian
    artist and psychiatric patient,
    brother of Dimitar Karakov 11,
    13, 101, 107–11, 115–6, 119 n.34
Kellogg, John Harvey (1852–1943)
    American businessman and
    physician
  electric light therapy 159–60
Khrushchev, Nikita (1894–1971) Soviet
    leader (1953–1964) 66, 224
  Khrushchev era 72, 224
  Khrushchev's Thaw 15, 224
Knobloch, Ferdinand (1916–2018) Czech
    psychiatrist
  on psychopathy 59
Knoblochová, Jiřina (1918–2015) Czech
    psychiatrist
  on psychopathy 59
Kobrinskii, AE (1915–1992) Soviet
    mechanical engineer 200, 204,
    207
Koch, Robert (1843–1910) German
    physician
  on electric lamps 158
Kolarov, Peter (1906–1996) Bulgarian
    Minister for National Health
    and Social Services
  compensation and incentives 112,
    113–14
  work therapy report 111–12, 117
Kolev, Tzvetan (1949–) Bulgarian artist
    103, 109, 111
Kosmodem'ianskaia, Zoia (1923–1941)
    Soviet partisan 89
Krafft-Ebing, Richard von (1840–1902)
    German psychiatrist 38
Kronfeld, Arthur (1886–1941) German
    psychiatrist
  *A Look into the Depth of the Soul: A
    Film about the Unconscious* (*Ein
    Blick in die Tiefen der Seele. Der
    Film vom Unbewussten*, 1923)
    32, 37–8, 43
  on hypnotism 37

  Zalkind's preface to Russian translation
    of *Hypnosis and Suggestion*
    (*Hypnose und Suggestion* (1924)
    43–4
Kruchenykh, Aleksei (1886–1968) Russian
    and Soviet poet 189
Kudrna, Josef (1920–1989) Czech
    politician
  on criminal recidivism 57
Kuffner, Karel (1858–1940) Czech
    psychiatrist
  Kuffner school 53
Kuleshov, Lev (1899–1977) Russian and
    Soviet film director 180, 184
Kulturfilm 32, 180, 184
  ethnographical films 13, 66, 182

Latvian Soviet Socialist Republic 7, 9
  Central Committee of the Latvian
    Communist Party 69
  forced incorporation into USSR 67
  House of Sanitary Enlightenment 65,
    68, 69, 71–2
  Russian and Latvian speakers 69, 80
    n.37
  Scientific Society of Dermato-
    Venereologists 71
  Laboratory for Medical and Biological
    Scientific Research into
    Technical and Military-Applied
    Sports 131
labour
  as analytic category 101–2
  forced labour 102
  heroes of 88–9
  mental illness 102
  in Soviet ideology 105–6, 117 n.1
  as therapy 101–17
  goals 107
law, lawyers 41
  Soviet anti-venereal disease law 76
  Soviet family law 72
Lebedinskii, Mark Samuilovich (1894/95–
    1980) Soviet psychotherapist
  on psychotherapists as 'teachers of life'
    124, 127
Lench, Leonid (1905–1991) Soviet writer
  'A Hypnotist's Séance' ('*Seans
    gipnotizera*', 1935) 44

Lenin, Vladimir (1870–1924) Soviet leader (1917–1924) 141
  Marxism-Leninism 14
  socialist hero 95–6 n.29
  theory of reflection 52
Leont'ev, Konstantin Leont'evich, Soviet engineer
  synaesthetic machine 217
Liébeault, Ambroise-Auguste (1823–1904) French physician
  'Nancy school' of hypnosis 31
Lifshits, (Professor) Semen Iakovlevich, Soviet hypnologist
  group hypnotherapy session 34
  on hypnotism and psychoanalysis 39
literature
  popular health 7
  self-help 12, 85
Litinetskii, Izot Borisovich (1912–1985) Soviet author 206–7, 214 n.62
lobeline (anti-smoking chemical) 146, 148
Löwenfeld, Leopold (1847–1923) German physician
  Hypnosis and Medicine (*Hypnotismus und Medizin*, 1922) 37
Lukanov, Karlo Todorov (1897–1982) Deputy Chairman of the Bulgarian Ministerial Council 113, 116
Lunacharskii, Anatolii (1875–1933) Soviet Commissar for Education (1917–1929) 87–8
Luriia, Aleksandr (1902–1977) Soviet psychologist
  'experimental unconscious' 40
  The Nature of Human Conflicts (*Priroda chelovecheskikh konfliktov*, 1932) 39
  research on hypnosis 39–40
  sensory swapping 221–2, 225
Lysenko, Trofim (1898–1976) Ukrainian and Soviet agronomist 6

Makarenko, Anton (1888–1939) Ukrainian and Soviet pedagogue 125
  on collective treatment 125

Malis, Georgii Iur'evich (1904–1962) Ukrainian and Soviet psychiatrist
  The Psychoanalysis of Communism (*Psikhoanaliz kommunizma*, 1924) 38
manufacturing
  plants and stress 86
Martynenko, A.A., sports psychologist
  on autosuggestion and reflexes 132–3
Marx, Karl (1818–1883) German philosopher
  on consciousness and social existence 6
  on work 105
Marxism
  communication 228
  scientific Marxism 10
Marxism-Leninism 14
  and work 101–2
  and work therapy 116
mass media 7, 9, 13, 86
  and sexual health 65–9, 74, 77
  and socialist heroism 88
materialism 6, 128
  and cinema 188
material turn (historiography) 16
Mayakovsky, Vladimir (1893–1930) Russian and Soviet artist 179, 180, 193 n.10, 193 n.13
  Shackled by Film (*Zakovannaia fil'moi*, 1918) 179
medicine
  expert knowledge and venereal disease 74–6
  folk medicine 74–5, 140
  history of 30, 36, 37, 157–8
    history of Soviet medicine 29–32, 37, 45 n.16, 122–3, 157–9
  medicalization 10–1
  physical 157
  and psychotherapy 122, 126
men, men's
  crisis of masculinity 72
  focus of sex education 72
  health 66, 89, 140, 146
  masculine cinema 184
  'New Soviet Man' **See under** humanity; New Soviet Person

menstruation 3, 164
mental
    characteristics 87, 125, 127, 130, 131, 144
    disability 101, 102, 106
    disorders 11, 38, 52, 53–5, 57, 59, 60, 101, 102, 111, 121, 125, 130, 131, 134
    experiences 5, 6
    health 8, 51, 56, 60, 83, 85, 86, 106
    healthcare 10, 103, 110, 111, 113, 116, 117, 118 n.4, 128
    inhibition 30, 32
    processes 8, 10, 34, 36, 37, 41, 49 n.101, 52, 53, 129, 208
    states 13
Mesmer, Franz Anton (1734–1815) Swabian physician 30
Mezhrabpom, Mezhrabpomfil'm (German-Russian film company 1928–1936) 37, 179, 180, 194 n.19
Miasishchev, Nikolaevich (1893–1973) Latvian and Soviet psychologist
    on psychotherapists as 'teachers of life' 124
Michurin, Ivan Vladimirovich (1855–1935) Russian and Soviet biologist 52
microbials 167–8
Mikoian, Anastas (1895–1978) Armenian and Soviet Commissar for Food Industry (1926–1938)
    Increased tobacco production 141
Miltiņš, Alfrēds (1939–) Latvian physician
    on venereal disease in foreign countries 73
mind, minds 2, 3, 5, 8, 31, 58, 130, 133
    and art 13
    mind-body 2, 3, 5, 6, 7, 14, 34, 52, 53, 54, 60, 83, 89, 91, 123, 127, 128, 133, 134, 225
    perfection of 1, 4, 5, 134
    and science 14
    self-control over 122, 129, 131, 134
    technologies of 3, 17, 83, 90, 101, 116, 117
    unconscious 7, 8, 10, 29, 30, 36–9, 40, 41, 42, 43, 44
        and 'double-ego' 47 n.59
        'experimental unconscious' 40
        post-hypnotic suggestion 43

mind control 199
    American understanding 200, 202, 205, 207
    Soviet understanding 200, 202
Minin, AV (1851–1909) Russian surgeon
    Minin lamp 160
M'Naghten rules 54
modernity 16, 84
    alternative modernity 5, 101
    illiberal modernity 10
    physical and mental consequences of 84–6
Moll, Albert (1862–1939) German psychiatrist
    on hypnotism 36–7
Molotov, Vyacheslav (1896–1986) Soviet Minister of Foreign Affairs (1939–1949, 1953–1956)
    'two worlds' 187
Morse code telephone 222–3, 225, 226
morphine 143, 148
Morzhov, Valentin (1957–) Russian prosthodontist 208
Moscow Hypnological Society 39
Mysliveček, Zdeněk (1881–1974) Czech psychiatrist
    holistic concept of mind and body 53
    on psychopathy 59

Nanii, P. I., Soviet researcher
    Nanii glass reflector 157
Neishtadt, Ia. E., Soviet microbiologist
    on bactericidal lamps 165, 166
    on microbial research 167
Neruda, Pablo (1904–1973) Chilian poet and politician
    on Lilya Brik 179
nerves 16, 141, 142, 146, 157, 200, 203, 230
    central nervous system 162, 165, 166
    nervizm 159
    nervous system 31, 34, 46 n.30, 53, 141, 157
    training of 121
nervous
    ailments 86, 91, 143, 146, 148, 164, 166
    framework in Soviet medicine 158, 164, 165
    and Freudian psychoanalysis 38
    health 163
    higher activity 53, 55, 60, 125, 127

neurology, neurologists 6, 30, 37, 42, 146, 229
  hospitals 85, 111–2, 114
  neurological hammer 143
  neurophysiology 13, 111
  neurosis, neurotic 11, 30, 58, 85, 87, 93 n.10, 107, 121, 125–7, 131, 134, 148
newspapers, magazines and pamphlets 66–8, 75, 218
  against smoking 147
  Bristol Daily Courier 207
  Daily News 207
  Homeland (*Vlasta*) 91
  Independent Newspaper (*Nezavisimaia gazeta*) 208
  Life of the Deaf (*Zhizn' glukhikh*) 217
  News (*Izvestiia*) 200, 204, 207
  Popular Electronics 198
  Science and Life (*Nauka i zhizn'*) 228
  Soviet Youth (*Padomju Jaunatne*) 75
  Soviet Youth (*Sovetskaia molodezh'*) 68, 69
  Struggle (*Cīņa*) 69
  Truth (*Pravda*) 228
  The Voice of Riga (*Rīgas Balss*) 65, 69
  Wausau Daily Herald 207
  Why Is Tobacco Dangerous? 141
Nicholas II (1868–1918) Russian Tsar 181
  The Russia of Nicholas II and Lev Tolstoy (*Rossiia Nikolaia i Lev Tolstoi*, 1928) 186
Nicholls, B. P., Canadian engineer 206
Nikolaev, A. P., Soviet hypnologist 39

Oderich, Peter (1933–1984) German psychologist
  Am I Living Right? (*Lebe ich richtig?* 1977) 85
'old life' 9, 181, 187
Omeliants, A. P., Soviet physician
  on lens technology and sun therapy 157
Ostrovskii, Nikolai (1904–1936) Ukrainian and Soviet writer
  How the Steel Was Tempered (*Kak zakalialas' stal'*, 1932) 88
Ottoman Empire 107, 118 n.5

Pastra Home for Men with Mental Disabilities and Idiocy 110–11
patients
  Aleksandr T. 70–1
  'Ania,' hypnosis patient of VV Sreznevskii 38–9
  Chistiakovich, AP., Soviet hypnosis patient in *To Your Health* 32–4
  Darisa T. 71
  in electric light therapy 161–2, 163–4, 169
  Leonid V. 70
  M., student, seen by SN Astakhov 126–7, 128–9
  Nadia, cochlear implant recipient 228
  P., medical student, 124–5
  parachutists 121
  R., teacher 121, 125, 130
Pavlov, Ivan (1849–1936) Russian and Soviet physiologist, 29, 62 n.7, 123
  on hypnosis 29
  on inhibition 31, 44
  Pavlovian behaviourist models 8, 10, 11, 44, 104–5, 116, 141
  Pavlovian theories of nervous activity 52–3
  Pavlovian turn in Soviet medicine (1948–1951) 158, 164, 165
  Pavlov's dogs and hypnosis 44
pedagogy
  and psychotherapy 12, 125
physical medicine 157–60, 165–6, 171
physiatry 160–1
physiology
  explanations of human behaviour 6
  explanations of hypnosis 31–2
  psychobiology 44
  psychophysiology 123, 127, 130
  theories of inhibition 8, 29–30, 32
planned economy
  and stress 86–7
  and work therapy 117
Platonov, Konstantin (1877–1969) Ukrainian and Soviet psychiatrist
  on Bernheim and the Nancy school 46 n.31
  foreword to *The Psychoanalysis of Communism* (*Psikhoanaliz kommunizma*, 1924) 38

on hypnosis and inhibition 36, 44
on hypnosis and reflexology 34
Hypnosis and Suggestion in Practical Medicine (*Gipnoz i vnushenie v prakticheskoi meditsine*, 1925) 38
on psychotherapy 133–4
on reflexology 31, 34, 38
'unified' interpretation of hypnosis 44
The Word as a Physiological and Therapeutic Factor (*Slovo kak fiziologicheskii i lechebnyi faktor* 1930) 31
Ponomareva, N. A., Soviet physician
on tsititon preparation 149
Preobrazhenskaya, Olga (1881–1971) Russian and Soviet film director
The Women of Ryazan' (*Baby riazanskie*, 1927) 177
preventative treatment 158, 165–166
Prutkov, Ivan Kuz'mich (1888–1943) Russian and Soviet writer
Hypnosis (*Gipnoz*, 1928) 40
psychiatry, psychiatrists 4, 7, 8, 9, 11, 13, 38, 41, 44, 51, 56–60, 101, 103, 104–6, 110, 115, 116, 117, 122, 124, 125, 146
evaluation 58–9
forensic 53–6
history in Bulgaria 9, 104–5, 118 n.5
hospitals 52, 53, 54, 56, 58, 62 n.6, 101, 102, 104, 106, 110–14, 116, 117
institutional care 106, 110, 116
medication 110
and religion 55
Sovietization 8
textbooks 52–3, 59, 106
psychoanalysis 10, 29, 37, 38, 39, 42, 43, 48 n.72, 122
experimental psychoanalysis 39
The Psychoanalysis of Communism (*Psikhoanaliz kommunizma*, 1924) 38
psycho-neuroses 30
psychology, psychologists 4, 9, 12, 37, 40, 43, 44, 51, 53–4, 59, 60, 83–8, 90, 142, 148, 233 n.15
psychological explanations of crime 59
psychological processes 5, 6

psychologization 11
self-help guidebooks 83, 85
textbooks 6
psychopathy, psychopathic 7, 58–60
psychophysiology 2, 3, 10, 11, 13, 31, 34, 37, 127, 130–1
mind-body dualism 2, 3, 5, 6, 7, 14, 34, 52, 53, 54, 60, 83, 89, 91, 123, 127, 128, 133, 134, 225
mindful body 6
psychosomatic
disease 85–7
psychotherapy, psychotherapists 10, 11, 12, 30, 31, 34, 39, 40, 44, 51, 85, 101–2, 105–6, 116, 121–35, 143, 145
autosuggestion 121–2, 129, 130, 132, 137 n.42, 148
Clinic song (*Kliniklied*) 87
collective (group) 143–4
discourse 127–30
hypnosis **See under** Hypnosis
hypnotherapeutic treatment 128–9
patients **See under** Patients
and pedagogy 12, 53
rational psychotherapy 122
and sport 131–3
as teachers of life 124, 130
in the 'West' 123, 126
Pudovkin, Vsevolod (1893–1953) Soviet film director 180
Deserter (*Dezertir*, 1932) 183

radio 7, 13, 65, 66–7, 69–71, 73, 74, 76, 77, 200, 203, 220, 231, 232 n.10
rational psychotherapy 122
Red Army 161
barracks 164–5
Central House of the Red Army 161
reflex, reflexes 141
and alcoholism 32
Bekhterev's theory of associative 31, 32
Pavlov's theory of conditioned 11, 31, 38, 139, 141, 145, 147
and social environment 6
and smoking 141–2, 145, 147
and sport 132
reflexology 150
and hypnosis 29, 32, 38

Platonov's *Hypnosis and Suggestion in Practical Medicine* (*Gipnoz i vnushenie v prakticheskoi meditsine*, 1925) 38
and smoking 11, 139, 142, 145, 147
sleep, reflexological 31
therapies 145, 148
in Zalkind's editing of Russian translation of Kronfeld's *Hypnosis and Suggestion* (*Hypnose und Suggestion* (1924), 43–4
religion
  Bulgarian Muslims 102
  Číhošt miracle 63 n.28
  Jehovah's Witnesses 55–6
  persecution 55–6
Reswick, James Bigelow (1922–2013) American mechanical engineer 205, 212 n.42
Rodchenko, Alexander (1891–1956) Soviet artist 189
Rokhlin, Leon Lazarevich (1903–1984) Soviet psychiatrist
  on work therapy 105
Rusk, Howard (1901–1989) American physician 203–4
Russia arm 198, 206, 207, 213 n.47
Russia, Imperial 6, 10, 105–6, 123
Russian (language) 199
Russian Revolution 2, 5, 140
Ruttmann, Walter (1887–1941) German cinematographer 180
  Berlin: Symphony of a City (*Berlin – Die Sinfonie der Großstadt*, 1927) 180, 183

science and technology 14–5
scientific government 4
Second World War (1939–1945) 67, 141, 203, 224
Seefeldt, Dieter. German physician
  Stress: Understanding – Recognizing – Overcoming (*Streß. Verstehen – Erkennen – Bewältigen*, 1989) 89–90, 91
Semashko, Nikolai (1874–1949) Soviet Commissar of Health (1918–1930) 220

anti-smoking campaign 140–1
Serafimov, Rumen (1952–) Bulgarian curator 103
sex
  abstinence 71–2
  causal sex 70–2, 76
  contraceptives 71, 72
  extramarital sex 66, 73
  and family 71–2
  homosexuality 66, 67, 73, 76
  population growth 73
  sex education 7, 67–70
  sex work 69, 73
  sexual health 69
    and the Cold War 73
  sexual morality 65, 69, 71, 76
Shklovsky, Viktor (1893–1984) Soviet literary theorist and writer 179, 186, 191
Shub, Esfir (1894–1959) Soviet film director 177, 184–9, 191, 192 n.1, 195 n.36
  compilation documentaries (*montazhnaia fil'ma*) 184
  The Fall of the Romanov Dynasty (*Padenie dinastii Romanovykh*, 1927) 186, 192 n.1
  The Great Way (*Velikii put'*, 1927) 186
  Komsomol: Patron of Electrification (*Komsomol: shef elektrofikatsii*, 1932) 187
  The Russia of Nicholas II and Lev Tolstoy (*Rossiia Nikolaia i Lev Tolstoi*, 1928) 186
  Today (*Segodnia*, 1930) 177, 187–9
Skorokhodora, Ol'ga (1911–1982) Soviet deaf-blind academic 226
Skriabin, Aleksandr (1872–1915) Russian composer 217
Slavchev, Slavi, Bulgarian institution director 114
Slobodianik, Aleksandr Pavlovich, Ukrainian psychiatrist
  on psychotherapy and pedagogy 125
  on the will 128
smoking
  aversion therapies 146
  campaigns, anti-smoking 140–1, 147
  carcinogenic dangers 146

cessation 11, 139
chemical dependence 141
chemicals, anti-smoking (atrophine, lobeline, tsititon /Tabex) 11, 146, 148
clinics 144, 148
collective (group) therapy 143–4
cytisine 146, 148–9
nicotine-replacement drugs 11, 140, 148
Pavlovian understanding of 141
in Revolutionary Russia 140–1
and willpower 129, 139
withdrawals 143
Sobchack, Vivian (1940–) American film theorist 183
society 2, 4, 6, 16, 18, 68, 74, 84, 105, 109, 116, 117 n.1, 125, 141, 142, 224
communist 54
improvement of 7, 10, 60, 86
industrial 12, 19 n.4, 85
problems of 8
socialist 16–17, 52, 55, 57, 60, 86, 90, 102, 103, 141, 224
Soviet 141, 224, 225
Society for the Settlement of Jewish Toilers on the Land (OZET – *Obshchestvo zemledel'tsev evreev trudiashchikhsia*) 179, 193 n.14
socialist
heroism 87–92, 96 n.29
labour 117 n.1
and gender 89
personality 54
society 16–17, 52, 55, 57, 60, 86, 90, 102, 103
Soiuzkino (All-Union Association of the Movie-Photo Industry, 1930–1933) 187
sound technology 220
Soviet
avant-garde 177–8
medicine 170
'New Soviet Person' 5, 6, 105, 122, 127, 224
psychiatry 52–3
self-improvement 125, 218
society 141, 224, 225
subjectivity 10–11
technology 207

Soviet-Afghan War (1979–1989)
'New Man' and 'New Woman' 1
Soviet Union, **See** Union of Soviet Socialist Republics
Sputnik One, Sputnik Two 198, 203, 209 n.6
Sreznevskii, Viacheslav Viacheslavovich (1880–1942) Soviet physiologist
'Ania,' hypnosis patient of, 38–9
on 'correct' interpretations of hypnosis 37
experiments with hypnosis 38–9
reflexologist 34
Stakhanov, Aleksei (1906–1977) Soviet coal miner
as 'New Soviet Person' 105
as socialist hero 5, 88
Stalin, Joseph (1878–1953) Soviet leader (1928–1953) 141
consciousness 6
cultural revolution 177
on deaf-mutes 228
death of 66
de-Stalinization 59
industrialization campaign 188
Stalinism 107
Stalinist state 125, 164
State Academy of Artistic Sciences (GAKhN – *Gosudarstvennaia akademiia khudozhestvennykh nauk*)
commission on hypnosis and suggestion 41
Stepanova, Varvara (1894–1958) Russian and Soviet artist 189, 192 n.1
Stoiko, A. G., Soviet neurologist and psychologist
on failures of tobacco therapies 142–143
on reflexology 144
stress 7, 8, 12, 83, 87, 89–92, 121, 146
expert discourse 85–6
and socialist ideology 86
Stupin S. S., Russian psychiatrist
on work therapy 106
suggestion 127, 137 n.42 **See also** hypnosis
autosuggestion 121–2, 130, 132, 137 n.42, 148

Hypnosis and Suggestion in Practical Medicine (*Gipnoz i vnushenie v prakticheskoi meditsine*, 1925) 38
and smoking therapy 143, 144
State Academy of Artistic Sciences' commission on hypnosis and suggestion 41
sun-lamps 15, 157, 158
Sollux lamp 160, 162, 164
surdotekhnika (deaf technology) 217, 218–24, 225, 227–31
Laboratory of *surdotekhnika* (1965–1979) 219, 220, 221–2, 223, 228, 230, 231, 233 n.15
Svilova, Elizaveta (1900–1975) Soviet film director 177
synaesthesia 16, 217, 218, 224–6
and consciousness 225

Tabex 11, 146, 148–9
Tarich, Yuri (1885–1967) Soviet film director 186
technology
and bodies 16–17, 218
as cause of stress 86–7
cochlear implant 227–8, 231
etymology 19 n.4–7
hearing aids 220, 226, 228
as historiographic category 2, 14–16
hypnosis as 'technology of the unconscious' 29, 42, 43, 44
Morse code telephone 222–3, 225, 226
and post-humanism 17
and science 14–15
and selves, 'cyborgs' 227
sound 220
superiority 207
'VIR' speech to image technology 223, 225, 229, 230
telephone, Morse code 222–3, 226
television 7, 13, 65–7, 69–70, 76, 85, 217, 225
Thalidomide 16, 198, 205, 210 n.8, 212 n.47
Therapy **See also** physical medicine, psychotherapy
aversion to smoking 146
electric light 158, 159, 160, 161, 162, 164, 165, 167, 169
and pedagogy 12

physical therapy 157, 158, 161
psychotherapy 10, 11, 129
and reflexology 145, 148
work therapy 102–3, 111–15, 118 n.4
therapeutics 11–12
Thomalla, Curt (1890–1939) German neurologist and screenwriter
A Look into the Depth of the Soul: A Film about the Unconscious (*Ein Blick in die Tiefen der Seele. Der Film vom Unbewussten*, 1923) 32, 37–8, 43
Todorov, Georgi (1958–) Bulgarian artist, caretaker of Nikola Kazakov 103, 109, 111, 115–16
Totev, Tsvetan, Bulgarian institution director 114
treatment, treatments 9, 11, 48 n.72, 54–5, 56, 87, 106, 110, 116, 158, 159, 162, 163, 164, 171, 203, 232 n.10
anti-smoking 143, 144, 146, 147, 149
hypnosis 30, 32, 39, 42
moral treatment 104, 105–6, 107, 122
preventative treatment 158, 165–6
psychotherapeutic 121–30, 134, 137 n.42, 143
venereal disease 66, 68, 69, 74–77
Tret'iakov Sergei (1892–1937) Soviet artist and writer 189, 191, 192 n.1
Autoanimals (*Samozveri*, 1926) 191
Trotsky, Lev (1879–1940) Soviet leader 'New Man' and 'New Woman' 1
Tsaneva, Lyuba (1956–) Bulgarian curator 103
Tserova Koria 'Home for the Mentally Retarded Deaf' 111
Tsiolkovskii, Konstantin (1857–1935) Russian-Soviet space engineer 220
Tsukerman, Veniamin Aronovich (1913–1993) Soviet physicist 218–19, 223, 228, 229, 230
cochlear implants 227–8
'VIR' speech to image technology 223
Tsukerman, Irina (1937–2018) Soviet engineer 219, 220, 222, 226, 228, 229, 231
cybernetics 226
treatment with Streptomycin 219, 232 n.10

Ulmanis, Kārlis (1877–1942) Latvian
    leader (1934–1940)
    May Coup 67
ultraviolet lamps 158, 159, 160, 161, 162,
    164, 165, 167, 169
    and gynaecological operations 164
    overexposure 169–70
unconscious 7, 8, 10, 36–9, 41 **See also**
    psychoanalysis
    and 'double-ego' 47 n.59
    'experimental unconscious' 40
    post-hypnotic suggestion 43
Union of Socialist Soviet Republics
    (USSR) 7, 67, 218
    All-Russian Society of the Deaf (VOG
        – *Vserossiiskoe obshchestvo
        glukhikh*) 217, 225, 230
    All-Union Conference on
        Psychotherapy 124
    All-Union Congress of OZET
        (Society for the Settlement of
        Jewish Toilers on the Land,
        *Obshchestvo zemledel'tsev evreev
        trudiashchikhsia*) 193 n.14
    All-Union Scientific Society of
        Neuropathologists and
        Psychiatrists (VNMONiP
        – *Vsesoiuznoe nauchnoe
        obshchestvo nevropatologov i
        psikhiatrov*) 124
    Central Committee, Party Control
        Commission of 231
    collapse 208, 231
    demographics and population 75
    Department of Sanitary Enlightenment
        146, 148
    Ministry of Health 68–9
United States of America (USA) 73, 94
    n.17, 130, 140, 146, 159, 187, 199,
    200, 205, 206, 220, 228, 232 n.10
    rivalry with USSR 15–16, 197–8,
        203–4, 206–7, 209 n.6, 211 n.24
Ushinskii, Anton (1824–1870) Russian
    pedagogue 125
    on childhood development 125

Vashkov, Vasilii Ignat'evich (1902–1976)
    Soviet microbiologist
    bactericidal lamp experiments 168

venereal disease **See** disease, venereal
Vermel', Samuil Borisovich (1868—1926)
    Soviet physician
    on physiatry 160–1
Vertov, Dziga (1896–1954) Soviet film
    director 182, 186, 188, 189, 191,
    192 n.1, 195 n.36, 196 n.51
    Cine-Eye (*kinoglaz*) theory 180, 184
    History of the Civil War (*Istoriia
        grazhdanskoi voiny*, 1921)
        192 n.1
    Man with a Movie Camera (*Chelovek s
        kinoapparatom*, 1929) 177, 180,
        191
    A Sixth Part of the World (*Shestaia
        chast' mira*, 1926) 182, 189
'VIR' speech to image technology 223,
    225, 229, 230
VKhUTEMAS (Higher Art and
    Technical Studios- *Vysshie
    Khudozhestvenno-Tekhnicheskie
    Masterskie*) 189
Vygotskii, Lev (1896–1934) Soviet
    psychologist
    'sensory swapping' 221, 225

Weitbrecht, Robert (1920–1983)
    American inventor 223
Weltfilm (German socialist film company)
    187, 195 n.39
Wiener, Norbert (1894–1964) American
    mathematician
    on cybernetics and bionic arms 204–5
willpower 6, 11, 123, 125, 127, 128, 134,
    228
    and hypnosis 128
    over mind and body 129, 134
    and smoking 139, 144, 145
women, women's
    anti-smoking campaigns 141, 142,
        145
    bodies 5, 6, 71, 73, 74, 162, 182
    cinema 15, 17, 182
    film 177, 181–3, 188, 189
    health 5, 7, 66, 69, 71, 72, 89
    labour 56
    motherhood and population 73
    'New Woman' 1, 10
    rights 56

work, **See** labour
World Health Organization (WHO) 84, 139
World War One (1914–1918) 10, 67
World War Two (1939–1945) **See** Second World War

Yaroslavsky, Yemelyan (1878–1943) Soviet leader 189
yoga 83, 90
Yugoslavia, Federal People's Republic of 10, 197
Yutkevich, Sergei (1904–1985) Soviet film director 186

Zalkind, Aron (1886–1936) Soviet neurologist 6
  edition of Russian translation of Kronfeld's *Hypnosis and Suggestion* (*Hypnose und Suggestion* (1924) 43–4
  opposition to hypnosis 42
  reflexes and social environment 6
  reflexology 44
Zhemchuzhnyi, Vitalii Leonidovich (1898–1966) Soviet film director 180
Zhukov, V., Latvian physician
  on venereal disease 65, 71
Zidarov, Filip (1952–) Bulgarian curator 103
Zolotniskii, Vladimir Nikolaevich (1853–1930) Soviet physician
  On the Danger of Smoking Tobacco (*O vrede kureniia tabaka*, 1921) 143
Zoshchenko, Mikhail (1894–1958) Soviet writer
  'Hypnosis' ('*Gipnoz*', 1926) 42–3

www.ingramcontent.com/pod-product-compliance
Lightning Source LLC
Chambersburg PA
CBHW071818300426
44116CB00009B/1363